ADVANCES IN

Surgery

Editor-in-Chief
John L. Cameron, MD

ELSEVIER

PHILADELPHIA LONDON TORONTO MONTREAL SYDNEY TOKYO

ADVANCES IN
Surgery

VOLUMES 1 THROUGH 39 (OUT OF PRINT)

VOLUME 43

1. Natural Orifice Translumenal Endoscopic Surgery: Current Status *by Denise W. Gee and David W. Rattner*

2. The Accuracy and Role of Cross-sectional Imaging in the Diagnosis of Acute Appendicitis *by Joshua D. Hawkins and Richard C. Thirlby*

3. Management of Pancreatic Serous Cystadenomas *by Jennifer A. Wargo, Carlos Fernandez-del-Castillo, and Andrew L. Warshaw*

4. Stem Cells and the Liver: Clinical Applications in Transplantation *by Jayme E. Locke, Michael J. Shamblott, and Andrew M. Cameron*

5. Is Intermittent Vasculogenic Claudication Still a Nonsurgical Disease? *by Spence M. Taylor*

6. Changes in Operative Case Experience for General Surgery Residents: Has the 80-Hour Work Week Decreased Residents' Operative Experience? *by John C. Kairys, Paul J. DiMuzio, Albert G. Crawford, Daniel J. Grabo, and Charles J. Yeo*

7. Laparoscopic Pancreatic Resections *by Attila Nakeeb*

8. The Role of Perioperative Hyperglycemia in Postoperative Infections *by Selwyn O. Rogers, Jr. and Michael J. Zinner*

9. Can Ileal Pouch Anal Anastomosis Be Used in Crohn's Disease? *by Myles R. Joyce and Victor W. Fazio*

10. Are Airbags Effective in Decreasing Trauma in Auto Accidents? *by Regan F. Williams and Martin A. Croce*

11. Posterior Retroperitoneoscopic Adrenalectomy *by Glenda G. Callender, Debra L. Kennamer, Elizabeth G. Grubbs, Jeffrey E. Lee, Douglas B. Evans, and Nancy D. Perrier*

VOLUME 42

VOLUME 41

VOLUME 40

Vice President, Continuity Publishing: Kimberly Murphy
Editor: Ruth Malwitz

Printed and bound by CPI Group (UK) Ltd, Croydon, CR0 4YY

Transferred to Digital Print 2011

Editorial Office:
Elsevier
1600 John F. Kennedy Blvd,
Suite 1800
Philadelphia, PA 19103-2899

International Standard Serial Number: 0065-3411
International Standard Book Number: 0-323-06823-5
978-0-323-06823-9

ADVANCES IN
Surgery

CONTRIBUTORS

ASHISH AGARWALA, DO, Department of Surgery, Virginia Commonwealth University School of Medicine, Richmond, Virginia

CHARLES M. BALCH, MD, FACS, Professor of Surgery, Dermatology and Oncology, Department of Surgery, Johns Hopkins Medical Institutions; Deputy Director of Clinical Trials and Outcomes Research, Director of the John Hopkins Clinical Research Network, John Hopkins Institute for Clinical and Translational Research, Baltimore, Maryland

CHAD G. BALL, MD, MSc, FRCSC, Department of Surgery, Indiana University School of Medicine, Indianapolis, Indiana

GEORGIA M. BEASLEY, MD, Deptartment of Surgery, Duke University Medical Center, Durham, North Carolina

MARTIN L. BLAKELY, MD, MS, Division of Pediatric Surgery, Department of Surgery, University of Tennessee Health Sciences Center, Memphis, Tennessee

NEFERTITI A. BROWN, MD, Resident, General Surgery; Research Fellow, Pancreaticobiliary Disease, Department of Surgery, SUNY Downstate Medical Center, Brooklyn, New York

MARCIA I. CANTO, MD, MHS, Associate Professor, Departments of Oncology and Gastroenterology, The Sol Goldman Pancreatic Cancer Research Center, The Johns Hopkins University School of Medicine, Baltimore, Maryland

SUSANNE CARPENTER, MD, Department of Surgery, Memorial Sloan-Kettering Cancer Center, New York, New York

MUHAMMAD A. CHAUDHRY, MD, Department of Nuclear Medicine, The Sol Goldman Pancreatic Cancer Research Center, The Sidney Kimmel Comprehensive Cancer Center, The Johns Hopkins Hospital, Baltimore, Maryland

YUMAN FONG, MD, Murray F. Brennan Chair in Surgery, Memorial Sloan-Kettering Cancer Center, New York, New York

MICHAEL GOGGINS, MD, Professor, Departments of Pathology, Oncology, and Gastroenterology, The Sol Goldman Pancreatic Cancer Research Center, The Johns Hopkins University School of Medicine, Baltimore, Maryland

ANKUSH GOSAIN, MD, PhD, Division of Pediatric Surgery, Department of Surgery, University of Tennessee Health Sciences Center, Memphis, Tennessee

STEPHEN R. GROBMYER, MD, Associate Professor of Surgery, Division of Surgical Oncology, Department of Surgery, University of Florida, Gainesville, Florida

BRUCE L. HALL, MD, PhD, MBA, Associate Chief of Surgical Services, Department of Surgery, John Cochran Veterans Affairs Medical Center; Professor, Department of Surgery, Washington University School of Medicine, Barnes Jewish Hospital; Professor Healthcare Management, Olin Business School, Washington University in St Louis; Senior Fellow, Center for Health Policy, Washington University in St Louis, St Louis, Missouri

BRIAN HIPSZER, PhD, Assistant Research Professor, Artificial Pancreas Center, Department of Anesthesiology, Jefferson Medical College, Thomas Jefferson University, Philadelphia, Pennsylvania

STEVEN N. HOCHWALD, MD, Edward M. Copeland, III Professor of Surgical Oncology, Associate Professor of Surgery, Molecular Genetics and Microbiology; Chief, Division of Surgical Oncology, University of Florida, Gainesville, Florida

THOMAS J. HOWARD, MD, FACS, Willis D. Gatch Professor of Surgery, Department of Surgery, Indiana University School of Medicine, Indianapolis, Indiana

RALPH H. HRUBAN, MD, Professor, Departments of Pathology and Oncology, The Sol Goldman Pancreatic Cancer Research Center, The Johns Hopkins University School of Medicine, Baltimore, Maryland

ANGELA M. INGRAHAM, MD, Division of Research and Optimal Patient Care, American College of Surgeons, Clinical Scholar in Residence, Chicago, Illinois; Department of Surgery, University of Cincinnati College of Medicine, Cincinnati, Ohio

JEFFREY I. JOSEPH, DO, Director of Research, Department of Anesthesiology; Director, Artificial Pancreas Center; Director, Anesthesiology Program for Translational Research, Jefferson Medical College, Thomas Jefferson University, Philadelphia, Pennsylvania

JOHN M. KELLUM, MD, Department of Surgery, Virginia Commonwealth University School of Medicine, Richmond, Virginia

ALISON P. KLEIN, PhD, Associate Professor; Director, The National Familial Pancreas Tumor Registry, Departments of Pathology and Oncology, The Sol Goldman Pancreatic Cancer Research Center, The Johns Hopkins University School of Medicine; Department of Epidemiology, Bloomberg School of Public Health, The Johns Hopkins University, Baltimore, Maryland

CLIFFORD Y. KO, MD, MS, MSHS, Clinical Director, American College of Surgeons National Surgical Quality Improvement Program, Chicago, Illinois; Professor of

Surgery, Department of Surgery, UCLA School of Medicine; Chief, Section of Colorectal Surgery, West Los Angeles, California

LEONIDAS G. KONIARIS, MD, Associate Professor, Division of Surgical Oncology, Department of Surgery, University of Miami Miller School of Medicine, Sylvester Comprehensive Cancer Center, Miami, Florida

BRIAN HUNG-HIN LANG, MS, FRACS, Chief of Endocrine Surgery, Division of Endocrine Surgery, Department of Surgery, University of Hong Kong Medical Centre, Queen Mary Hospital, Pokfulam, Hong Kong SAR, China

STEVEN D. LEACH, MD, Department of Surgery, The Sol Goldman Pancreatic Cancer Research Center, The Sidney Kimmel Comprehensive Cancer Center, The Johns Hopkins Hospital, Baltimore, Maryland

RYAN M. LEVY, MD, Cardiothoracic Surgery Resident, Heart, Lung & Esophageal Surgery Institute, Department of Surgery, Division of Thoracic and Foregut Surgery, University of Pittsburgh, Pittsburgh, Pennsylvania

ERIC H. LIU, MD, Assistant Professor of Surgery, Division of Surgical Oncology & Endocrine Surgery, Department of Surgery, Vanderbilt University Medical Center, Nashville, Tennessee

JAMES D. LUKETICH, MD, Henry T. Bahnson Professor of Cardiothoracic Surgery; Director, Heart, Lung and Esophageal Surgery Institute; Chief, Division of Thoracic and Foregut Surgery, Department of Surgery, University of Pittsburgh, Pittsburgh, Pennsylvania

GENEVIEVE B. MELTON, MD, MA, Assistant Professor, Department of Surgery; Faculty Fellow, Institute for Health Informatics, Minneapolis, Minnesota

NIPUN B. MERCHANT, MD, Associate Professor of Surgery, Division of Surgical Oncology & Endocrine Surgery, Department of Surgery, Vanderbilt University Medical Center, Nashville, Tennessee

SUBHASIS MISRA, MD, Fellow, Division of Surgical Oncology, Department of Surgery, University of Miami Miller School of Medicine, Sylvester Comprehensive Cancer Center, Miami, Florida

FREDERICK L. MOFFAT, MD, Professor, Division of Surgical Oncology, Department of Surgery, University of Miami Miller School of Medicine, Sylvester Comprehensive Cancer Center, Miami, Florida

DAVID G. NESCHIS, MD, Department of Surgery, University of Maryland School of Medicine, Baltimore, Maryland

NINH T. NGUYEN, MD, Professor of Surgery and Chief, Division of Gastrointestinal Surgery, University of California, Irvine Medical Center, Orange, California

XUAN-MAI T. NGUYEN, PhD, Research Analyst, University of California, Irvine Medical Center, Orange, California

JOHN A. OLSON Jr, MD, PhD, Deptartment of Surgery, Duke University Medical Center, Durham, North Carolina

ALEXANDER A. PARIKH, MD, Assistant Professor of Surgery, Division of Surgical Oncology & Endocrine Surgery, Department of Surgery, Vanderbilt University Medical Center, Nashville, Tennessee

KAREN E. RICHARDS, BS, Administrative Director, American College of Surgeons, National Surgical Quality Improvement Program (ACS NSQIP), Chicago, Illinois

THOMAS M. SCALEA, MD, R Adams Cowley Shock Trauma Center and Department of Surgery, University of Maryland School of Medicine, Baltimore, Maryland

RICHARD SCHULICK, MD, PhD, Professor of Surgery and Oncology, John L. Cameron Professor; Chief, Division of Surgical Oncology; Director, Hepatopancreatobiliary Surgery Fellowship, Departments of Oncology and Surgery, The Sol Goldman Pancreatic Cancer Research Center, The Johns Hopkins University School of Medicine, Baltimore, Maryland

DON J. SELZER, MD, Associate Professor, Department of Surgery, Indiana University School of Medicine; Staff General Surgeon, Clarian Health Partners, Indianapolis, Indiana

OSCAR K. SERRANO, MD, Department of Surgery, The Sol Goldman Pancreatic Cancer Research Center, The Sidney Kimmel Comprehensive Cancer Center, The Johns Hopkins Hospital, Baltimore, Maryland

TAIT SHANAFELT, MD, Associate Professor of Medicine, Department of Medicine, Mayo Clinic, Rochester, Minnesota

MANISHA SHENDE, MD, Assistant Professor of Surgery, Heart, Lung & Esophageal Surgery Institute, Department of Surgery, Division of Thoracic and Foregut Surgery, University of Pittsburgh, Pittsburgh, Pennsylvania

JOHNATHAN SLOAN, MD, Surgical Resident, University of California, Irvine Medical Center, Orange, California

NAVEENRAJ L. SOLOMON, MD, Fellow, Division of Surgical Oncology, Department of Surgery, University of Miami Miller School of Medicine, Sylvester Comprehensive Cancer Center, Miami, Florida

WILLIAM M. STONE, MD, FACS, Associate Professor of Surgery, Chief, Division of Vascular Surgery, Mayo Clinic, Phoenix, Arizona

ANTHONY Y. TSAI, MD, Chief Resident, General Surgery Residency, Department of Surgery, Indiana University School of Medicine, Indianapolis, Indiana

REGAN F. WILLIAMS, MD, Division of Pediatric Surgery, Department of Surgery, University of Tennessee Health Sciences Center, Memphis, Tennessee

JOSEPH WIZOREK, MD, Assistant Professor of Surgery, Heart, Lung & Esophageal Surgery Institute, Department of Surgery, Division of Thoracic and Foregut Surgery, University of Pittsburgh, Pittsburgh, Pennsylvania

MICHAEL E. ZENILMAN, MD, Clarence and Mary Dennis Professor and Chairman, Department of Surgery, SUNY Downstate Medical Center, Brooklyn, New York

ADVANCES IN
Surgery

CONTENTS VOLUME 44 • 2010

Laparoscopic Gastric Bypass or Gastric Banding: Which Operation is Best?
Ninh T. Nguyen, Johnathan Sloan, and Xuan-Mai T. Nguyen

Prevention, Detection, and Management of Leaks Following Gastric Bypass for Obesity
Ashish Agarwala and John M. Kellum

Distinguishing Acute from Ruptured Appendicitis Preoperatively in the Pediatric Patient
Ankush Gosain, Regan F. Williams, and Martin L. Blakely

Screening Criteria for Breast Cancer

Subhasis Misra, Naveenraj L. Solomon, Frederick L. Moffat, and Leonidas G. Koniaris

Laparoscopic and Thoracoscopic Esophagectomy

Ryan M. Levy, Joseph Wizorek, Manisha Shende, and James D. Luketich

Biomedical and Health Informatics for Surgery

Genevieve B. Melton

Real-Time Glucose Monitoring in the Hospital: Future or Now?

Jeffrey I. Joseph and Brian Hipszer

Minimally Invasive Thyroid and Parathyroid Operations: Surgical Techniques and Pearls

Brian Hung-Hin Lang

What's New in Neoadjuvant Therapy for Breast Cancer?

Georgia M. Beasley and John A. Olson Jr

Advances in Surgery 44 (2010) 1-27

ADVANCES IN SURGERY

ELSEVIER
MOSBY

Single-Port Laparoscopic Surgery

Anthony Y. Tsai, MD[a,*], Don J. Selzer, MD[b,c]

[a]General Surgery Residency, Department of Surgery, Indiana University School of Medicine, 545 Barnhill Drive #203, Indianapolis, IN 46202, USA
[b]Department of Surgery, Indiana University School of Medicine, 545 Barnhill Drive #507, Indianapolis, IN 46202, USA
[c]Department of Surgery, Clarian Health Partners, 545 Barnhill Driver #507, Indianapolis, IN 46202, USA

The field of laparoscopic or minimally invasive surgery (MIS) has come a long way from Kelling's [1] description of its use in a dog in 1901 in Dresden. Although laparoscopy was initially popularized by gynecologists, it did not gain wide spread use until the advent of the transistor chip and a video camera was attached to the end of the laparoscope. Originally termed video-laparoscopy, general surgeons used this tool to remove uninflamed gallbladders at the end of the 1980s. As video imaging systems improved and new instruments were developed, applications of laparoscopy spread until essentially all operations performed with a large laparotomy could be completed with MIS tools.

As surgeons and industry continue to push the boundaries of MIS, new and controversial approaches such as natural orifice translumenal endoscopic surgery (NOTES) and single-incision or single-port laparoscopic surgery are being explored with the goal of reduced surgical morbidity. NOTES was first introduced as an "incision-free" approach to help minimize the pain associated with laparoscopic port incisions. NOTES combines technology from both laparoscopy and flexible endoscopy and is performed by intentionally penetrating a hollow viscus. The endoscope is then passed through the enterotomy into the peritoneal cavity for diagnostic or therapeutic intent. Proponents suggest NOTES improves cosmesis, diminish discomfort, reduce infection rates from skin flora (eg, methicillin-resistant *Staphylococcus*), and increase collaboration among several disciplines (ie, endoscopists, laparoscopists, surgeons of various specialties, engineers, and the industry). The most compelling argument in favor of NOTES is the development of better instrumentation that will benefit all of medicine.

Similar to NOTES, single-incision laparoscopy aims at minimizing the number of abdominal wall incisions. The fundamental idea is to allow all of the laparoscopic instruments to enter through one skin incision. When compared with standard laparoscopy, the benefits of single-incision

*Corresponding author. *E-mail address*: antsaipa@gmail.com.

0065-3411/10/$ – see front matter
doi:10.1016/j.yasu.2010.05.017

laparoscopy seem similar to NOTES. However, unlike NOTES, an abdominal incision is still required, frequently near the umbilicus. In addition, single-incision laparoscopy avoids the potential risk of intraperitoneal sepsis from intentional organ perforation. Finally, single-incision laparoscopic instruments are more readily adapted from standard laparoscopic equipment and are even currently available for use.

First clinical use of a single-opening approach to laparoscopic surgery was reported in human subjects as early as 1969 by Wheeless [2] who successfully performed single-puncture tubal ligation with a laparoscope. As he and other gynecologists continued to push the envelope on the approach (they performed the first single-port appendectomies in 1992), the general surgery community began to adopt the concept in the early 1990s. Despite its early use, the approach was slow to gain acceptance until recently. This could be explained by surgeons overcoming the learning of standard laparoscopy and the advent of improved instrumentation. Nevertheless, since the approach has received renewed attention, it has been used to complete various procedures including: cholecystectomy, colectomy, splenectomy, adrenalectomy, inguinal hernia repair, and even bariatric surgery. Recently, urologists have made their own contributions by combining it with robotic assistance and experimenting with prostatectomy, nephrectomy, and pyeloplasty. Although single-port pioneers, gynecologists were slow to do more advanced procedures. However, hysterectomy and salpingectomy are now being attempted with this approach.

NOMENCLATURE

Unlike NOTES, there is no consensus on the nomenclature for the developing field of single-incision surgery. Also unlike NOTES, there have been no national organizations like the Natural Orifice Surgery Consortium for Assessment and Research (NOSCAR) to organize, champion, and implement recommendations such as *The ASGE/SAGES Working Group on Natural Orifice Translumenal Endoscopic Surgery* white paper [3].

Whereas methodology and access techniques are similar, various acronyms are used to represent this technique (Box 1). The lack of consensus on a nomenclature has allowed individuals and companies to trademark a name in hopes that it will be widely accepted. This led to more acronyms than actual differences in techniques and added to the confusion. One of the more commonly used names is Single-Incision Laparoscopic Surgery (SILS), trademarked by Covidien, Inc Ethicon EndoSurgery, Inc proposed the name Single-Site Laparoscopy (SSL). Drexel University has also trademarked its own name, calling this technique Single-Port Access (SPA) [4–6]. Certain groups advocate particular names for various reasons. Similarities to NOTES have led to names like Natural Orifice Trans-Umbilical Surgery (NOTUS) [7] and Embryonic NOTES (E-NOTES) [8,9] denoting the umbilicus as a natural orifice. Other names have also revolved around the umbilical access such as One-Port Umbilical Surgery (OPUS) [10] and Trans-Umbilical Endoscopic Surgery (TUES) [11,12], advocated by the Chinese laparoscopic community.

Box 1: Single-incision surgery acronyms

SILS Single-incision laparoscopic surgery
SSL Single-site laparoscopy
SPA Single-port access surgery
OPUS One-port umbilical surgery
TUES Transumbilical endoscopic surgery
NOTUS Natural orifice transumbilical surgery
E-NOTES Embryonic NOTES
SLAPP Single laparoscopic port procedure
SPLS Single-port laparoscopic surgery
SPL Single-port laparoscopy
SLIT Single laparoscopic incision transabdominal surgery
SIMPL Single-instrument port laparoscopic surgery
SPICES Single-port incisionless conventional equipment-using surgery
LESS Laparo-endoscopic single-site surgery

The names are also not very well defined, leading to liberal use of the acronyms with some describing procedures that are not true single-incision laparoscopic procedures (eg, using Single-Instrument Port Laparoscopic Surgery or SIMPL for a procedure with one camera port and one instrument port). Additional suggestions include Single-Laparoscopic Port Procedure (SLAPP), Single-Port Laparoscopic Surgery (SPLS), Single-Port Laparoscopy (SPL), Single-Laparoscopic Incision Transabdominal (SLIT) surgery, and Single-Port Incisionless Conventional Equipment-using Surgery (SPICES).

The need for a consensus and oversight, as was done for the NOTES by NOSCAR, is obvious. For this reason, a recently convened consortium at the Cleveland Clinic had suggested the term Laparo-Endoscopic Single-Site (LESS) surgery to describe single-incision laparoscopic operations. Whether the surgical community will adopt this acronym, remains to be seen. For the purposes of this text, the acronym LESS will be used.

DEVICES

LESS tools are similar to standard laparoscopic instruments. Ports are used to maintain pneumoperitoneum and a channel through which instruments can be inserted and exchanged. Laparoscopes and other instruments still consist of long, thin shafts with handles on one end that drive the actuators at the other end. However, modifications have been made to each of these components to better suit their role in LESS. Some of these modifications are simplistic while others are intricate and complex. As one might expect, more complex the modifications result in more expensive equipment. Cost has led many to continue using standard laparoscopic instrumentation as often as possible–potentially sacrificing visualization, dexterity, and safety.

Ports

TriPort or QuadPort

The TriPort (Advanced Surgical Concepts, Wicklow, Ireland), initially introduced as the R-Port, has two components: an outer multichannel valve and a fascial retractor with an inner and outer ring connected by a retractable sleeve. The TriPort has two 5-mm channels, one 12-mm channel, and two channels for insufflation or desufflation. The QuadPort has 4 legs: one 5 mm, two 10 mm, and one 15 mm in diameter. Each port is covered with a simple valve of thermoplastic elastomer that maintains pneumoperitoneum. Lubrication with mineral oil, iodine solution, or other lubricants is required to minimize friction between the instruments and the elastomer. The TriPort is deployed into the abdomen by loading the inner ring with a nonbladed introducer and the inner ring is expanded once it is pushed out of the introducer. This is done through a small fasciotomy ranging in size from 1.5 to 4.5 cm (TriPort to QuadPort). Once the inner ring is inside the abdomen, slack in the plastic sleeve is removed and the rings form a tight seal around the incisional opening while retracting it open similarly to a wound protector. Once in place, the multi-instrument access port accommodates up to three (TriPort) or four (QuadPort) instruments to be used simultaneously (Fig. 1).

Besides allowing for multiple instruments, the TriPort can be safely introduced through controlled deployment. It can also be easily removed and replaced as in the case of specimen removal as the current formation of this device allows the entire diaphragm that contains the channels to be removed and replaced. A fourth benefit of the TriPort system is an ability to adapt to abdominal walls of various thicknesses up to 10 cm. Plastic valves and a low profile allow passage of prebent instruments and provide a wider field of view once the laparoscope is inserted through one of the valves. Similarly, the short channels afford greater angle of distraction compared with standard

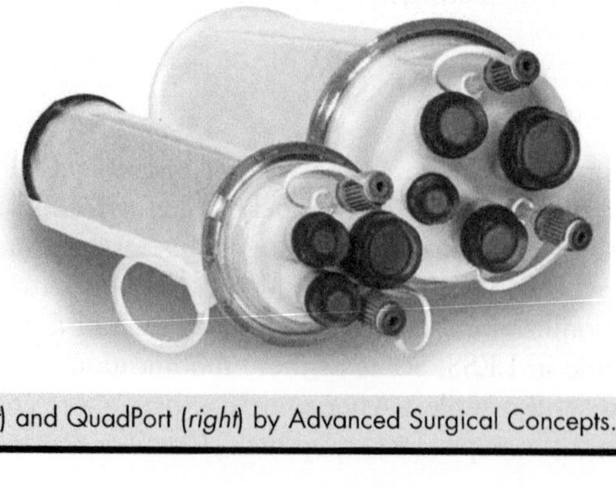

Fig. 1. TriPort (*left*) and QuadPort (*right*) by Advanced Surgical Concepts.

rigid trocars, increasing the achievable triangulation between the instruments. The dependence on the rings to anchor the TriPort in place allows for incisions of various sizes from 12 to 25 mm depending on the needs of the procedure.

The main drawback of the TriPort design is the gel valves. They have been known to come apart from the significant torque of the instruments requiring replacement of the entire device. Moreover, the addition of a lubricant with passage of each instrument is a significant impediment to efficiency. Finally, initial configurations of the port required removing the entire port for removal of a specimen or introduction of a device like an adjustable gastric band. Reinsertion of the port proved to be quite difficult. More recently, the multichannel valve has been made removable. Once the valve is removed, reinsertion is easy but seal maintenance remains inconsistent.

The larger QuadPort is now commercially available from Advanced Surgical Concepts with one 5-mm port, two 10-mm ports, and one 15-mm port, allowing up to four instruments to be used through a single incision between 2.5 cm to 6.5 cm in length.

AirSeal

AirSeal (SurgiQuest, Orange, CT, USA) ports employ an alternative technology to maintain a stable pneumoperitoneum. Instead of a mechanical barrier, as in traditional laparoscopic ports, AirSeal ports use an innovative pressure barrier to prevent gas loss by using insufflated carbon dioxide gas to create an invisible pressure barrier within the open lumen of the cannula. Since the air pressure is higher within the port, intra-abdominal gas is prevented from leaking out. This "invisible" seal effectively creates a dynamic equilibrium separating the intra-abdominal gas from the ambient room air. A filter recirculates the insufflated carbon dioxide, removing smoke and debris at the same time. Additionally, the pressure seal can also be overcome by increased abdominal wall pressure such as coughing or patient-initiated respiration (Fig. 2).

Benefits are created by the lack of a physical barrier through which instruments must pass to enter the peritoneum. While improving visibility by eliminating laparoscope smudging, the lack of mechanical barrier also allows for insertion of multiple instruments and increased freedom of movement. It also permits extracorporeal knot tying without gas loss, and enhanced specimen extraction.

Some of the drawbacks of the AirSeal port include the relatively long fulcrum of the 12-mm port that limits the range of distraction and the noise associated with the pressure barrier. The necessity of the generator unit adds cost to the procedure and requires additional space on the booms, not to mention the noise it generates. The lack of a mechanical barrier translates into less anchoring of the instruments, allowing them to move around inside the channel. The greatest drawback of the AirSeal system is that it has yet to be released for commercial use.

SILS port

Another LESS port is the SILS port (Covidien, Inc, Norwalk, CT, USA). It's made with an elastic polymer in a dumbbell shape. The port fits a 2.5 cm

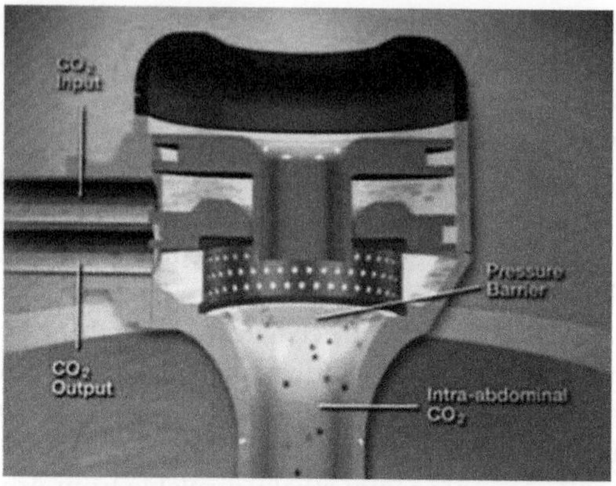

Fig. 2. AirSeal port by SurgiQuest with pressure barrier.

incision and allows for three custom-made trocars of up to 12 mm in size with one three-way stopcock for the purpose of insufflation or smoke evacuation. The elastic material allows the port to conform to the shape of the abdominal wall to maintain pneumoperitoneum as well as access of multiple cannulas of different sizes (Fig. 3).

One benefit of the SILS port configuration is the removable caps on the cannulas make small specimen retrieval easier. Specimen larger than the port, however, will still require removal of the entire device. However, access to this device is wide given the presence of Covidien, Inc in the surgical marketplace. Moreover, the port is durable and withstands significant torque.

On the other hand, the SILS port has only one length and therefore has a limited range of abdominal wall thickness that it will accommodate. Removal and reinsertion is challenging and has a steeper learning curve than some of the other port choices. Finally, the use of standard laparoscopic ports inside the elastic channel prevents use of some newer prebent instruments and creates

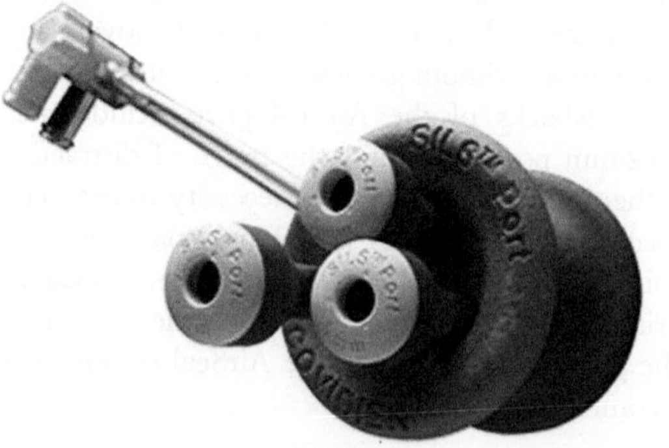

Fig. 3. Single-Incision Laparoscopic Surgery (SILS) port by Covidien, Inc made of elastic polymer.

more material that can cause bumping of the extra-corporeal instrument components.

Uni-X port

Originally invented by Dr Gregory Piskun from Pnavel Systems, Inc (Pnavel Systems, Brooklyn, NY, USA; subsequently acquired by Covidien, Inc in 2008), the Uni-X Single-Port Access Laparoscopic System consists of a single multicannula laparoscopic port and a variety of curved laparoscopic instruments. The port is cone-shaped with a built-in port for insufflation and three 5-mm cannulas for instrumentation. The shape affords a shorter fulcrum than a standard laparoscopic trocar (Fig. 4). However, fascial fixation sutures are required to maintain it in position. The lack of larger cannulas limits the use of larger instruments such as staplers.

Several case reports using the Uni-X port have been published showing its feasibility [13,14,15]. Unfortunately, Uni-X has yet to reach the marketplace.

GelPoint

The GelPort (or Alexis [r]) (Applied Medical, Rancho Santa Margarita, CA, USA) is commonly used in hand-assisted laparoscopy and has been used in single-incision laparoscopic procedures as described by Merchant and colleagues [16]. This eventually led to the creation of the GelPoint system. The GelPoint uses identical technology as the GelPort. The major advantage

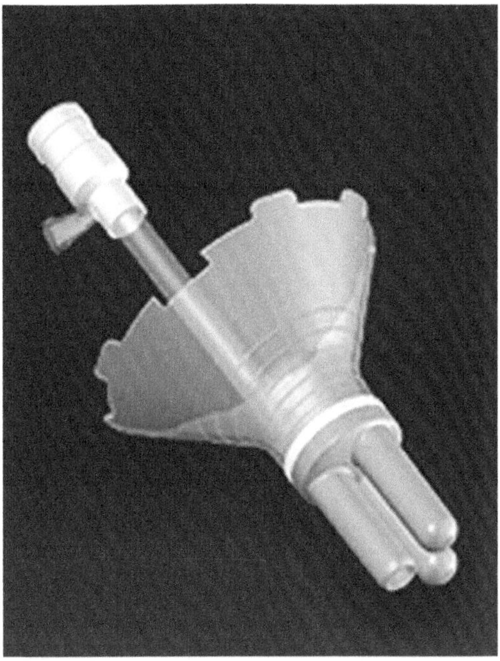

Fig. 4. Uni-X Port (Pnavel Systems, now part of Covidien, Inc.)

is that it provides a "flexible fulcrum" for the manipulation of the laparoscope and instruments, even without trocars. When used without trocars, extracorporeal instrument crowding is minimized. As in hand-assisted laparoscopy, GelPoint, easily maintains pneumoperitoneum despite multiple instrument reinsertions. It also permits 360 degrees of visualization and field of access (Fig. 5). However, the minimum incisional size required is 2.5 cm and a larger incision may be required thereby abating the benefits of single-incision laparoscopic surgery.

SSL port

The SSL Access System (Ethicon Endo-Surgery, Inc, Cincinnati, OH, USA) is a newly developed low-profile access system with detachable seal cap with separate wound retractors. The sealed cap can accommodate two 5-mm and one 10-mm instruments and its unique 360 degree rotation allows for quick reorientation of instrumentation. Its low profile accommodates straight, bent, or curved instruments. The removable cap allows for easier retrieval of specimen without removing the wound retractor while the rigid body provides a fulcrum for instrumentation (Fig. 6).

TransEnterix SPIDER

A promising new development is the SPIDER (Single-Port Instrument Delivery Extended Reach) Surgical System by TransEnterix, Inc (Research Triangle

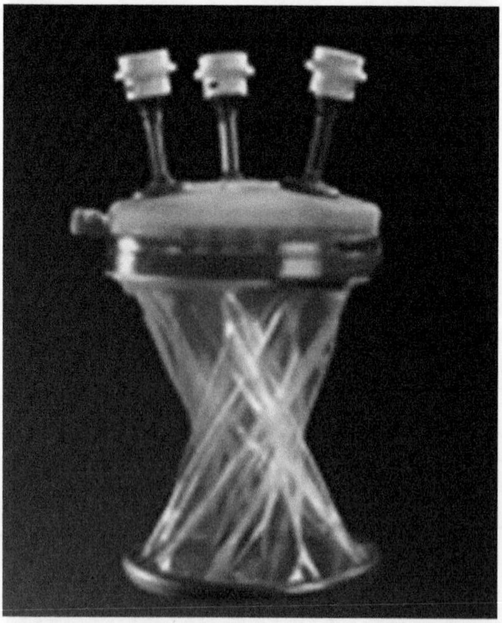

Fig. 5. GelPoint by Applied Medical with Alexis wound retractor and self-retaining 5 mm trocars.

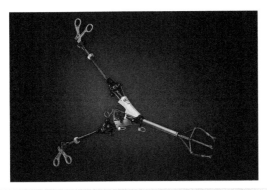

Fig. 6. SPIDER (Single-Port Instrument Delivery Extended Research) by TransEnterix Inc (Research Triangle Park, NC, USA) has a single port housing four working channels (two static and two flexible). External crowding is minimized and internal triangulation is achieved through flexible instruments and internal tubing. *Reprinted from* TransEnterix, Inc; with permission.

Park, NC, USA). It contains a single-port housing four working channels: two static and two flexible (Fig. 7). This device was developed by a cardiologist who transferred the technology of directable catheters from endovascular procedures to a port with directable channels. This entire elegant device can be inserted through a single incision, whether percutaneous or transluminal. Once inside the abdominal cavity, two channels superiorly and inferiorly accommodate rigid laparoscopes and instruments less than 6 mm in diameter. Two instrument delivery tubes (IDTs), positioned laterally, are deployed outward and used to guide flexible surgical instruments to the surgical site. They can then be actuated to provide movement in all three dimensions and allow a wide-angled approach to the desired organ, simulating triangulation of traditional laparoscopy. Three additional ports are available for smoke evacuation or insufflation and a support arm accessory is included to stabilize the device. Pryor and colleagues [17] have demonstrated in swine models that the SPIDER

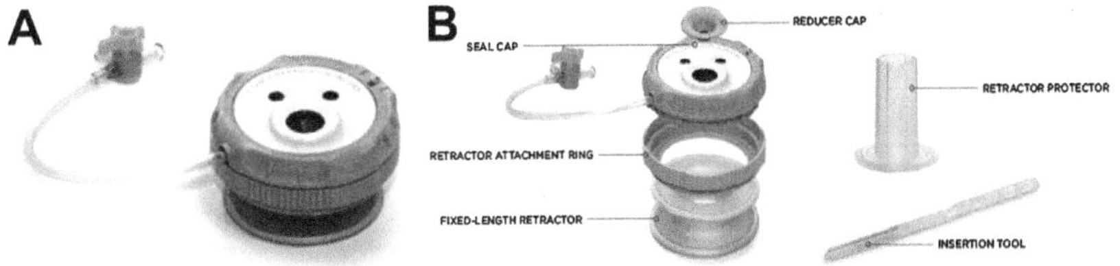

Fig. 7. SSL Access System (*Courtesy* Ethicon Endo-Surgery, Inc) (*A*) the assembled view, and (*B*) detached view with removable seal cap, attachment ring, and retractor on left, retractor protector, and insertion tool on right.

system resulted in less inflammation and tissue trauma at the trocar sites compared with standard trocars when performing cholecystectomy. This theoretically minimizes the risk of infection, delayed healing, and herniation caused by seroma formation and fat necrosis resulting from traumatized tissue.

Laparoscope

Several laparoscope options are available for one-incision laparoscopic procedures. Simple procedures requiring small changes in the field of view may suffice with a standard 30 or 45 degree 5-mm laparoscope. In other cases, the preferred umbilical location for the solitary incision requires a longer reach to the surgical field, hence necessitating longer laparoscopes or even a flexible tip scope to minimize clashing of the instruments. Changing the light cord adapter on the laparoscopes from a perpendicular projection to a parallel or in-line projection minimizes crowding with other instruments.

EndoEYE

EndoEYE laparoscope (Olympus Surgical & Industrial America Inc, Center Valley, PA, USA) represents a more advanced option. With a distally mounted charged-couple device (CCD) chip that provides high image quality and a one-piece design, EndoEYE minimizes clutter and external instrument crowding. It comes in 5-mm and 10-mm sizes, although the high-definition option is not available on the more commonly used 5-mm scope (Fig. 8). The flexible tip option allows for adjustability in the positioning of the scope to improve visualization and minimize sword-fighting effect (Fig. 9).

Endoscopes

In an attempt to provide even more flexibility to the video imaging source, surgeons have also used double-channel flexible endoscopes (KARL STORZ GmbH & Co KG, Tuttlingen, Germany, and Olympus America, Inc, Center Valley, PA, USA) with LESS procedures. Flexible endoscopic tools and newer techniques such as hydrodissection with subserosal saline injection were used [18,19]. Distance from the surgical field is less of an issue with the endoscopes and the built-in suction and irrigation are helpful to improve visibility. The flexibility of the endoscope increases the degree of freedom of movement.

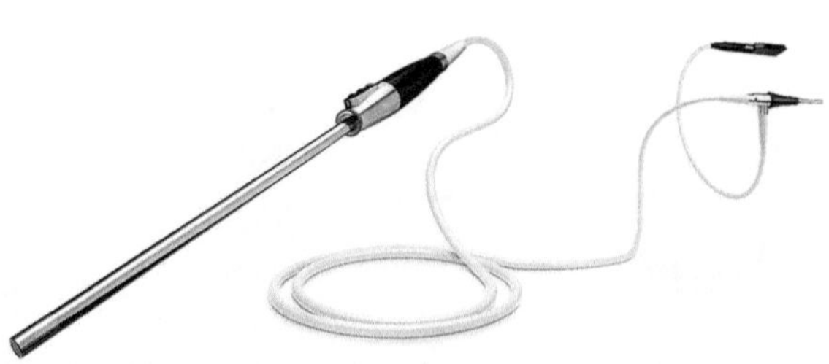

Fig. 8. EndoEYE laparoscope (Olympus Surgical & Industrial America Inc) with the rigid tip shown. Note the in-line cord insertion and streamline design of the control buttons.

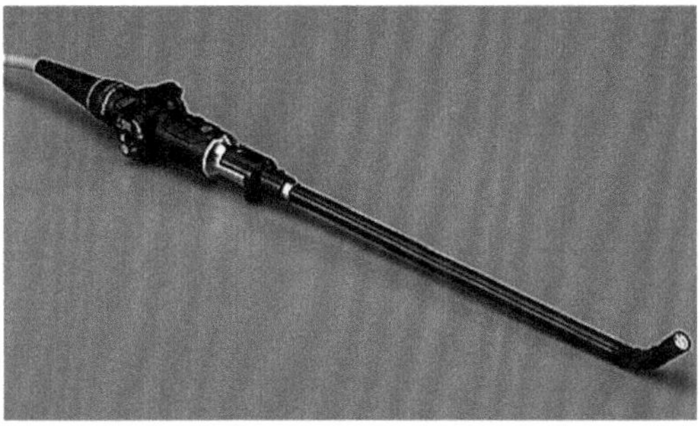

Fig. 9. The flexible tip option for the EndoEYE laparoscope. The CCD chip is mounted distally to provide high image quality.

However, the flexibility afforded by the lack of rigidity also removes the ability to fine-tune the scope's position and field of view whether an abdominal wall port is used or not. In addition, in-line instrumentation with flexible instruments and triangulation are challenging especially in complicated procedures. Sterilization of instruments and parts is also an issue as the endoscopes are not designed for sterile procedures.

Instrumentation

Standard rigid laparoscopic instruments have been used with success. In other cases, curved or flexible instruments in addition to laparoscopes are used to minimize the crowding of the instruments and improve triangulation. There are instruments that have varying degrees of flexibility and freedom. In fact, although not commercially available yet, many surgeons are developing prebent instruments.

Roticulator

Covidien, Inc (Norwalk, CT, USA) manufactures an array of instruments with an articulating (or "roticulating") tip that has 80 degrees of articulation and 360 degree rotation of jaws. The 5-mm instruments include a grasper, dissector, and scissors of standard length (31 cm). The company also makes longer 5 mm-scissors (45 cm) and 2-mm, standard length (33-cm) scissors for selected cases (Fig. 10). These instruments were actually developed over 10 years ago but have found a new use with the gaining popularity of LESS procedures. A more recent development from Covidien, Inc is a roticulating suturing device. The EndoStitch is a 10-mm instrument also developed over 10 years ago. It facilitates intracorporeal laparoscopic suturing. Although some surgeons feel the use of EndoStitch in standard laparoscopy sacrifices the accuracy and safety of standard needle and suture, it addresses the most difficult task in LESS procedures: intracorporeal tying. Covidien, Inc has recently made efforts to create a roticulating EndoStitch. It remains a 10-mm instrument and, therefore, limits some of the flexibility of LESS ports.

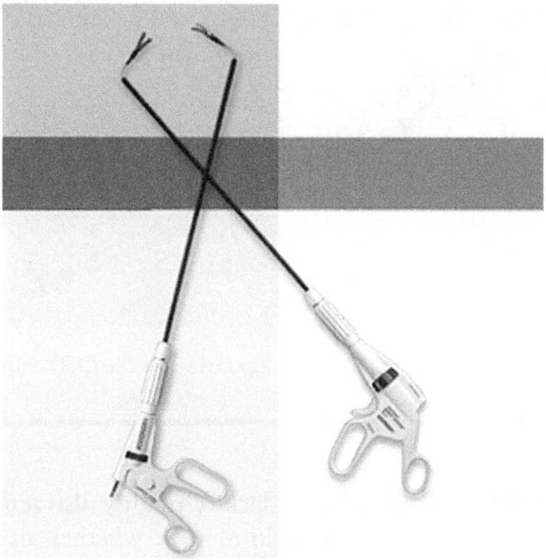

Fig. 10. Roticulator instruments with reticulating tips.

RealHand

Novare Surgical Systems, Inc (Cuperlino, CA, USA), developed the RealHand product line that includes a dissector, flexible graspers, needle holder, scissors, and hook-spatula cautery. This design offers seven degrees of freedom of movement and greater control and instrument dexterity (Fig. 11). They are designed to mirror the surgeon's hand movements. That is, if the surgeon's hand moves in one direction, the flexible tip follows in the same direction. However, the same freedom is lost when the handle is in proximity to other instruments. Working at an angle requires continued deflection of the wrist leading to surgeon fatigue and some discomfort. However, newer models have included a locking mechanism to hold the articulation in place. It requires two hands to activate the locking mechanism.

Autonomy Laparo-Angle

CambridgeEndo (Framingham, MA, USA) developed the Autonomy Laparo-Angle technology. It also offers seven degrees of freedom of movement. The

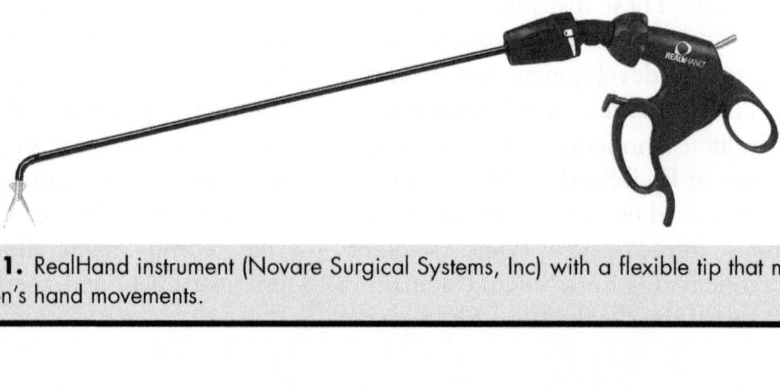

Fig. 11. RealHand instrument (Novare Surgical Systems, Inc) with a flexible tip that mirrors surgeon's hand movements.

distal tips have near 90 degrees of articulation mapping the handle motion and 360 degrees of axial rotation controlled by a knob in the handle. It is currently the only handle that locks at any angle and still able to rotate. In addition, the lock is activated with the ipsilateral hand (Fig. 12). All 5 mm in size, available products include a needle holder, dissector, hook electrocautery, dissector, and grasper in both the standard (33 or 34 cm) and longer (44 or 45 cm) lengths. The handle is unlike any other encountered in laparoscopy and therefore requires a learning curve. Once the learning curve is overcome, the instrument is much easier to use but still not intuitive.

Unfortunately, with any instrument, working through a solitary incision will always lead to extracorporeal interference with other instruments. This is minimized by using alternate length instruments (eg, a standard length instrument with one of longer length). It's also reduced with a combination of one flexible instrument used with one rigid instrument. Use of more than one flexible instrument is mentally challenging and increases wrist fatigue. Unfortunately, new articulating instruments deflect when force is applied and therefore limit their use when torque is required.

S-Portal single-port access

KARL STORZ Endoskope (Tuttlingen, Germany) is the first company to develop reusable instrumentation for LESS procedures. Although no product is currently available commercially in the United States, premanufactured models consist of a combination of a multichannel ports and bent instruments that can be inserted through the ports. The two ports are called Endocone and X-cone. The instruments consist of either a rigid shaft with bends at predetermined locations or a completely malleable shaft that can take any configuration and maintain an element of rigidity once placed in a specific form (Fig. 13).

Developing technology

To overcome the loss of triangulation and the presence of extracorporeal crowding created by LESS ports, the novel idea of intracorporeal deployable

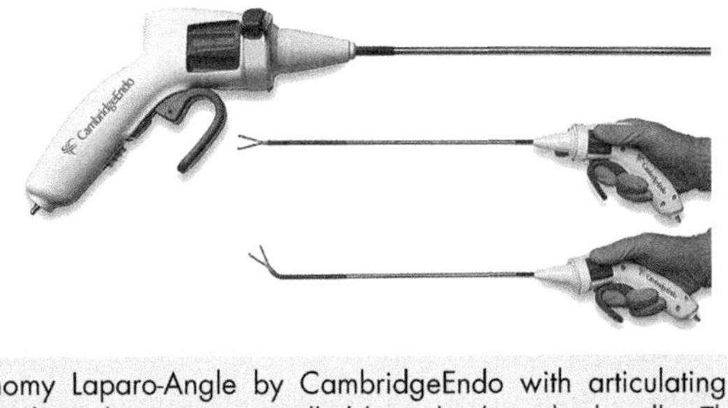

Fig. 12. Autonomy Laparo-Angle by CambridgeEndo with articulating tip mapping the handle motion and axial rotation controlled by a knob in the handle. The angle of the tip can be locked.

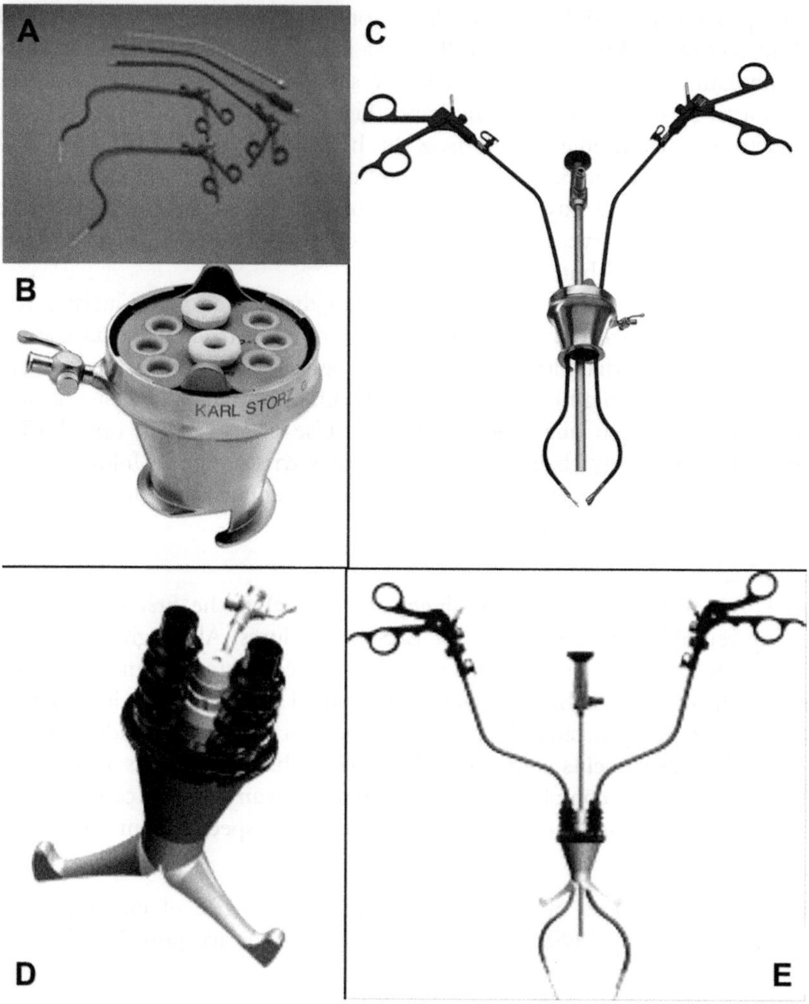

Fig. 13. S-Portal Single Port Access by KARL STORZ Endoscopy. (*A*) Prebent instruments. (*B*) Endocone port. (*C*) Endocone with prebent instruments and camera inserted. (*D*) X-cone port. (*E*) X-cone port with precurved instruments. *Courtesy of* KARL STORZ Endoscopy-America, Inc, © 2010 photo; with permission.

instruments was explored. Researchers at Columbia University (New York, NY, USA) designed a novel stereoscopic three-dimensional imaging device that collapses for abdominal insertion and has two motorized, remote controlled cameras with five degrees of freedom. Clipped to the peritoneal cavity, this robotic imaging device provides three-dimensional imaging of one or two areas. Alternatively, it shows a pair of two-dimensional views of separate abdominal fields. These images are provided while freeing a port lumen for insertion of other instruments [20,21]. University of Nebraska independently developed a mobile camera robotic system called Mobile Adjustable-focus Robotic Camera (MARC) that deploys through an access port and maneuvers throughout the abdomen. With MARC, researchers successfully completed a laparoscopic cholecystectomy in a porcine and canine model [22,23].

Similarly, Raman and colleagues [24] from the University of Texas (UT Southwestern Medical Center and UT Arlington) developed a magnetic anchoring and guidance system (MAGS). MAGS includes a magnetic platform that controls a miniature commercial camera. The camera is inserted through a conventional 15-mm port, and it is controlled by external magnets. A magnet-attached baseplate incorporates retractors and dissectors in a similar matter allowing for external maneuvering. Whereas the usefulness of a magnet system is limited by thickness of the abdominal wall and interference with other metallic instruments, it may prove useful in selected cases.

Other technologies in development include a robotically controlled camera holder, ViKY (Vision Kontrol for endoscopY; ViKY Ste Endocontrol-Medical SAS 38,000, Grenoble, France).

CURRENT APPLICATIONS

Biliary surgery

Laparoscopy first revolutionized the field of general surgery after the introduction of laparoscopic cholecystectomy more than two decades ago [25]. Although skepticism initially predominated, the benefits of a shorter recovery time and reduced postoperative pain were attractive to patients. By the mid 1990s, it became the gold standard for treatment of gallstone disease. It is now one of the most commonly performed surgeries with approximately 500,000 cases performed each year in the United States [26–28]. As patients began to request less invasive procedures, technology and equipment improved. Surgeons modified the procedure from the traditional four-port cholecystectomy to three ports and then two ports [29–32].

In 1997, Navarra and colleagues [33] reported the first successful LESS cholecystectomy. Thirty patients underwent the procedure with two 10-mm ports inserted through a single umbilical incision. In 1999, a similar umbilical approach was provided by Piskun and Rajpal [34]. Two 5-mm ports and two intra-abdominal stay sutures were used. The specimen was removed by joining the 5-mm fasciotomies. Cuesta and colleagues [35] fixed the fundus of the gallbladder using a 1-mm Kirschner wire introduced at the subcostal line. No complications were reported. When compared with patients that underwent a standard laparoscopic cholecystectomy, LESS patients exhibited lower pain scores and required fewer postoperative analgesics [36].

Other variations in technique include the use of commercially available devices like the TriPort and 12-mm AirSeal. In both, transabdominal sutures provided retraction of the gallbladder. Zhu [11] successfully completed a cholecystectomy with a novel trichannel port that accommodates one 5-mm and two 3-mm instruments [37].

Foregut surgery

Once considered an extremely challenging laparoscopic procedure, cholecystectomy is now considered commonplace. However, procedures that require intracorporeal suturing with either extra- or intracorporeal tying raise the bar for technical difficulty. This is equally true for LESS procedures. As a result, foregut procedures, that generally require suturing, are less commonly reported in the literature. However, several groups report the successful completion of bariatric procedures. Insertion of an adjustable gastric band and sleeve gastrectomy were first performed using multiple ports inserted through a single umbilical [38,39] or epigastric incision [40,41]. Recently, single-incision laparoscopic Roux-en-Y gastric bypass was reported by Huang and colleagues [42]. The patient was discharged on postoperative day two. Multiple groups in the United States and abroad are currently amassing large series of LESS bariatric procedures, including gastric bypass. However, there has yet to be a randomized and controlled comparison of standard laparoscopy to LESS in bariatric patients.

Colorectal and intestinal surgery

Similar to standard laparoscopy, appendectomy was the first general surgery procedure attempted with the LESS approach. Laparoscopic appendectomy has slowly gained favor with decreased pain, fewer postoperative complications, shorter hospitalization, earlier ambulation, earlier return to normal activity and work, and better cosmesis [43]. Single-incision laparoscopic appendectomy became more popular as people became aware of the benefits of laparoscopy and attempted to reduce the number of ports from the conventionally used three-port system [44], or decrease size of the used ports (sometimes called minilaparoscopy) [45,46].

The earliest reporting of LESS appendectomy was in 1992 by Pelosi and Pelosi [47]. Twenty-five cases were performed using an operative laparoscope inserted through a single port. In 1998, Esposito [48] demonstrated a one-port appendectomy in the pediatric population. The appendix was grasped through a 10-mm telescope and delivered outside of the abdomen. Then, the appendectomy was performed similar to an open procedure. There was no intra- or perioperative mortality or morbidity. The mean length of hospital stay was 2 days. A follow-up study published by the same group in 2002 showed a conversion rate of 15.3% in the study population of 55 patients. Half of the conversions were made to the standard laparoscopic approach and the other half were made to open surgery. Six (11%) wound related complications were noted in this cohort [49]. In 2002, D'Alessio and colleagues [50] reported their experience with 116 pediatric patients undergoing a one-port transumbilical laparoscopic-assisted appendectomy (TULAA). Their technique was similar to Esposito. An 11-mm laparoscope with a 5-mm working channel was used through an 11-mm Hasson trocar. The appendix was grasped and delivered through the umbilical incision. The appendectomy was then performed in an open fashion. Success rate of using one trocar was 77.3% with 18.7% requiring additional trocars and 4% converted to an open operation. No mortalities or complications were noted and the mean hospital stay was 3.5 days.

Several other groups have published modifications of the standard laparoscopic approach to assist with the appendectomy. Ates and colleagues [51] used one 11-mm port with one or two working channels with the appendix retracted with a percutaneous suture. Roberts [52] described the "puppeteer technique." Retraction and dissection were facilitated with a loop placed inside the abdomen.

Whereas the laparoscopic approach to colorectal surgery is slow in gaining popularity, the exploration of the single-incision approach is evident here as well. Several groups have successfully completed various partial colectomies. Bucher and colleagues [37] performed a sigmoid colectomy with multiple ports placed through a single umbilical incision. A right hemicolectomy was completed by Remzi and colleagues [13] with a Uni-X Single-Port inserted in a 3.5 cm umbilical incision. Rieger and Lam [53] also completed a series of right hemicolectomies with multiple trocars inserted through an umbilical incision ranging from 2.5 to 4.5 cm. Merchant and Lin [54] performed a right hemicolectomy in one patient with a GelPort inserted through a 2.5 cm incision. In all cases, the anastomosis were performed in an extracorporeal fashion. Procedure indications included benign and malignant diseases.

Meckel's diverticulum is another intestinal pathology successfully addressed by LESS. This was completed through an umbilical incision with a single trocar. The terminal ileum was delivered from the abdomen, and the operation was completed with an extracorporeal diverticulectomy or intestinal resection and anastomosis [55,56].

Hernia repair

The first reported single-incision laparoscopic inguinal hernia repair was described in 2005 by Chawla and colleagues [57] from India. A 10-mm laparoscope and additional instruments were inserted through a 2 to 2.5-cm incision located over the inguinal ring. An external mechanical retractor apparatus provided retraction. In a randomized and controlled study comparing the procedure to a traditional approach, the novel technique demonstrated less postoperative pain, an earlier return to work, and better cosmesis. There was no difference in time of operation and comorbidities. Others have attempted a LESS approach of the more popular forms of the laparoscopic inguinal hernia repairs. Totally extraperitoneal (TEP) inguinal hernia repair has been successfully performed through single incision through a port device [58,59], a modified GelPort [13], and with a combination of one 10-mm trocar and two adjacent 5-mm ports [60]. Transabdominal preperitoneal (TAPP) inguinal hernia repair was accomplished with the Uni-X Single-Port System [14], Tri-Port [61], and modified GelPort [62].

Solid organ surgery

Hirano and colleagues [63] reported the first laparoscopic single-incision adrenalectomy in 1992. A 4.5-cm skin incision was used in a majority of patients

(98.1%, n = 54) with limited complications (11.1% morbidity, 1.9% mortality). Walz and Alesina [64] accomplished a similar approach through a 1.5-cm incision. Merchant and colleagues [13] used a GelPort, and Castellucci and colleagues [4] successfully performed adrenalectomies with three 5-mm trocars via a single 2-cm supraumbilical incision. Cindolo and colleagues [65] were able to remove a 4-cm nonfunctional left adrenal mass with a TriPort and 5-mm instruments inserted through a 3-cm subcostal incision.

Recently, LESS splenectomy was completed with a single transumbilical incision. The majority of cases were performed with multiple trocars inserted through the same incision [66–68]. The spleen was typically placed in an endobag and morcellated before it was removed through a 1.5- to 2-cm incision. In one case, an 8-cm Pfannenstiel incision was required for a large specimen [67].

Other procedures

Various groups have reported cases of gastrostomy-tube placement, enterolysis, intussusception reduction, thoracoscopic lung biopsy, and thoracoscopic decortication attempted through single incisions [68,69].

Urology

Urethropexy was the first urological procedure performed with the LESS approach. This was accomplished using a needle suspension technique in four patients. All four patients were discharged the following day with minimal pain [70]. While single-incision nephrectomies were performed with laparoscopic assistance as early as 1996 [71], true LESS nephrectomies were not reported until 2007 [72]. Since then, various LESS urological procedures were completed. Tracy and colleagues [73] and Canes and colleagues [74] published reviews on the topic (Table 1).

Gynecology

Wheeless [2] reported the first single-incision tubal ligations in 1969. Subsequently, more than 3000 cases were completed using a single transumbilical trocar. At times, procedures were completed under local anesthesia [75,76]. In 1991, Pelosi and Pelosi [77] reported total hysterectomy with bilateral salpingo-oophorectomy (BSO) using a single-puncture technique through the umbilicus. The same group subsequently used the same approach to perform a sling procedure for stress incontinence [78], interstitial ectopic pregnancy removal [79], and myomectomy during pregnancy [80]. Others have experimented with simple procedures such as single-port ovarian cystectomy. One case report was performed on a 2-month-old infant using a Wolf cerebral endoscope (Panoview telescope, Richard Wolf, Knittlingen, Germany). In this case, a 6-cm cyst was delivered from the abdomen and the procedure was completed in an extracorporeal fashion [81]. In addition, LESS procedures have been completed with robotic assistance [82].

Table 1
Reports of urologic single-port laparoscopic surgery

Procedure	First report	Author	Number of cases	Port selection	Incision size	Other approaches
Simple nephrectomy	2007	Raman et al. [72]	3	Multitrocar, umbilical	2 to 4.5 cm	Flank incision [83], balloon dissection [83], R-port [84]
Ureterolithotomy	2008	Rane et al. [10]	1	R-port, umbilical	1.5 cm	—
Radical nephrectomy	2008	Ponsky et al. [85]	1	GelPort, paramedian	7 cm	Umbilical R-port [86], umbilical Uni-X port [15]. Umbilical Robotic GelPort [87]
Orchidectomy	2008	Rane et al. [10]	1	R-port, umbilical	1.2 cm	—
Orchidopexy	2008	Rane et al. [10]	1	R-port, umbilical	1.2 cm	Multitrocar [88]
Prostatectomy	2008	Desai et al. [89]	3	R-port, transvesical	2.5 cm	Robotic [90], transumbilical [91]
Urethropexy	1994	Knapp et al. [70]	4	10 mm port, suprapubic	1 to 2 cm	—
Bladder augmentation	2009	Sotelo et al. [91]	1	R-port, umbilical	6 cm	—
Live-donor nephrectomy	2008	Gill et al. [9]	4	R-port, umbilical	4 to 5 cm	QuadPort [92]
Sacrocolpopexy	2008	Kaouk et al. [15]	4	Uni-X port, umbilical	1.5 cm	—
Renal biopsy	2008	Kaouk et al. [15]	1	Uni-X port, umbilical	1.5 cm	Umbilical R-port [86], Umbilical Robotic GelPort [87]
Renal cryotherapy	2008	Kaouk et al. [15]	4	Uni-X port, umbilical or flank	1.5 cm	—
Pyeloplasty	2008	Desai et al. [84]	3	Umbilical R-port	2.5 cm	Umbilical Uni-X port [15]. Umbilical Robotic GelPort [87]

TECHNICAL CHALLENGES

Triangulation

Considered one of the cardinal rules of standard laparoscopy, instrument triangulation allows for effective retraction and tissue dissection along proper anatomic planes. With LESS, this becomes much more difficult even with flexible-tip or curved instruments. Crossing instruments often becomes necessary to achieve the necessary retraction even though it is a frowned-upon move in standard laparoscopy (Figs. 14 and 15). Such deviations from traditional laparoscopy have curbed surgeons' enthusiasm for adopting this new approach. Much of future technological development focuses on improving this aspect of the procedure. Some of the ideas include innovative port designs such as the TransEnterix SPIDER or prebent instruments to increase the angle of approach to the tissue.

Retraction and exposure

Effective traction and counter-traction is reduced by the lack of triangulation. Certain laparoscopic procedures also require two or more retractors, requiring modification in technique. Sutures have been used in various forms to replace one of the required ports. This can be an intra-abdominal suture used as a sling, a percutaneous suture affixed to an intra-abdominal object, or inline suture retraction through one of the ports. However, retraction of the liver during foregut surgery remains a significant obstacle for mainstream acceptance of these LESS procedures.

Inline vision

In laparoscopy, depth perception is removed by the reduction of two convergent optical fields into one, and is compensated by the coupling of action and perception of depth. Not only does this require mental rewiring and altered hand-eye coordination, uninhibited movements of the instruments are also essential.

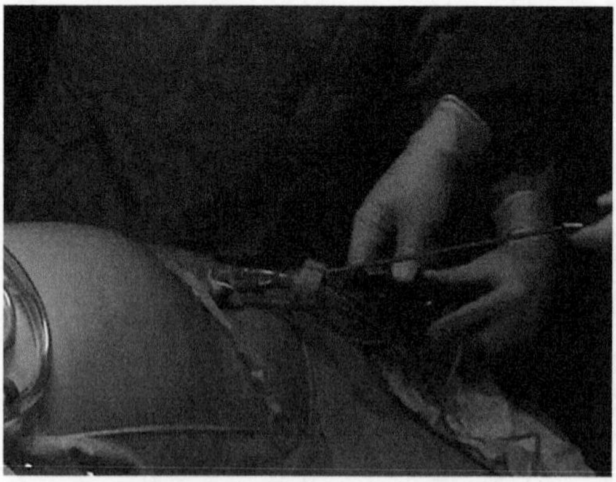

Fig. 14. External view of a LESS procedure without intracorporeal crossing of instruments leading to crowding and awkwardness of instrument handling.

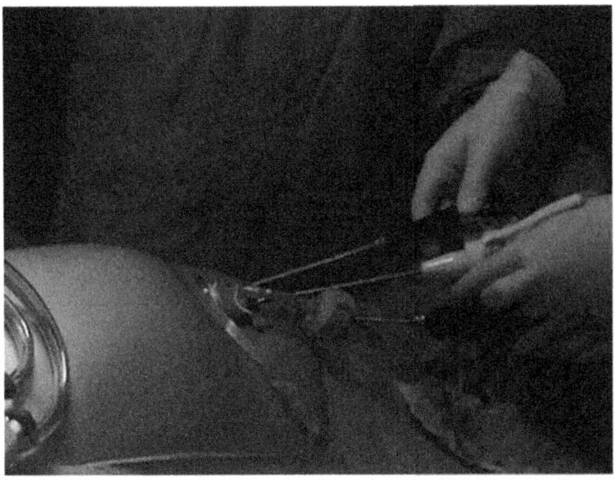

Fig. 15. External view of a LESS procedure with intracorporeal crossing of instruments to minimize external crowding and create internal triangulation.

In-line vision during LESS removes some of the visual cues that are helpful in the perception–action coupling. The juxtaposition of the instruments to the camera may also hamper the freedom of movements. Flexible laparoscopes have been used to combat this problem. Instead of moving the entire laparoscope to change the point of view, two adjustment knobs are used to achieve the same purpose which is less intuitive and prolongs the learning-curve required.

Instrument crowding

Inserting four instruments through the same incision creates interference of instruments with one another. This is accentuated by the standard laparoscope's light cable projecting at 90 degrees from the lens. Moreover, bulkier handles used on flexible tip instruments create significant problems. The limitation on range of motion increases the technical challenge and learning curve for these procedures. Although this has led to the use of light-cord adapters and creative designs of more streamline laparoscopes such as the EndoEYE (see previous discussion), further adjustments are required by the camera holder to choose alternate camera position and angle to avoid instrument clashing. Using instruments of different lengths has been helpful in addressing this issue. Alternating flexible and standard, fixed instruments have also addressed this issue. Finally, intracorporeal crossing of instruments reduces extracorporeal instrument clashing. However, this adds additional complexity to the procedures. As the surgeon moves his left-handed instrument, the instrument on the right side of the screen responds. Some groups have demonstrated that the da Vinci robot can address this issue with great success. The robot's computer can be adjusted to switch the movements of the right and left hands, overcoming confusing the situation.

Ergonomics

With standard laparoscopy, part of the port site selection is determined by locations that will allow comfortable hand positioning during the case. This flexibility is taken away in the LESS approach. In addition, technical adjustments to avoid instrument crowding and lack of triangulation sometimes require the surgeon and the assistant to maintain uncomfortable positions throughout the procedure. As the laparoscopic instruments become more sophisticated to address the various issues of LESS, ergonomic placements of the knobs and triggers become even more important. These factors can potentially affect the durability of the surgeon in performing the procedure, and may ultimately affect the safety of the approach.

Patient-related limitations

Most of the entry sites for single-incision surgery have been done through the umbilicus, removing the flexibility in port site selection afforded in standard laparoscopy. This limits the type of patients suitable for the procedure such as patients with previous incision at the umbilicus, and tall or obese patients with surgical site distant from the umbilicus such as the upper gastrointestinal tract or pelvis. Familiarity in standard multiport laparoscopy is essential in this case to properly select a patient with the appropriate body habitus.

Instrumentation

It is clear that the development of instrumentation is still in its infant stage. More streamlined and lower profile instruments are required to minimize external crowding. Newer technology is also required to decrease the external maneuvering necessary for internal movements. Current flexible-tip instruments tend to dissipate retraction or dissection forces at the tip, reducing their effectiveness. Tactile feedback is also decreased in such instruments. More logical cable placements for the laparoscope will be helpful to increase external working space. Technology such as the EndoEYE, where the camera chip is located at the tip of the instrument, is one such advancement that reduces bulk. Further innovations to creatively solve the limitations of single-incision approach and miniaturization of the equipments will make the operation less challenging.

Cost and safety

With the development of any new technology, there comes the expected increase in price tag associated with purchase of new instruments and console, servicing, and training. As some of the equipments become more sophisticated, they become more expensive compared with standard laparoscopic instruments. In the case of robotics, costs rapidly climb. Whether the added cost of instrumentation is balanced by a decreased length of stay and a more rapid return to activity remains to be determined.

Development of new instrumentation may address technical issues of LESS procedure, but the safety of the LESS approach must be studied. This is potentially difficult as the procedures have not been standardized and variations of the approach carry their own inherent risks. Yet, the safety of patients is paramount and demands that LESS procedures are proven safe before they are accepted by the surgical community. Even then, the minimum number of procedures one needs perform to overcome the learning curve needs to be determined.

SUMMARY

Laparoscopic surgery performed through a single-incision is gaining popularity. The demand from the public for even less invasive procedures will motivate surgeons, industry, and academic centers to explore the possibilities and refine the technology. Although the idea seems quite attractive, there are several technological obstacles that are yet to be conquered by improved technology or additional training. The question of safety has yet to be answered and will require well-designed randomized control trials. Opponents to the approach argue that the size of the single incision (see Table 1) is frequently larger than all the standard laparoscopy incisions combined. On the other hand, proponents remember a similar argument from traditional open surgeons during the initial development of laparoscopy. That argument was quickly discredited when the immediate benefits of laparoscopy were compared with patients undergoing surgery with small laparotomy incisions.

During the development of a new technique, the learning curve exposes patients to risk and society to expense. LESS pioneers appear to have reached a level of comfort with technology and techniques that paves the way for scientific scrutiny. Perhaps, the surgical community will capitalize on this situation with randomized, controlled studies and sound evidence to support or refute the benefits of LESS. If we do not seize this opportunity, patient demand and industry's dual edge message of financial success versus fear of losing referrals will lead to a scenario similar to the development of laparoscopic cholecystectomy in the 1990s.

Regardless of its future, the surgical community will still benefit from a renewed excitement as surgeons aim to continually reduce the amount of pain and trauma our patients must endure. In addition, technological advances on instrumentation will benefit the field of laparoscopy and improve patient care.

References

[1] Kelling G. Ueber die Besichtigung der Speiseroehre und des Magens. The 73rd Congressional meeting of German naturalists and scientists. Verhandlungen der Gesellschaft 1901;117–9.

[2] Wheeless C. A rapid, inexpensive, and effective method of surgical sterilization by laparoscopy. J Reprod Med 1969;3(5):65–9.

[3] Rattner D, Kalloo A, ASGE/SAGES Working Group. ASGE/SAGES working group on natural orifice translumenal endoscopic surgery. October 2005. Surg Endosc 2006;20: 329–33.

[4] Castellucci SA, Curcillo PG, Ginsberg PC, et al. Single port access adrenalectomy. J Endourol 2008;22(8):1573–6.

[5] Podolsky ER, Rottman SJ, Curcillo PG 2nd. Single Port Access (SPA) gastrostomy tube in patients unable to receive percutaneous endoscopic gastrostomy placement. Surg Endosc 2009;23(5):1142–5.

[6] Podolsky ER, Rottman SJ, Poblete H, et al. Single port access (SPA) cholecystectomy: a completely transumbilical approach. J Laparoendosc Adv Surg Tech A 2009;19(2): 219–22.

[7] Nguyen NT, Reavis KM, Hinojosa MW, et al. Laparoscopic transumbilical cholecystectomy without visible abdominal scars. J Gastrointest Surg 2009;13(6):1125–8.

[8] Desai MM, Stein R, Rao P, et al. Embryonic natural orifice transumbilical endoscopic surgery (E-NOTES) for advanced reconstruction: initial experience. Urology 2009;73(1):182–7.

[9] Gill IS, Canes D, Aron M, et al. Single port transumbilical (E-NOTES) donor nephrectomy. J Urol 2008;180(2):637–41 [discussion: 641].

[10] Rane A, Rao P, Rao P. Single-port-access nephrectomy and other laparoscopic urologic procedures using a novel laparoscopic port (R-port). Urology May 12 2008;72:260–3, 2009.

[11] Zhu J. Scarless endoscopic surgery: NOTES or TUES. Surg Endosc 2007;21:1898–9.

[12] Zhu JF, Hu H, Ma YZ, et al. Transumbilical endoscopic surgery: a preliminary clincal report. Surg Endosc 2009;23(4):813–7.

[13] Remzi FH, Kirat HT, Kaouk JH, et al. Single-port laparoscopy in colorectal surgery. Colorectal Dis 2008;10(8):823–6.

[14] Kroh M, Rosenblatt S. Single-port, laparoscopic cholecystectomy and inguinal hernia repair: first clinical report of a new device. J Laparoendosc Adv Surg Tech A 2009;19(2):215–7.

[15] Kaouk JH, Haber GP, Goel RK, et al. Single-port laparoscopic surgery in urology: initial experience. Urology 2008;71(1):3–6.

[16] Merchant AM, Cook MW, White BC, et al. Transumbilical Gelport access technique for performing single incision laparoscopic surgery (SILS). J Gastrointest Surg 2009;13(1): 159–62.

[17] Pryor AD, Tushar JR, Dibernardo LR. Single-port cholecystectomy with the TransEnterix SPIDER: simple and safe. Surg Endosc 2010;24(4):917–23.

[18] Afthinos JN, Forrester GJ, Binenbaum SJ, et al. Single-incision laparoscopic cholecystectomy using flexible endoscopy: saline infiltration gallbladder fossa dissection technique. Surg Endosc Mar 19 2009.

[19] Binenbaum SJ, Teixeira JA, Forrester GJ, et al. Single-incision laparoscopic cholecystectomy using a flexible endoscope. Arch Surg 2009;144(8):734–8.

[20] Fowler DL, Hu T, Nadkarni T, et al. Initial trial of a stereoscopic, insertable, remotely controlled camera for minimal access surgery. Surg Endosc 2010;24(1):9–15.

[21] Miller A, Allen P, Fowler D. In-vivo stereoscopic imaging system with 5 degrees-of-freedom for minimal access surgery. Stud Health Technol Inform 2004;98:234–40.

[22] Rentschler ME, Dumpert J, Platt SR, et al. Mobile in vivo camera robots provide sole visual feedback for abdominal exploration and cholecystectomy. Surg Endosc 2006;20(1):135–8.

[23] Joseph JV, Oleynikov D, Rentschler M, et al. Microrobot assisted laparoscopic urological surgery in a canine model. J Urol 2008;180(5):2202–5.

[24] Raman JD, Scott DJ, Cadeddu JA. Role of magnetic anchors during laparoendoscopic single site surgery and NOTES. J Endourol 2009;23(5):781–6.

[25] Reynolds W Jr. The first laparoscopic cholecystectomy. JSLS 2001;5(1):89–94.

[26] Sain AH. Laparoscopic cholecystectomy is the current "gold standard" for the treatment of gallstone disease. Ann Surg 1996;224(5):689–90.

[27] Mosimann F. Laparoscopic cholecystectomy has become the new gold standard for the management of symptomatic gallbladder stones. Hepatogastroenterology 2006;53(69): 1, preceding I; author reply 1 p preceding I.

[28] Begos DG, Modlin IM. Laparoscopic cholecystectomy: from gimmick to gold standard. J Clin Gastroenterol 1994;19(4):325–30.

[29] Bakr AA. A new modified layout for laparoscopic cholecystectomy. JSLS 1997;1(3):281–3.

[30] Leggett PL, Bissell CD, Churchman-Winn R, et al. Three-port microlaparoscopic cholecystectomy in 159 patients. Surg Endosc 2001;15(3):293–6.

[31] Roll S, Azevedo JL, Gorski W, et al. Two-port technique for laparoscopic cholecystectomy using a microendoscope. Endoscopy 1997;29(7):S43.

[32] Poon CM, Chan KW, Lee DW, et al. Two-port versus four-port laparoscopic cholecystectomy. Surg Endosc 2003;17(10):1624–7.

[33] Navarra G, Pozza E, Occhionorelli S, et al. One-wound laparoscopic cholecystectomy. Br J Surg 1997;84(5):695.
[34] Piskun G, Rajpal S. Transumbilical laparoscopic cholecystectomy utilizes no incisions outside the umbilicus. J Laparoendosc Adv Surg Tech A 1999;9(4):361–4.
[35] Cuesta MA, Berends F, Veenhof AA. The "invisible cholecystectomy": a transumbilical laparoscopic operation without a scar. Surg Endosc 2008;22(5):1211–3.
[36] Bresadola F, Pasqualucci A, Donini A, et al. Elective transumbilical compared with standard laparoscopic cholecystectomy. Eur J Surg 1999;165(1):29–34.
[37] Bucher P, Pugin F, Morel P. Transumbilical single incision laparoscopic sigmoidectomy for benign disease. Colorectal Dis 2009;12(1):61–5.
[38] Saber AA, El-Ghazaly TH. Early experience with single-access transumbilical adjustable laparoscopic gastric banding. Obes Surg 2009;19(10):1442–6.
[39] Saber AA, Elgamal MH, Itawi EA, et al. Single incision laparoscopic sleeve gastrectomy (SILS): a novel technique. Obes Surg 2008;18(10):1338–42.
[40] Nguyen NT, Hinojosa MW, Smith BR, et al. Single laparoscopic incision transabdominal (SLIT) surgery-adjustable gastric banding: a novel minimally invasive surgical approach. Obes Surg 2008;18(12):1628–31.
[41] Reavis KM, Hinojosa MW, Smith BR, et al. Single-laparoscopic incision transabdominal surgery sleeve gastrectomy. Obes Surg 2008;18(11):1492–4.
[42] Huang CK, Houng JY, Chiang CJ, et al. Single incision transumbilical laparoscopic Roux-en-Y gastric bypass: a first case report. Obes Surg 2009;19(12):1711–5.
[43] Sauerland S, Lefering R, Neugebauer EA. Laparoscopic versus open surgery for suspected appendicitis. Cochrane Database Syst Rev 2004;4:CD001546.
[44] Rao MM, Rao RK. Two-port and single port laparoscopic appendicectomy. J Indian Med Assoc 2004;102(7):360, 362, 364.
[45] Croce E, Olmi S, Azzola M, et al. Laparoscopic appendectomy and minilaparoscopic approach: a retrospective review after 8-years' experience. JSLS 1999;3(4):285–92.
[46] Lee PI, Chi YS, Chang YK, et al. Minilaparoscopy to reduce complications from cannula insertion in patients with previous pelvic or abdominal surgery. J Am Assoc Gynecol Laparosc 1999;6(1):91–5.
[47] Pelosi MA, Pelosi MA. Laparoscopic appendectomy using a single umbilical puncture (minilaparoscopy). J Reprod Med 1992;37:588–94.
[48] Esposito C. One-trocar appendectomy in pediatric surgery. Surg Endosc 1998;12(2):177–8.
[49] Rispoli G, Armellino MF, Esposito C. One-trocar appendectomy. Surg Endosc 2002;16(5):833–5.
[50] D'Alessio A, Piro E, Tadini B, et al. One-trocar transumbilical laparoscopic-assisted appendectomy in children: our experience. Eur J Pediatr Surg 2002;12(1):24–7.
[51] Ates O, Hakguder G, Olguner M, et al. Single-port laparoscopic appendectomy conducted intracorporeally with the aid of a transabdominal sling suture. J Pediatr Surg 2007;42(6):1071–4.
[52] Roberts KE. True single-port appendectomy: first experience with the "puppeteer technique". Surg Endosc 2009;23(8):1825–30.
[53] Rieger NA, Lam FF. Single-incision laparoscopically assisted colectomy using standard laparoscopic instrumentation. Surg Endosc 2010;24(4):880–90.
[54] Merchant AM, Lin E. Single-incision laparoscopic right hemicolectomy for a colon mass. Dis Colon Rectum 2009;52(5):1021–4.
[55] Clark JM, Koontz CS, Smith LA, et al. Video-assisted transumbilical Meckel's diverticulectomy in children. Am Surg 2008;74(4):327–9.
[56] Cobellis G, Cruccetti A, Mastroianni L, et al. One-trocar transumbilical laparoscopic-assisted management of Meckel's diverticulum in children. J Laparoendosc Adv Surg Tech A 2007;17(2):238–41.

[57] Chawla S, Lal P, Ganguly PK, et al. Endoscope-assisted inguinal hernia repair. JSLS 2005;9(1):42–6.
[58] Agrawal S, Shaw A, Soon Y. Single-port laparoscopic totally extraperitoneal inguinal hernia repair with the TriPort system: initial experience. Surg Endosc 2010;24(4):952–6.
[59] Jacob BP, Tong W, Reiner M, et al. Single incision total extraperitoneal (one SITE) laparoscopic inguinal hernia repair using a single access port device. Hernia 2009;13(5):571–2.
[60] Filipovic-Cugura J, Kirac I, Kulis T, et al. Single-incision laparoscopic surgery (SILS) for totally extraperitoneal (TEP) inguinal hernia repair: first case. Surg Endosc 2009;23(4):920–1.
[61] Menenakos C, Kilian M, Hartmann J. Single-port access in laparoscopic bilateral inguinal hernia repair: first clinical report of a novel technique. Hernia 2010;14(3):309–12.
[62] Tai HC, Lin CD, Wu CC, et al. Homemade transumbilical port: an alternative access for laparoendoscopic single-site surgery (LESS). Surg Endosc 2010;24(3):705–8.
[63] Hirano D, Minei S, Yamaguchi K, et al. Retroperitoneoscopic adrenalectomy for adrenal tumors via a single large port. J Endourol 2005;19(7):788–92.
[64] Walz MK, Alesina PF. Single access retroperitoneoscopic adrenalectomy (SARA)–one step beyond in endocrine surgery. Langenbecks Arch Surg 2009;394(3):447–50.
[65] Cindolo L, Gidaro S, Tamburro FR, et al. Laparo-endoscopic single-site left transperitoneal adrenalectomy. Eur Urol 2010;57(5):911–4.
[66] Barbaros U, Dinccag A. Single incision laparoscopic splenectomy: the first two cases. J Gastrointest Surg 2009;13(8):1520–3.
[67] Dutta S. Early experience with single incision laparoscopic surgery: eliminating the scar from abdominal operations. J Pediatr Surg 2009;44(9):1741–5.
[68] Ponsky TA, Diluciano J, Chwals W, et al. Early experience with single-port laparoscopic surgery in children. J Laparoendosc Adv Surg Tech A 2009;19(4):551–3.
[69] Rothenberg SS, Shipman K, Yoder S. Experience with modified single-port laparoscopic procedures in children. J Laparoendosc Adv Surg Tech A 2009;19(5):695–8.
[70] Knapp PM Jr, Siegel YI, Lingeman JE. Laparoscopic retroperitoneal needle suspension urethropexy. J Endourol 1994;8(4):279–84.
[71] Repassy DL, Frang D, Jako GJ. Minimal and direct access surgery in urology. Diagn Ther Endosc 1996;3(2):99–105.
[72] Raman JD, Bensalah K, Bagrodia A, et al. Laboratory and clinical development of single keyhole umbilical nephrectomy. Urology 2007;70(6):1039–42.
[73] Tracy CR, Raman JD, Cadeddu JA, et al. Laparoendoscopic single-site surgery in urology: where have we been and where are we heading? Nat Clin Pract Urol 2008;5(10):561–8.
[74] Canes D, Desai MM, Aron M, et al. Transumbilical single-port surgery: evolution and current status. Eur Urol 2008;54(5):1020–9.
[75] Wheeless CR Jr. Outpatient laparoscope sterilization under local anesthesia. Obstet Gynecol 1972;39(5):767–70.
[76] Wheeless CR Jr, Thompson BH. Laparoscopic sterilization. Review of 3600 cases. Obstet Gynecol 1973;42(5):751–8.
[77] Pelosi MA, Pelosi MA 3rd. Laparoscopic hysterectomy with bilateral salpingo-oophorectomy using a single umbilical puncture. N J Med 1991;88(10):721–6.
[78] Pelosi MA. Single puncture laparoscopic sling procedure. J Am Assoc Gynecol Laparosc 1994;1(4, Part 2):S28.
[79] Pelosi MA. Successful laparoscopic removal of an interstitial ectopic pregnancy. J Am Assoc Gynecol Laparosc 1994;1(4, Part 2):S28.
[80] Pelosi MA, Pelosi MA 3rd, Giblin S. Laparoscopic removal of a 1500-g symptomatic myoma during the second trimester of pregnancy. J Am Assoc Gynecol Laparosc 1995;2(4):457–62.
[81] Kosumi T, Kubota A, Usui N, et al. Laparoscopic ovarian cystectomy using a single umbilical puncture method. Surg Laparosc Endosc Percutan Tech 2001;11(1):63–5.

[82] Escobar PF, Fader AN, Paraiso MF, et al. Robotic-assisted laparoendoscopic single-site surgery in gynecology: initial report and technique. J Minim Invasive Gynecol 2009;16(5):589–91.

[83] Msezane LP, Mushtaq I, Gundeti MS. An update on experience with the single-instrument port laparoscopic nephrectomy. BJU Int 2009;103(10):1406–8 [discussion: 1408–9].

[84] Desai MM, Rao PP, Aron M, et al. Scarless single port transumbilical nephrectomy and pyeloplasty: first clinical report. BJU Int 2008;101(1):83–8.

[85] Ponsky LE, Cherullo EE, Sawyer M, et al. Single access site laparoscopic radical nephrectomy: initial clinical experience. J Endourol 2008;22(4):663–6.

[86] Desai MM, Berger AK, Brandina R, et al. Laparoendoscopic single-site surgery: initial hundred patients. Urology 2009;74(4):805–12.

[87] Stein RJ, White WM, Goel RK, et al. Robotic laparoendoscopic single-site surgery using GelPort as the access platform. Eur Urol 2010;57(1):132–7.

[88] de Lima GR, da Silveira RA, de Cerqueira JB, et al. Single-incision multiport laparoscopic orchidopexy: initial report. J Pediatr Surg 2009;44(10):2054–6.

[89] Desai MM, Aron M, Canes D, et al. Single-port transvesical simple prostatectomy: initial clinical report. Urology 2008;72(5):960–5.

[90] Kaouk JH, Goel RK, Haber GP, et al. Robotic single-port transumbilical surgery in humans: initial report. BJU Int 2009;103(3):366–9.

[91] Sotelo R, Astigueta JC, Carmona O, et al. [Laparo-endoscopic single site (LESS)]. Actas Urol Esp 2009;33(2):172–81 [in Spanish] [discussion: 110–72].

[92] Ganpule AP, Dhawan DR, Kurien A, et al. Laparoendoscopic single-site donor nephrectomy: a single-center experience. Urology 2009;74(6):1238–40.

Advances in Surgery 44 (2010) 29–47
ADVANCES IN SURGERY

ELSEVIER
MOSBY

Combating Stress and Burnout in Surgical Practice: A Review

Charles M. Balch, MD[a,*], Tait Shanafelt, MD[b]

[a]Johns Hopkins Medical Institutions, Department of Surgery, 1515 Orleans St. Cancer Research Building II, Room 507, Baltimore, MD 21231, USA
[b]Mayo Clinic, Department of Medicine, 200 First Street South West, Rochester, MN 55905, USA

Surgeons work hard, work long hours, deal regularly with "life and death" situations with their patients, and make substantial personal sacrifices to practice in their chosen field. These attributes of surgery, along with the rigors and length of training for this profession, attract individuals of a particular character sharing an unwritten but clearly understood code of rules, norms, and expectations. This code includes coming in early and staying late, working nights and weekends, performing a high volume of procedures, meeting multiple simultaneous deadlines, and keeping emotions or personal problems from interfering with work. While these characteristics of surgeons should be celebrated, there is a fine line separating dedication from unhealthy overwork that, if unchecked, could lead to counterproductive, unhealthy, or even self-destructive behavior, which may ultimately affect patient care [1,2]. Indeed, studies show that a substantial proportion of surgeons experience distress or burnout, which can have negative repercussions for themselves, their families, their colleagues, and their patients.

Burnout is a syndrome of emotional exhaustion and depersonalization that leads to decreased effectiveness at work [3]. Burnout can affect both physicians' satisfaction with their work and the quality of medical care that they provide [4–7]. Burnout is markedly more common among physicians than depression, substance abuse, or suicide. As a clinical syndrome, burnout is characterized by emotional exhaustion, depersonalization, and a decreased sense of personal accomplishment [8,9]. This syndrome primarily affects individuals, such as doctors, nurses, and social workers, whose work involves constant demands and intense interactions with people having physical and emotional needs. There are 2 common symptoms of burnout: treating patients and colleagues as objects rather than human beings, and feeling emotionally depleted. Other symptoms and signs of burnout include physical exhaustion, poor judgment, cynicism, guilt, ineffectiveness, and a sense of depersonalization in relationships with coworkers or patients [2,8,10,11]. Burnout has also been associated with

*Corresponding author. *E-mail address*: balchch@jhmi.edu.

0065-3411/10/$ – see front matter
doi:10.1016/j.yasu.2010.05.018

poor health, including headaches, sleep disturbances, depression, hypertension, anxiety, alcoholism, and myocardial infarction [2,8–10,12–15].

One of the tragic paradoxes of burnout is that those who are most susceptible seem to be the most dedicated, conscientious, responsible, and motivated. Individuals with these traits are often idealistic and have perfectionist qualities, which may lead them to submerse themselves in their work and devote themselves to it until they have nothing left to give. Thus, commitment to patients, attention to detail, and recognition of the responsibility associated with patients' trust, the very traits that define a good surgeon, place them at a greater risk for burnout [11,16].

SOME CAUSES OF BURNOUT

Several studies have explored the potential causes of physician burnout [8–10,13,14,17]. These studies suggest that a lack of autonomy, difficulty in balancing personal and professional life, excessive administrative tasks, and high patient volume are the greatest sources of stress. The manner in which these and other work characteristics affect a given individual is complex and depends on their personal responsibilities (eg, relationships, age of children, other interests), personality, health, and enthusiasm for work. Nonetheless, there appear to be some common themes that affect a larger number of individuals. A partial list of potential contributing causes includes (1) length of training, (2) a mentality of delayed gratification, (3) insufficient protected research time and funding, (4) long working hours, (5) imbalance between career and family, (6) hostile workplace environment, and (7) gender and age-related issues [2].

Long hours and lack of control over one's schedule during medical school, residency, and fellowship may also inculcate surgeons (and physicians from other medical specialties) with a set of habits that are counterproductive to achieving a balanced and full life, once training is completed [18–20]. During this time, a coping strategy that puts personal life on hold seems to foster a mentality of delayed gratification (ie, "things will get better when I finish residency") that many physicians carry with them into practice [9,11,12,19,21]. Once developed, many physicians maintain this strategy of delayed gratification after completing residency or fellowship, and rather than cultivating their personal relationships and interests these physicians find themselves perpetually delaying this task to the future (eg, until after establishing their practice, until after becoming an associate professor, and so forth). In fact, many physicians seem to believe that they cannot simultaneously have a fulfilling personal and professional life, and may maintain a strategy that puts their personal life on hold until they retire or leave the practice of medicine [9,11,12,21].

Although the total number of hours worked by surgeons has not been found to be an independent predictor of burnout in most studies, the vast majority of them work more than 60 h/wk [17]. For example, in the study by Kuerer and colleagues [22], 89% of surgical oncologists worked more than 50 h/wk, while 60% and 24% worked more than 60 h/wk and 70 h/wk, respectively. This work profile contrasts with other occupations, because according to the United States Bureau of Labor Statistics the average American workweek is 34.5 h/wk [23].

THE AMERICAN COLLEGE OF SURGEONS BURNOUT SURVEY

Because of the importance of burnout as a form of distress, a survey of the membership of the American College of Surgeons (ACS) was commissioned by the ACS Governor's Committee on Physician Competency and Health in 2008 to determine the incidence of burnout among American surgeons and to evaluate the personal and professional characteristics associated with surgeon burnout. Of the approximately 64,300 fellows and associate fellows (surgeons in their first year of practice) in the ACS at the time of the survey, approximately 24,000 surgeons had an e-mail address on record, which they were permitted to use for purposes of correspondence with the college and formed the study sample. Among these surgeons, 7905 (32%) returned surveys. Their personal and professional characteristics are shown in Table 1 and their workload (hours and nights on call per week) is shown in Fig. 1. This responding sample of nearly 8000 surgeons represents the largest study of burnout among physicians that has ever been reported. In this article, the investigators summarize some of the previous publications that describe the survey results and focus on several important issues, including the association of burnout with medical errors, depression, and suicide ideation [5,15,17].

Overall results

There was a high rate of burnout among American surgeons, with nearly 40% meeting the criteria for burnout (Table 2). Factors independently associated with burnout on multivariate analysis are shown in Table 3. Overall, 32% of the surgeons had high emotional exhaustion, 26% demonstrated high depersonalization, and 13% had a low sense of personal accomplishment (Table 2) [17]. Consistent with these results, 28% of surgeons had a mental quality of life (QOL) score more than 0.5 SD below the population norm, a decrement shown to be clinically meaningful [24], while 11% had a physical QOL score more than 0.5 SD below the population norm. Younger surgeons and those with children between the ages of 5 and 21 years were at higher risk, and so were surgeons whose compensation was based entirely on billing/productivity and those who spent more nights on call per week. Area of subspecialization was also associated with burnout, with higher risk among trauma, urology, otolaryngology, vascular, and general surgeons. However, the number of hours worked was not associated with burnout, despite the surgeons working a median of 60 h/wk and 30% of them working more than 70 h/wk.

Approximately 30% of the study participants were screened positive for depression (Table 2). Given the sensitivity (96%) and specificity (57%) of the screening instrument used [25,26], this finding implies that between 10% and 15% of respondents would have met the criteria for major depressive disorder at the time of the survey if they had undergone a full psychiatric assessment.

Career satisfaction

Nearly three-fourths of surgeons would become a surgeon again, but only half would recommend that their children should become a physician (Table 2). Burnout was the single greatest predictor of career dissatisfaction among

Table 1
Personal and Professional Characteristics of the 2008 American College of Surgeons Survey (Data from reference 17)

		N (%) or Median (Q1, Q3)[3] N = 7905
AGE	Median	51 years (43, 59)
GENDER	Male	6815 (86.7%)
	Female	1043 (13.3%)
RELATIONSHIP STATUS	Missing	6
	Single	678 (8.6%)
	Married	6950 (88%)
	Partnered	221 (2.8%)
	Widowed or widower	50 (0.6%)
EVER GONE THROUGH A DIVORCE	Missing	58
	Yes	1671 (21.3%)
	No	6176 (78.7%)
PARTNER OR SPOUSE WORK OUTSIDE HOME[1]	Yes	3700 (51.6%)
	No	3471 (48.4%)
PARTNER OR SPOUSE CURRENT PROFESSION[2]	Surgeon	335 (9.2%)
	Physician but not surgeon	830 (22.7%)
	Other health care professional (e.g. nurse, therapist)	1060 (29%)
	Non-medical professional (e.g. engineer, business)	1033 (28.3%)
	Other	397 (10.9%)
HAVE CHILDREN	missing	1
	Yes	6917 (87.5%)
	NO	987 (12.5%)
SURGICAL SPECIALTY	Missing	44
	Cardiothoracic	489 (6.2%)
	Colorectal	302 (3.8%)
	Dermatologic	2 (0%)
	General	3233 (41.1%)
	Neuro	184 (2.3)
	Otolaryngology	371(4.7%)
	Ob/Gyn	105 (1.3%)
	Oncologic	407 (5.2%)
	Ophthalmologic	181 (2.3%)
	Orthopedic	155 (2.0%)
	Pediatric	243 (3.1%)
	Plastic	458 (4%)
	Transplant	123 (1.6%)
	Trauma	345 (4.4%)
	Urologic	315 (4%)
	Vascular	463 (5.9%)
	Other	485 (6.2%)
YEARS IN PRACTICE	Median	18.5 (9, 27)
	<10 years	1987 (25.7%)
	10-19 years	2209 (28.3%)
	20-30 years	2467 (31.6%)
	>30 years	1132 (14.5%)

(*continued on next page*)

Table 1
(continued)

		N (%) or Median (Q1, Q3)[3] N = 7905
HOURS WORKED PER WEEK	Median	60 (50, 70)
	<40 hrs	666 (8.5%)
	40-49 hrs	800 (10.3%)
	50-59 hrs	1410 (18.2%)
	60-69 hrs	2539 (32.6%)
	70-79 hrs	1048 (13.4%)
	≥80 hrs	1336 (17.1%)
HOURS PER WEEK IN OPERATING ROOM	Median	16 (10, 24)
# NIGHTS ON CALL PER WEEK	Median	2 (1, 4)
PRIMARY PRACTICE SETTING	Missing	9
	Private practice	4240 (53.7%)
	Academic Medical Center	2272 (28.8%)
	Veterans hospital	155 (2%)
	Active military practice	114 (1.4%)
	Not in practice or retired	290 (3.7%)
	Other	825 (10.4%)
PRIMARY METHOD DETERMINING COMPENSATION	Missing	179
	Salaried, no incentive pay	1674 (21.7%)
	Salaried, bonus pay based on billing	2372 (30.7%)
	Incentive pay based entirely on billing	2934 (38%)
	Other	746 (9.7%)
% TIME DEDICATED TO NON-PATIENT CARE ACTIVITIES	missing	57
	0%	384 (4.9%)
	<10%	2273 (29%)
	10-20%	2539 (32.4%)
	21-30%	1204 (15.3%)
	31-50%	805 (10.3%)
	>50%	643 (8.2%)

[1]Only asked of surgeons indicating they currently are married or partnered.
[2]Only asked of surgeons indicating their spouse currently working outside the home.
[3]Q1 is the lower 25th percentile and Q3 is the upper 75th percentile.

surgeons, and accounted for more of the variation in satisfaction with career and specialty choice than any other personal or professional factor [17]. Factors that are independently associated with career and specialty choice satisfaction on multivariate analysis are shown in Table 4. Personal characteristics associated with a greater satisfaction with overall career choice (being a physician) were older age and the absence of burnout.

Professional characteristics associated with greater satisfaction with overall career choice were absence of burnout, area of specialization, having higher academic rank among academic surgeons, being in active military practice,

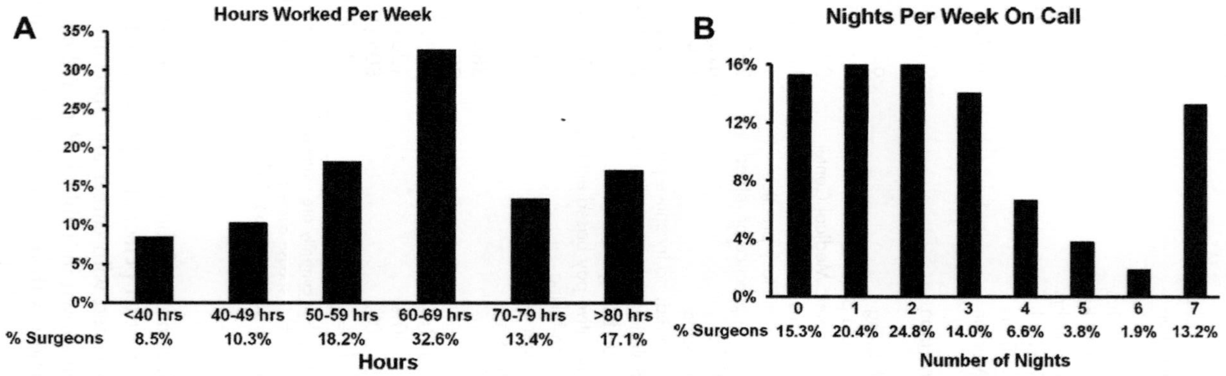

Fig. 1. Hours worked and call schedule of American surgeons. (*A*) Distribution of average hours worked per week. (*B*) Distribution of nights on call. *From* Shanafelt TD, et al. Burnout and Career Satisfaction Among American Surgeons. Ann Surg 2009;250:466; with permission.

Table 2
Burnout, Depression, and Career Satisfaction among the 7905 Members of the American College of Surgeons Who Participated in the Survey Study (Data from reference 17)

	N (%) or median
Burnout indices[1]	
Emotional exhaustion	
Median score	19.0
% Low score	3667 (47.2%)
% Moderate score	1639 (21.1%)
% High score	2464 (31.7%)
Depersonalization	
Median score	5.0
% Low score	4079 (52.6%)
% Moderate score	1657 (21.4%)
% High score	2020 (26%)
Personal accomplishment	
Median score	42.0
% High score	5056 (65.7%)
% Moderate score	1656 (21.5%)
% Low score	982 (12.8%)
Burned out[2]	3083 (39.6%)
Depression	
Screen positive for depression	2349 (30%)
Career satisfaction	
Would become physician again (career choice)	5548 (70.5%)
Would become a surgeon again (specialty choice)	5823 (74.0%)
Would you recommend your children pursue a career as a physician/surgeon?	3462 (50.5%)
Work schedule leaves enough time for personal/family life	2856 (36.4%)

[1]Participants with high scores on the Emotional Exhaustion (score ≥27) and Depersonalization (score ≥10) subscales or low scores on the Personal Accomplishment subscale (score ≤33) are considered to have symptoms of burnout.
[2]High score on Emotional Exhaustion and/or Depersonalization subscales.

and spending more working hours in the operating room (see Table 4). Having more nights on call per week was associated with a lower satisfaction with overall career choice. Similar to satisfaction with overall career choice, personal characteristics associated with a greater satisfaction with specialty choice (being a surgeon) were older age and the absence of burnout.

Depression and suicide ideation

Suicide ideation (SI) was reported by 501 (6.4%) surgeons in the ACS survey during the previous 12 months [15,17]. SI was 1.5 to 3.0 times more common among surgeons than the general population in the age groups 45 to 54 years (7.6% vs 5.0%, $P = .008$), 55 to 64 years (6.9% vs 2.3%, $P < .001$), and 65 years and older (2.7% vs 1.2%, $P = .023$). The prevalence of SI was highest among surgeons aged 45 to 54 years and did not differ by sex. Being married (odds ratio [OR] 0.561, $P < .0001$) and having children (OR 0.668, $P = .0011$) were associated with a lower likelihood of SI, whereas risk was higher among those

Table 3
Factors independently associated with burnout on multivariate logistic analysis

Characteristics and associated factors	OR[a]	*P* value
Subspecialty choice[b]	1.2–1.6	All ≤.013
Youngest child aged between </= 21 y	1.54	<.001
Compensation = incentive pay, based entirely on billing	1.37	<.001
Spouse works as other health care professional (nurse, pharmacist, and so forth)	1.23	.004
Number of nights on call per week (each additional night)	1.05	<.001
Number of years in practice (each additional year)	1.03	<.001
Hours worked per week (each additional hour)	1.02	p<0.001
Age (each additional year older)	0.96	<.001
Has children	0.82	.006
>50% time dedicated to non–patient care (research, administration)	0.81	.035

Abbreviation: OR, odds ratio.

[a]OR>1 indicates increased risk of burnout; OR<1 indicates lower risk of burnout.

[b]Trauma (OR = 1.56), urology (OR = 1.48), otolaryngology (OR = 1.33), vascular (OR = 1.36), general (OR 1.17).

Modified from Shanafelt TD, Bechamps G, Russell T, et al. Burnout and career satisfaction among American surgeons. Ann Surg 2009;250:467; with permission.

who had gone through a divorce (OR = 1.6, $P<.0001$). Although SI was more common among 8% of surgeons working 40 h/wk or more (OR 2.071, $P=.001$), no further stratification of risk was observed by the number of hours worked for the remaining 92% of surgeons working 40 h/wk or more. Surgeons with SI reported a greater frequency of overnight call (mean 3 d/wk vs 2.6 d/wk, $P=.0001$). The perception of having made a major medical error in the last 3 months was associated with a 3-fold increased risk of SI in 16.2% of surgeons who reported a recent error as compared with 5.4% of surgeons not reporting an error ($P<.0001$). No difference in SI was observed by subspecialty discipline, hours per week spent in the operating room, percentage of time dedicated to non–patient care activities (eg, research, administration), method of compensation, or years in practice, with the exception of lower risk among those who had been in practice for more than 30 years [15,17].

SI was strongly correlated with measures of distress and QOL [15]. Symptoms of depression were endorsed by 390 of 501 (77.8%) surgeons with SI compared with 1938 (26.7%) without SI ($P<.0001$). SI demonstrated a large positive correlation with each domain of burnout. For each 1-point higher score on the emotional exhaustion (OR = 1.069, $P<.0001$) or depersonalization (OR 1.109, $P<.001$) subscale or each 1-point lower score on the personal accomplishment (OR 1.057, $P<.001$) subscale, surgeons were 5.7% to 10.9% more likely to report SI. The aggregate effect of the relationship between burnout and SI is large because the score in emotional exhaustion subscale ranges from 0 to 54; in depersonalization subscale from 0 to 33; and in personal accomplishment subscale from 0 to 48. Of note, the prevalence of SI increased with the severity of burnout, independent of the symptoms of depression. Although SI also demonstrated a strong

Table 4
Factors independently associated with satisfaction with specialty and career choice on multivariate analysis

Characteristics and associated factors	OR[a]	*P* value
Satisfaction with Overall Career Choice (Being a Physician)		
Absence of burnout	4.59	<.001
Subspecialty[b]	1.4–2.6	All ≤.020
Higher academic rank[c]	1.36	0.020
Active military practice	1.85	.014
Age (each additional year older)	1.03	<.001
Hours per week in operating room (each additional hour)	1.01	<.001
Number of nights on call per week (each additional night)	0.97	.005
Satisfaction with Overall Specialty Choice (Surgery)		
Absence of burnout	4.12	<.001
Subspecialty[d]	1.8–2.2	All ≤.002
Higher academic rank[e]	1.31–1.37	All ≤.018
Age (each additional year older)	1.03	<.001
Hours per week in operating room (each additional hour)	1.01	.033
Number of nights on call per week (each additional night)	0.95	<.001
Private practice	0.71	<.001
Subspecialty choice being vascular surgery	0.71	.002

Abbreviation: OR, odds ratio.

[a]OR>1 indicates greater satisfaction with career/specialty choice; OR<1 indicates lower satisfaction with career/specialty choice.

[b]Otolaryngology (OR = 2.57), transplant (OR = 2.18), plastic (OR = 2.18), ophthalmology (OR = 2.10), orthopedic (OR = 1.98), pediatric (OR = 1.87), urology (OR = 1.90), trauma (OR = 1.69), neuro (OR = 1.62), oncologic (OR = 1.46).

[c]Full professor (OR = 1.31), associate professor (OR = 1.37).

[d]Transplant (OR = 2.24), pediatric (OR = 1.81).

[e]Associate professor (OR = 1.37), full professor (OR = 1.31).

Modified from Shanafelt TD, Bechamps G, Russell T, et al. Burnout and career satisfaction among American surgeons. Ann Surg 2009;250:467; with permission.

inverse association with mental QOL (OR for each 1-point higher score = 0.906, $P<.0001$), the association with physical QOL was small (OR for each 1-point higher score = 0.986, $P = .029$) [15].

Although the relationship between SI and depression is well recognized [27,28], the association between SI and burnout has only begun to be defined. In a recent study of medical students in the United States, burnout had a substantial dose-response relationship with SI that persisted on multivariable analysis, controlling for symptoms of depression [29]. Of note, the relationship between SI and burnout was reversible in this longitudinal study in which recovery from burnout decreased the likelihood of subsequent SI [29]. The findings of this study suggest that burnout and depression are independently associated with SI whereby the consequences of burnout may be particularly important among individuals with underlying depression. In the ACS study on surgeons in United States, SI was also markedly increased among surgeons who perceived that they had made a major medical error in the last 3 months, highlighting the personal consequences of medical errors on physicians [15,30].

Despite the prevalence of SI, surgeons experiencing SI may be reluctant to seek help. Although surgeons with SI were more likely to have sought psychiatric or psychological help in the last 12 months than those without (26.0% vs 5.8%, $P < .0001$), they were also more likely to report that they were reluctant to seek professional help because of the concern that it could affect their license to practice medicine (60.1% vs 37.4%, $P < .0001$) [15]. Similarly, although surgeons with SI were more likely to have used antidepressant medication in the last 12 months (21.8% vs 4.8%, $P < .0001$), they were also more likely to have used self-prescribed medication (15.7% vs 6.9%, $P = .0059$) [15].

Medical errors

Beyond potentially dire personal consequences, physician distress may have an effect on quality of care [5,18,31–33]. Increasing evidence suggests that physician burnout can adversely affect patient safety and quality of patient care, and can even contribute to medical errors [5]. Research has found strong associations between physician burnout/dissatisfaction and medical errors [4–7], prescribing habits [34,35], patient compliance [36], patient's satisfaction with their medical care [37,38], and medical malpractice suits [39]. These findings underscore the fact that surgeons' mental health and professional burnout matter not only to the individual surgeons and their family but also to their patients, colleagues, societies, hospitals, and government agencies tasked with promoting quality of care [1,9]. In addition to its potential effect on patient safety, physician burnout should also be of concern to health care organizations because workers who are less satisfied tend to be less productive, and eventually may decide to quit for a different practice opportunity or take an early retirement [11,40]. Medical errors and decreased patient satisfaction associated with the medical care provided by burned-out physicians may also increase the threat of malpractice litigation, hence physician burnout also poses a substantial risk to the economic well-being of health care organizations [41].

In the ACS survey, 700 (8.9%) participating surgeons reported that they had made a major medical error in the last 3 months (Table 5) [5]. Surgeons reporting errors had an average age slightly lower than those not reporting errors (49 vs 52 years, $P \leq .0001$), worked an average of 4.6 hours more in a week (63.5 vs 58.9 hours, $P < .0001$), spent an additional hour per week in the operating room (18.2 vs 17.1 hours, $P = .0098$), and had slightly more nights on call per week (2.8 vs 2.6 nights, $P = .0001$). In the self-report, surgeons perceived a lapse in judgment as the greatest contributing factor to recent major medical errors that they reported, with lesser numbers reporting a system issue, stress/burnout, lapse in concentration, or fatigue as the greatest contributing factor (see Table 5).

Reporting a perceived error during the last 3 months had a strong association with mental QOL, all 3 domains of burnout, and the likelihood of being screened positive for symptoms of depression (Table 6) [5]. For example, reporting a major medical error in the last 3 months was associated with a 7-point increase (59% of

Table 5
Perceived medical errors by responding surgeons

		No. of physicians who answer the questions
Made major medical error in last 3 months	Missing information	6
	Yes	700 (8.9%)
	No	7199 (91.1%)
Greatest contributing factor in medical error	Lapse in judgment	217 (31.8%)
	A system issue	103 (15.1%)
	Degree of stress or burnout	89 (13%)
	Lapse in concentration	89 (13%)
	Degree of fatigue	47 (6.9%)
	Lack of knowledge	31 (4.5%)
	Others	107 (15.7%)

From Shanafelt TD, Balch CM, Bechamps G, et al. Burnout and medical errors among surgeons. Ann Surg 2010;251(6):997; with permission.

the standard deviation, ie, a large effect size) in emotional exhaustion on the Maslach Burnout Inventory and roughly a doubling in the risk of being screened positive for depression (27.5% vs 54.9%; $P<.0001$). Reported errors were also related to career satisfaction. Surgeons reporting recent errors were less likely to report that they would become a physician (60% vs 71.6%, $P<.0001$) or a surgeon (58.4 vs 75.5%, $P<.0001$) again and were also less likely to recommend their children to pursue a career as a physician or surgeon (40.8 vs 51.4%, $P<.0001$) [5]. Higher levels of burnout were also associated with an increased likelihood of reporting an error in the last 3 months (Fig. 2). Each 1-point increase in depersonalization (scale range 0–33) was associated with an 11% increase in the likelihood of reporting an error, whereas each 1-point increase in emotional exhaustion (scale range 0–54) was associated with a 5% increase. The personal accomplishment domain (scale range 0–48) of burnout was inversely correlated with reporting errors, in which each 1-point increase in score (ie, an indicator of lower burnout) was associated with a 3.6% decrease in the likelihood of reporting an error.

A multivariate analysis showed that both burnout and depression were strongly associated with perceived medical errors, after controlling for other personal and professional characteristics (Table 7). Older surgeons were less likely to report errors (approximately 15% had decreased likelihood for each additional 10 years of age), similar to those who spent less than 50% of their time in clinical practice. Practice characteristics such as the number of nights on call per week, practice setting, method of compensation, and number of hours worked were not associated with reported errors, after controlling for other factors.

PERSONAL WELLNESS

Personal growth and renewal involves optimizing meaning, both at work and in personal life. Strategies that may help increase wellness for individual surgeons include participating in research, continuing educational activities

Table 6
Distress among surgeons reporting perceived errors versus those not reporting errors

	Metric (scale)	Did not report errors (N = 7199)	Reported errors (N = 700)	Effect size as % of standard deviation	*P* value
Burnout					
Emotional exhaustion	MBIEE (0–54), mean	20.3	27.5	59%	<.0001
Depersonalization	MBIDP (0–33), mean	6.3	10.3	71%	<.0001
Personal accomplishment	MBIPA (0–48), mean	40.8	39.1	27%	<.0001
QOL					
Mental QOL	SF-12 (0–100)	49.5	42.5	71%	<.0001
Physical QOL	SF-12 (0–100)	53.5	53.8	5%	.0135
Depression	% of physicians who screen positive for depression	27.5%	54.9%	–	<.0001
Would become physician again (career choice)	% Yes	71.6%	60.0%	–	<.0001
Would become a surgeon again (specialty choice)	% Yes	75.5%	58.4%	–	<.0001
Would recommend their children to pursue a career as a physician/surgeon	% Yes	51.4%	40.8%	–	<.0001

Abbreviations: MBIDP, Maslach Burnout Inventory-depersonalization; MBIEE, Maslach Burnout Inventory-emotional exhaustion; MBIPA, Maslach Burnout Inventory-personal accomplishment; SF-12, medical outcomes study 12-item short form.

From Shanafelt TD, Balch CM, Bechamps G, et al. Burnout and medical errors among surgeons. Ann Surg 2010;251(6):998; with permission.

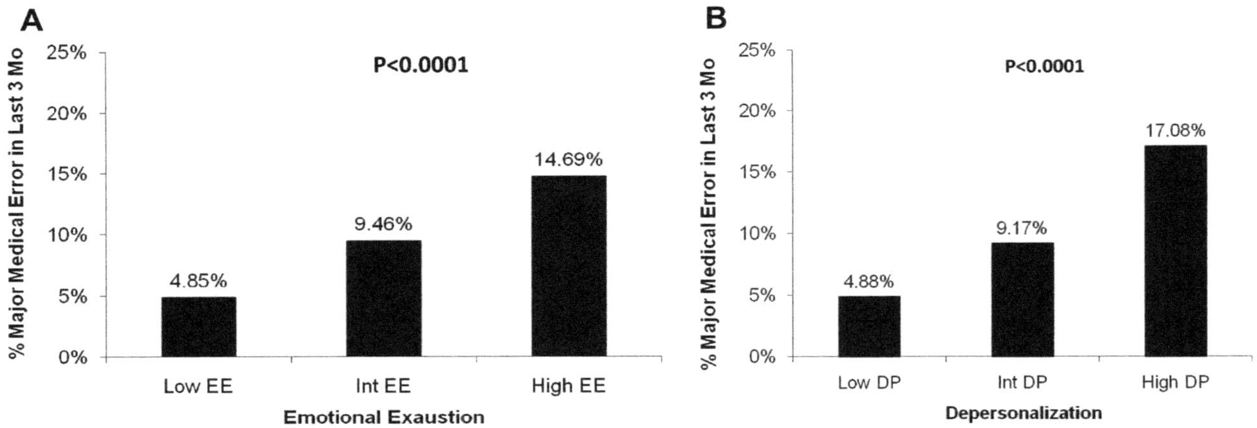

Fig. 2. Report of making a recent medical error by degree of burnout. (*A*) Report of making a recent medical error because of degree of emotional exhaustion. According to the standardized scoring system for health care professionals, surgeons with emotional exhaustion scores less than or equal to 18, 19 to 26, and greater than 27 are considered to have low, intermediate (Int), and high degrees of burnout, respectively. (*B*) Report of making a recent medical error by degree of depersonalization. According to the standardized scoring system for health care professionals, surgeons with depersonalization scores less than 5, 6 to 9, and greater than 10 are considered to have low, intermediate (Int), and high degrees of burnout, respectively. (*From* Shanafelt TD, Balch CM, Bechamps G, et al. Burnout and medical errors among surgeons. Ann Surg 2010;251(6):999; with permission.)

Table 7
Factors independently associated with perceived medical errors on multivariate analysis

Characteristics and associated factors[c]	OR[a]	*P* value
Burnout	1.993	<.0001
Retired	0.229	.0407
Plastic surgeon	0.269	<.0001
>50% time dedicated to nonpatient care (research, administration)	0.587	.0191
Age[b]	0.984	.001
Screened positive for depression	2.108	<.0001

[a]OR>1 indicates increased risk of perceived medical error; OR<1 indicates lower risk of perceived medical error.
[b]Each 1-year change.
[c]Nonsignificant factors: hours worked per week, number of hours per week in operating room, number of nights on call per week, primary method of compensation (eg, salaried, incentive-based pay, mixed), years in practice, practice setting, academic rank, relationship status, having children, age of children, gender.
From Shanafelt TD, Balch CM, Bechamps G, et al. Burnout and medical errors among surgeons. Ann Surg 2010;251(6):999; with permission.

outside of work, paying particular attention to important personal relationships, spiritual practices, recognizing the importance of one's work, cultivating personal interests outside of work, and creating a balance between personal and professional life [8,9,12,14,21,42].

There are serious consequences of burnout that can adversely affect one's personal and/or professional life as a surgeon (Table 8) (2). The best way for physicians to prevent burnout is to actively nurture and protect their personal and professional well-being on physical, emotional, psychological, and spiritual levels throughout their professional life cycle, from medical school to retirement. It is a challenge not only for individual physicians in their own

Table 8
Consequences of Physician Stress and Burnout

- Personal:
  - Depression
  - Anxiety
  - Suicide
  - Broken relationships with family, friends and colleagues
  - Addiction to alcohol and/or drug
  - Marital dysfunction and divorce
  - Early retirement
- Professional:
  - disengagement
  - poor judgment in patient care decision-making
  - hostility towards patients
  - medical errors
  - adverse patient events
  - diminished commitment and dedication to optimal patient care
  - difficult relationships with co-workers

lifestyles but also for the profession and the organizations in which physicians work [10]. Physicians have their own combination of activities that can be self-renewing and energizing, that no doubt change as they go through phases of career and seasons of life. What is required is a new way of thinking about one's personal energy, that is, work is not merely a domain of energy expenditure but also of energy renewal [9,10]. Physicians can learn to receive support, healing, and meaning while giving of themselves in each professional activity of the day.

Box 1: Steps to promote personal well-being[a]

1. Identify personal and professional values and priorities
   - Reflect on personal values and priorities.
   - Strive to achieve balance between personal and professional lives.

     Make a list of personal values and priorities; rank them in order of importance.

     Make a list of professional values and priorities: rank them in order of priorities.

     Integrate these 2 lists.

     Identify areas of conflict where personal and professional goals may be incompatible.
   - Based on priorities, determine how conflicts should be managed.
2. Enhance areas of work that are most personally meaningful
   - Identify areas of work that are most meaningful to you (patient care, patient education, medical education, participation in clinical trials, research, administration).
   - Find out how you can reshape your practice to increase your focus in this or these area or areas.
   - Decide if improving your skills in a specific area would decrease your stress at work, or if seeking additional training in this or other areas would be helpful for you.
   - Identify opportunities to reflect with colleagues about stressful and rewarding aspects of practice.
   - Periodically reassess what you enjoy most about your work.
3. Identify and nurture personal wellness strategies that are of importance to you
   - Protect and nurture your relationships.
   - Nurture religion/spirituality practices.
   - Develop hobbies and use vacations to encourage nonmedical interests.
   - Ensure adequate sleep, exercise, and nutrition.
   - Define and protect time for personal reflection, at least monthly.
   - Obtain a personal primary care provider and seek regular medical care.

[a] *Adapted from* Shanafelt TD. Finding meaning, balance, and personal satisfaction in the practice of oncology. J Support Oncol 2005;3(2):157–62.

Personal wellness strategies

The first step to promoting personal satisfaction is honest self-appraisal to determine whether one has adopted a mentality of perpetual delayed gratification in one's personal and professional life. Individuals should then identify personal and professional goals, so that they can begin to make choices that can help them to achieve these objectives. To translate these concepts into an actionable plan, the authors have proposed a 5-step process that involves: (1) identifying values, (2) career shaping/optimization, (3) identification and management of

Box 2: Personal wellness strategies[a]

Items listed under each category are intended to provide examples rather than being an inclusive list

1. Cultivating relationships
   - spouse/other significant people
   - children
   - friends
2. Personal reflection activities
   - journaling
   - reflection or storytelling groups
   - experiencing the arts (theater, music, poetry, and so forth)
3. Spiritual practices
   - services
   - religious practice
   - meditation
   - personal awareness and growth
4. Self-care
   - exercise
   - adequate sleep
   - nutrition
   - medical care including preventive care
   - vacations
5. Hobbies and personal interests
   - reading
   - arts
   - activities (eg, cooking, hiking, fishing, sporting events)
   - community service (eg, coaching, civic activities, tutoring, scouts)
   - travel

[a] *Adapted from* Shanafelt TD. A Career in Surgical Oncology: Finding meaning, balance, and personal satisfaction. Ann Surg Oncol 2007;15(2):400–6.

practice-specific stressors, (4) achieving balance between personal and professional goals, and (5) nurturing personal wellness strategies (Box 1) [14,43].

Although identifying personal values and protecting personal time is necessary to achieve work-life balance, time away from work should be more than simply a chance to rest for another workday. Caring for self, cultivating relationships, and nurturing personal interests is what makes time away from work meaningful and provides individuals the opportunity for achievement and personal growth outside of work. Although innumerable activities can be valuable in this regard, prior studies suggest that the strategies used by individual physicians often share common themes (Box 2) [12,43,44].

SUMMARY

The practice of surgery offers the potential for tremendous personal and professional satisfaction [1,21,42]. Few careers provide the opportunity to have such a profound effect on the lives of others and to derive meaning from work. Surgeons choose this arduous task to change the lives of individuals facing serious health problems, to experience the joy of facilitating healing, and to help support those patients for whom medicine does not yet have curative treatments. Despite its virtues, a career in surgery brings with it significant challenges, which can lead to substantial personal distress for the individual surgeons and their family. By identifying the priorities of their personal and professional life, surgeons can identify values, choose the optimal practice type, manage the stressors unique to that career path, determine the optimal personal work-life balance, and nurture their personal wellness. Being proactive is better than reacting to burnout after it has damaged one's professional life or personal wellness.

Studies like the ACS survey can benefit surgeons going through a personal crisis by helping them to know that they are not alone and that many of their colleagues face similar issues. It is important that surgeons do not make the mistake of thinking: "I must not be tough enough," or "no one could possibly experience what I am going through." The available evidence suggests that those surgeons most dedicated to their profession and their patient may very well be most susceptible to burnout. Silence on career distress, as a strategy, simply does not work among professionals whose careers, well-being, and level of patient care may be in jeopardy.

Additional research in these areas is needed to elucidate evidence-based interventions to address physician distress at both the individual and organizational level to benefit the individual surgeon and the patient they care for. Surgeons must also be able to recognize how and when their personal distress affects the quality of care they provide (both in the delivery of care and in the emotional support of patients and their families).

There is no single formula for achieving a satisfying career in surgery. All surgeons deal with stressful times in their personal and professional life and must cultivate habits of personal renewal, emotional self-awareness, connection with colleagues, adequate support systems, and the ability to find meaning in work to combat these challenges. As surgeons, we also need to set an example of good health to our patients and future generations of surgeons. To provide the best care for our patients, we need to be alert, interested in our work, and ready to provide for our patient's needs. Maintaining these values and healthy habits is the work of a lifetime [2].

References

[1] Balch CM, Copeland E. Stress and burnout among surgical oncologists: a call for personal wellness and a supportive workplace environment. Ann Surg Oncol 2007;14(11): 3029–32.

[2] Balch CM, Freischlag JA, Shanafelt TD. Stress and burnout among surgeons: understanding and managing the syndrome and avoiding the adverse consequences. Arch Surg 2009;144(4):371–6.

[3] Maslach C, Jackson S, Leiter M. Maslach burnout inventory manual. 3rd edition. Palo Alto (CA): Consulting Psychologists Press; 1996.

[4] Shanafelt TD, Bradley KA, Wipf JE, et al. Burnout and self-reported patient care in an internal medicine residency program. Ann Intern Med 2002;136(5):358–67.

[5] Shanafelt TD, Balch CM, Bechamps G, et al. Burnout and medical errors among American surgeons. Ann Surg 2010;251(6):995–1000.

[6] West CP, Huschka MM, Novotny PJ, et al. Association of perceived medical errors with resident distress and empathy: a prospective longitudinal study. JAMA 2006;296(9):1071–8.

[7] Firth-Cozens J, Greenhalgh J. Doctors' perceptions of the links between stress and lowered clinical care. Soc Sci Med 1997;44(7):1017–22.

[8] Meier DE, Back AL, Morrison RS. The inner life of physicians and care of the seriously ill. JAMA 2001;286(23):3007–14.

[9] Shanafelt TD, Sloan JA, Habermann TM. The well-being of physicians. Am J Med 2003;114(6):513–9.

[10] Spickard A Jr, Gabbe SG, Christensen JF. Mid-career burnout in generalist and specialist physicians. JAMA 2002;288(12):1447–50.

[11] Campbell DA Jr, Sonnad SS, Eckhauser FE, et al. Burnout among American surgeons. Surgery 2001;130(4):696–702 [discussion: 702–5].

[12] Shanafelt TD. Finding meaning, balance, and personal satisfaction in the practice of oncology. J Support Oncol 2005;3(2):157–62, 164.

[13] Shanafelt TD, Novotny P, Johnson ME, et al. The well-being and personal wellness promotion strategies of medical oncologists in the North Central Cancer Treatment Group. Oncology 2005;68(1):23–32.

[14] Shanafelt T, Chung H, White H, et al. Shaping your career to maximize personal satisfaction in the practice of oncology. J Clin Oncol 2006;24(24):4020–6.

[15] Shanafelt T, Balch CM, Dyrbye L. Suicide ideation among American surgeons. Arch Surg, in press.

[16] Arigoni F, Bovier PA, Mermillod B, et al. Prevalence of burnout among Swiss cancer clinicians, paediatricians and general practitioners: who are most at risk? Support Care Cancer 2009;17(1):75–81.

[17] Shanafelt TD, Balch CM, Bechamps GJ, et al. Burnout and career satisfaction among American surgeons. Ann Surg 2009;250(3):463–71.

[18] Kellerman SE, Herold J. Physician response to surveys. A review of the literature. Am J Prev Med 2001;20(1):61–7.

[19] Panagopoulou E, Montgomery A, Benos A. Burnout in internal medicine physicians: differences between residents and specialists. Eur J Intern Med 2006;17(3):195–200.

[20] Embriaco N, Azoulay E, Barrau K, et al. High level of burnout in intensivists: prevalence and associated factors. Am J Respir Crit Care Med 2007;175(7):686–92.

[21] Shanafelt T. A career in surgical oncology: finding meaning, balance, and personal satisfaction. Ann Surg Oncol 2008;15(2):400–6.

[22] Kuerer HM, Eberlein TJ, Pollock RE, et al. Career satisfaction, practice patterns and burnout among surgical oncologists: report on the quality of life of members of the Society of Surgical Oncology. Ann Surg Oncol 2007;14(11):3043–53.
[23] Kirkland K. On the decline in average weekly hours worked. Mon Labor Rev 2000;26:31.
[24] Sloan JA, Cella D, Hays RD. Clinical significance of patient-reported questionnaire data: another step toward consensus. J Clin Epidemiol 2005;58(12):1217–9.
[25] Spitzer RL, Williams JB, Kroenke K, et al. Utility of a new procedure for diagnosing mental disorders in primary care. The PRIME-MD 1000 Study. JAMA 1994;272(22):1749–56.
[26] Whooley MA, Avins AL, Miranda J, et al. Case-finding instruments for depression. Two questions are as good as many. J Gen Intern Med 1997;12(7):439–45.
[27] Kessler RC, Berglund P, Borges G, et al. Trends in suicide ideation, plans, gestures, and attempts in the United States, 1990–1992 to 2001–2003. JAMA 2005;293(20):2487–95.
[28] Kessler RC, Borges G, Walters EE. Prevalence of and risk factors for lifetime suicide attempts in the national comorbidity survey. Arch Gen Psychiatry 1999;56(7):617–26.
[29] Dyrbye LN, Thomas MR, Massie FS, et al. Burnout and suicidal ideation among U.S. medical students. Ann Intern Med 2008;149(5):334–41.
[30] Waterman AD, Garbutt J, Hazel E, et al. The emotional impact of medical errors on practicing physicians in the United States and Canada. Jt Comm J Qual Patient Saf 2007;33(8):467–76.
[31] Olkinuora M, Asp S, Juntunen J, et al. Stress symptoms, burnout and suicidal thoughts in Finnish physicians. Soc Psychiatry Psychiatr Epidemiol 1990;25(2):81–6.
[32] Guntupalli KK, Fromm RE Jr. Burnout in the internist-intensivist. Intensive Care Med 1996;22(7):625–30.
[33] Keller KL, Koenig WJ. Management of stress and prevention of burnout in emergency physicians. Ann Emerg Med 1989;18(1):42–7.
[34] Grol R, Mokkink H, Smits A, et al. Work satisfaction of general practitioners and the quality of patient care. Fam Pract 1985;2(3):128–35.
[35] Melville A. Job satisfaction in general practice: implications for prescribing. Soc Sci Med Med Psychol Med Sociol 1980;14A(6):495–9.
[36] DiMatteo MR, Sherbourne CD, Hays RD, et al. Physicians' characteristics influence patients' adherence to medical treatment: results from the Medical Outcomes Study. Health Psychol 1993;12(2):93–102.
[37] Haas JS, Cook EF, Puopolo AL, et al. Is the professional satisfaction of general internists associated with patient satisfaction? J Gen Intern Med 2000;15(2):122–8.
[38] Linn LS, Brook RH, Clark VA, et al. Physician and patient satisfaction as factors related to the organization of Internal Medicine Group practices. Med Care 1985;23(10):1171–8.
[39] Jones JW, Barge BN, Steffy BD, et al. Stress and medical malpractice: organizational risk assessment and intervention. J Appl Psychol 1988;73(4):727–35.
[40] Kent GG, Johnson AG. Conflicting demands in surgical practice. Ann R Coll Surg Engl 1995;77(Suppl 5):235–8.
[41] Grunfeld E, Whelan TJ, Zitzelsberger L, et al. Cancer care workers in Ontario: prevalence of burnout, job stress and job satisfaction. CMAJ 2000;163(2):166–9.
[42] Kuerer HM, Breslin T, Shanafelt TD, et al. Road map for maintaining career satisfaction and balance in surgical oncology. J Am Coll Surg 2008;207(3):435–42.
[43] Weiner EL, Swain GR, Wolf B, et al. A qualitative study of physicians' own wellness-promotion practices. West J Med 2001;174(1):19–23.
[44] Quill TE, Williamson PR. Healthy approaches to physician stress. Arch Intern Med 1990;150(9):1857–61.

Advances in Surgery 44 (2010) 49–57
ADVANCES IN SURGERY

ELSEVIER
MOSBY

Laparoscopic Gastric Bypass or Gastric Banding: Which Operation is Best?

Ninh T. Nguyen, MD*, Johnathan Sloan, MD, Xuan-Mai T. Nguyen, PhD

Division of Gastrointestinal Surgery, University of California, Irvine Medical Center, Orange, CA, USA

Roux-en-Y gastric bypass has long been the bariatric procedure of choice for the treatment of morbid obesity. This operation consists of constructing a small gastric pouch (30 mL), bypassing the majority of the stomach, duodenum, and proximal jejunum and performing reconstruction with a 75 to 150 cm jejunal Roux limb. The mechanisms for weight loss are restrictive and malabsorptive, however, recent data have been reported that support the metabolic effects of the Roux-en-Y gastric bypass [1–3]. The laparoscopic approach to gastric bypass was first reported in 1994 but was not widely disseminated until 1999 [4]. By 2004, the number of laparoscopic gastric bypass operations exceeded that of open gastric bypass operations [5]. In June of 2001, the Food and Drug Administration approved the laparoscopic adjustable gastric banding system (Lap-Band, Allergan Inc, Irvine, CA, USA) for use as a less invasive surgical alternative for the treatment of morbid obesity. The gastric banding procedure consists of placing an adjustable gastric band around the gastric cardia using a pars flaccida technique and implanting a port subcutaneously over the rectus fascia. Unlike the gastric bypass, gastric banding can be adjusted at follow-up visits. Over the past several years, laparoscopic adjustable gastric banding has gained popularity. From 2004 to 2007, there was a 329% increase in the number of gastric banding procedures performed in the Unites States [6]. At the current time, laparoscopic gastric bypass and laparoscopic gastric banding are the two most commonly performed operations worldwide for the treatment of morbid obesity. The availability of different surgical options for treatment of a single condition begs the question of which operation is best. Multiple retrospective studies have reported on the outcome of gastric bypass versus gastric banding [7–13]. However, there have been only 2 prospective, randomized trials to date comparing laparoscopic gastric bypass versus gastric banding [14,15]. This article summarizes the current available literature on the outcomes of gastric bypass versus gastric banding with regards

*Corresponding author. Department of Surgery, 333 City Boulevard West, Suite 850, Orange, CA 92868. *E-mail address*: ninhn@uci.edu.

0065-3411/10/$ – see front matter
doi:10.1016/j.yasu.2010.05.005

to safety, perioperative and long-term morbidity, weight loss efficacy, and improvement of comorbidities.

BYPASS VERSUS BAND: COMPARATIVE STUDIES

There have been multiple retrospective studies comparing the outcomes of gastric bypass versus gastric banding [7–13]. Baseline patient characteristics and outcomes from these comparative studies are summarized in Table 1. Five of the seven comparative studies examined laparoscopic gastric bypass versus laparoscopic gastric banding for all participants, whereas 2 of 7 studies evaluated outcomes for gastric bypass versus gastric banding only in a subset of subjects with super obesity (body mass index [BMI] >50 kg/m^2).

Safety and perioperative morbidity

Laparoscopic gastric bypass and laparoscopic gastric banding are safe procedures and both are associated with low perioperative morbidity. Laparoscopic gastric bypass appears to have a higher rate of early complications compared with laparoscopic gastric banding. The early complication rate after gastric bypass among these studies ranged from 5.2% to as high as 18%, and the early complication rate after gastric banding ranged from 0.6% to 18%. In a large comparative study of gastric bypass versus gastric banding, Jan and colleagues [11] reported an early complication rate of 15% after gastric bypass and 8% after gastric banding. Among these comparative studies, early minor complications after gastric bypass included wound infection, renal insufficiency, urinary tract infection, and dehydration. Early major complications after gastric bypass included gastrointestinal leak, intra-abdominal abscess, intestinal obstruction, gastrointestinal and intra-abdominal hemorrhage, deep venous thrombosis, and pneumonia. Early minor complications after gastric banding included dehydration, wound infection, urinary tract infection, food impaction, and renal insufficiency. Early major complications after gastric banding included band obstruction, gastric perforation, intra-abdominal bleeding, pulmonary embolism, band and port infection, congestive heart failure, myocardial infarction, and pneumonia. The 30-day mortality rate is low for both procedures. In the 4 studies with more than 100 subjects in each treatment arm, Cottam and colleagues [8] and Kim and colleagues [10] reported zero mortality for gastric bypass and gastric banding, whereas Mognol and colleagues [7] reported a mortality rate of 0.9% after gastric bypass and 0.6% after gastric banding. Lastly, Jan and colleagues [11] reported a 0.2% mortality rate after both gastric bypass (n = 492) and gastric banding (n = 406).

Late morbidity

Among these comparative studies, late complication after gastric bypass has ranged from 0.4% to as high as 28.0% and late complication after gastric banding has ranged from 3.7% to as high as 78%. Jan and colleagues [11] reported late complications after gastric bypass in 23% of 492 subjects and in 19% of 406 subjects after gastric banding. In a prospective, comparative analysis of gastric bypass versus gastric banding in the super obese (BMI >50 kg/m^2), Bowne and

Table 1
Characteristics and outcomes of laparoscopic gastric bypass versus gastric banding: retrospective comparative studies

Author (y)	Arm	N	Age (y)	BMI (kg/m^2)	LOS (d)	Early comp (%)	Late comp (%)	Mortality (%)	% EWL (<2 y)	% EWL (2–3 y)	% EWL (≥4 y)
Mognol [7]	Bypass	111	40	59	8	10.0	16.2	0.9	70	73	—
(2005)	Band	179	40	54	2	2.8	24.5	0.6	46	46	
Cottam [8]	Bypass	181	43	47	—	—	—	0.0	83	74	—
(2006)	Band	208	42	47				0.0	51	51	
Bowne [9]	Bypass	46	43	57	3.5	17.0	28.0	0.0	52	—	—
(2006)	Band	60	42	55	1.8	18.0	78.0	0.0	31		
Kim [10]	Bypass	232	39	47	—	5.2	0.4	0.0	64	68	—
(2006)	Band	160	42	47		0.6	3.7	0.0	41	48	
Jan [11]	Bypass	492	44	49	2.5	14.8	23.3	0.2	70	66	63
(2007)	Band	406	47	41	1.1	7.9	18.9	0.2	39	39	35
Puzziferri [12]	Bypass	958	43	51	—	—	—	—	75	75	—
(2008)	Band	560	45	49					41	44	
Riele [13]	Bypass	53	38	51	5.0	15.1	7.6	0.0	62 (M)	60 (M)	—
(2008)	Band	53	40	51	2.0	7.5	3.8	0.0	34 (M)	43 (M)	

All data are given as mean values.
Abbreviations: comp, complications; EWL, excess weight loss; LOS, length of stay; M, median value.

colleagues [9] reported late complications in 28% after gastric bypass and in 78% after gastric banding. Late complications after gastric bypass included internal hernia, marginal ulceration, ulcer perforation, anastomotic stricture, vitamin deficiency, incisional hernia, iron-deficiency anemia, gastrogastric fistula, and intestinal obstruction. Late complications after gastric banding included band slippage, band erosion, pouch dilation, port rotation, tubing breakage, esophageal dilation, small bowel obstruction, and incisional hernia.

Weight loss

All comparative studies to date have consistently shown better weight loss after gastric bypass compared with gastric banding [7–13]. For short-term weight loss (<2-year follow-up), all 7 comparative studies found better weight loss after gastric bypass. In a subset of super obese subjects, Bowne and colleagues [9] reported 52% excess weight loss (EWL) after gastric bypass and 31% after gastric banding. Six of the seven comparative studies reported on medium-term weight loss (2–3 year follow-up) and all 6 studies continued to show better weight loss after gastric bypass [7–10,12,13]. Kim and colleagues [10] reported 68% EWL after gastric bypass compared with 48% EWL after gastric banding at 2 years. In a large comparative study of gastric bypass (n = 958) versus gastric banding (n = 560), Puzziferri and colleagues [12] similarly reported a 75% EWL after gastric bypass and a 44% EWL after gastric banding at a 2-year follow-up. In another study, Riele and colleagues [13] reported a median value of 60% EWL after gastric bypass and 43% EWL after gastric banding. Only 1 of the 7 studies reported on long-term weight loss outcome. Jan and colleagues [11] reported better long-term weight loss after gastric bypass compared with gastric banding (63% vs 35% EWL, respectively) at a 4-year follow-up.

BYPASS VERSUS BAND: PROSPECTIVE, RANDOMIZED TRIALS

At this time, there have been only 2 prospective, randomized trials published comparing the outcomes of gastric bypass versus gastric banding [14,15]. The characteristics and outcomes from these two studies are summarized in Table 2.

In the first study, published in 2007, Angrisani and colleagues [14] reported the outcomes of a randomized trial comparing laparoscopic gastric bypass versus laparoscopic gastric banding in a cohort of 51 subjects. Twenty-four subjects were randomized to gastric bypass and 27 subjects were randomized to gastric banding. The mean BMI was 43 kg/m^2 for both groups. The mean operative time was significantly longer for the gastric bypass group (220 vs 60 minutes, respectively). There were no perioperative mortalities. Conversion to laparotomy occurred in 4.2% of subjects in the gastric bypass group. The rate of early complication was 4.2% in the gastric bypass group (jejunal perforation) and 0.0% in the gastric banding group. Long-term weight loss at 5 years was 67% EWL after gastric bypass and 48% EWL after gastric banding [14].

The second randomized trial was recently reported in 2009 by Nguyen and colleagues [15]. This trial is the largest to date comparing the outcomes of

Table 2
Characteristics and outcomes of laparoscopic gastric bypass versus gastric banding: prospective, randomized trials

Author (y)	Arm	N	Age (y)	BMI (kg/m^2)	Early comp (%)	Late comp (%)	Mortality (%)	% EWL (<2 y)	% EWL (2–3 y)	% EWL (≥4 y)
Angrisani [14] (2007)	Bypass	24	33	44	4.2	4.2	0	51	67	67
	Band	27	35	43	0.0	7.6	0	35	47	48
Nguyen [15] (2009)	Bypass	111	41	48	21.6	39.6	0	64	68	68
	Band	86	45	46	7.0	11.6	0	37	42	45

All data are given as mean values.
Abbreviations: comp, complications; M, median value.

gastric bypass versus gastric banding. Besides weight loss outcome, changes in quality of life and costs were also evaluated. In this trial, 250 subjects with a BMI between 35 to 60 kg/m^2 were randomized to undergo either laparoscopic gastric bypass or gastric banding. After exclusions, data from 86 subjects in the gastric banding group and 111 subjects in the gastric bypass group were evaluable. With regard to baseline characteristics, preoperative BMI was higher in the gastric bypass group than in the gastric banding group (48 vs 46 kg/m^2, respectively), whereas mean age was higher in the band group than in the bypass group (45 vs 41 years, respectively). With regard to perioperative outcomes, gastric bypass was associated with a longer operative time and higher intraoperative blood loss. Intensive-care-unit stay was required in 2.7% of subjects in the gastric bypass group compared with 1.2% of subjects in the gastric banding group. The length of hospitalization was shorter in the gastric banding group than in the gastric bypass group (1.5 vs 3.1 days, respectively). The time to return to normal activities of daily living and return to work was significantly shorter after gastric banding compared with gastric bypass. With regard to operative safety, perioperative complications were fewer after gastric banding compared with gastric bypass. Early major and minor complications occurred in 21.6% of subjects after gastric bypass and in 7% of subjects after gastric banding. Major complications in the gastric bypass group included gastrointestinal hemorrhage and early postoperative bowel obstruction. The most common early minor complication in the gastric bypass group was wound infection, and dehydration was the most common reason for readmission. Major complications in the gastric banding group included band obstruction and postoperative renal insufficiency. Late complications also occurred more frequently in the gastric bypass group than in the gastric banding group (39.6% vs 11.6%, respectively). Late complications after gastric bypass included anastomotic stricture (14.3%), marginal ulceration, and iron deficiency anemia. In contrast, most late complications in the gastric band group were related to the gastric band (obstruction, slippage, or erosion) or port-related complications. With regard to weight loss, the

EWL was 68.9% after gastric bypass (n = 94) and 41.8% after gastric banding (n = 79) at a 2-year follow-up. The EWL was 67.5% after gastric bypass (n = 81) and 41.5% after gastric banding (n = 62) at a 3-year follow-up. The EWL was 68.4% after gastric bypass (n = 71) and 45.4% after gastric banding (n = 30) at a 4-year follow-up [15]. With regard to quality of life, both gastric bypass and gastric banding subjects had a depressed quality of life perioperatively as reflected in low scores in 7 of 8 heath domains on the Short Form-36 (SF-36) quality-of-life questionnaire. By 12 months after surgery, the SF-36 scores for all 8 health domains in both groups significantly improved and were comparable with that of norms in the United States. Lastly, with regard to costs, gastric bypass was associated with higher cost ($12,310 for gastric bypass vs $10,766 for gastric banding) because of the longer intraoperative time and longer length of hospitalization in the gastric bypass group.

BYPASS VERSUS BAND: SYSTEMATIC REVIEW

There have been several meta-analyses and systematic reviews of bariatric operations; however, only 1 study limited the review to comparative studies of gastric bypass versus gastric banding. The difficulties in comparing the outcomes of different operations using the published literature of individual studies of band versus bypass include the differences in baseline characteristics of the study population between different centers, variability in follow-up of study subjects, and differences in the definition and reporting of outcomes among different investigators and institutions. Tice and colleagues [16] reviewed 13 retrospective comparative studies and 1 prospective randomized trial comparing gastric bypass versus gastric banding. In summary, they found that operating room time and length of hospital stay were shorter for those undergoing gastric banding. Operative mortality was less than 0.5% for both operations. Perioperative complications were higher after gastric bypass than after gastric banding (9% vs 5%, respectively), whereas long-term reoperation rates were lower after gastric bypass than after gastric banding (16% vs 24%, respectively). Weight loss outcomes consistently favored gastric bypass. The median absolute difference in EWL between the 2 groups at 1 year was 25%.

DISCUSSION

The previously mentioned data from multiple retrospective comparative studies and 2 prospective randomized trials may be useful for patients and surgeons in deciding the optimal procedures for the treatment of morbid obesity. To decide upon the optimal operation, one must decide what the most important outcome parameters are. If low risk for perioperative complication is the most important objective, gastric banding is associated with a lower rate of perioperative complication and often associated with lower severity of complication. In the Angrisani trial, there was a 4.2% rate of major complication related to a jejunal perforation [14]. In the Nguyen trial, the rate of early complication was significantly higher after gastric bypass, although there were no leak complications in the gastric bypass group [15]. Therefore, gastric banding is an attractive option for high-risk patients, such as the elderly or transplant patients on immunosuppressive agents. If long-term weight loss is the most important outcome objective, then gastric bypass is the operation of choice. All retrospective comparative studies and the 2 randomized trials showed superior weight loss after gastric bypass [7–15]. At a 5-year follow-up, Angrisani and colleagues [14] reported better weight loss after gastric bypass compared with gastric banding (67% vs 47%, respectively). Nguyen and colleagues [15] also found that weight loss was superior after gastric bypass at a 4-year follow-up (68% bypass vs 45% banding). In attempting to identify preoperative factors that may be predictive of weight loss, Nguyen and colleagues [15] found better weight loss for patients receiving gastric bypass and gastric banding who had a BMI less than 50 kg/m^2 compared with patients with a BMI greater than or equal to 50 kg/m^2. In a comparative study of gastric bypass versus gastric banding in super-morbidly obese patients (BMI >50 kg/m^2), Bowne and colleagues [9] similarly reported better weight loss after gastric bypass compared with gastric banding (52% vs 31% EWL, respectively) at a median follow-up time of 16.2 months. Another preoperative factor that has been shown to be predictive of weight loss is male gender. Nguyen and colleagues [15] found that men who underwent gastric banding were significantly more likely to have poor or failure of weight loss (defined as losing <20% EWL). Of the 21 men who underwent gastric banding, 33% of subjects loss less than 20% EWL at follow-up. Bueter and colleagues [17] similarly reported a large variability in postoperative weight loss in 85 subjects who underwent gastric banding, and they also found that male gender was a predictor of weight loss failure with an odds ratio of 3.9. Lastly, if reversal of comorbidities is the main outcome objective, gastric bypass has been shown to induce better remission of type 2 diabetes. In a systematic review and meta-analysis of 621 bariatric studies, 888 treatment arms, and 135,246 subjects, Buchwald and colleagues [18] reported that 78.1% of subjects with diabetes had complete resolution of diabetes. Diabetes resolution was greatest for subjects undergoing biliopancreatic diversion/duodenal switch (95%) followed by gastric bypass (80%), and the lowest resolution was seen after gastric banding (57%). However, 1 recent study reported that improvement of diabetes was similar between the 2 groups, although weight loss was better in the gastric bypass group [19]. Parikh and colleagues [19] reported that the proportion of subjects requiring oral hypoglycemics at 2 years postoperatively was 34% for gastric banding and 13% for gastric bypass.

SUMMARY

Data from the available published literature support that laparoscopic gastric bypass and laparoscopic adjustable gastric banding are safe and effective bariatric procedures for the treatment of morbid obesity. Compared with gastric bypass, gastric banding is commonly associated with a shorter operative time and length of hospital stay, and lower perioperative morbidity. However, the medium- and long-term weight losses were consistently and dramatically better after gastric bypass. The 2 preoperative factors predictive of poor weight loss in patients with gastric banding were male gender and patients with a BMI greater than or equal to 50 kg/m^2. With this knowledge, the final decision regarding gastric bypass versus gastric banding will rely on an in-depth discussion between patients and surgeons with regard to perioperative and late complication data, long-term weight loss and variability of weight loss between the 2 operations, as well as the data regarding the rate for remission of comorbidities between the 2 operations. At the current time, there is ample evidence for surgeons and patients to make a well-informed decision with regard to which operation is best for the individual patient.

References

[1] Smith BR, Hinojosa MW, Reavis KM, et al. Remission of diabetes after laparoscopic gastric bypass. Am Surg 2008;74:948–52.

[2] Rubino F, Gagner M. Potential of surgery for curing type 2 diabetes mellitus. Ann Surg 2002;236:554–9.

[3] Rubino F, Forgione A, Cummings DE, et al. The mechanism of diabetes control after gastrointestinal bypass surgery reveals a role of the proximal small intestine in the pathophysiology of type 2 diabetes. Ann Surg 2006;244:741–9.

[4] Nguyen NT, Root J, Zainabadi K, et al. Accelerated growth of bariatric surgery with the introduction of minimally invasive surgery. Arch Surg 2005;140:1198–202.

[5] Nguyen NT, Silver M, Robinson M, et al. Result of a national audit of bariatric surgery performed at academic centers: a 2004 University Health System Consortium Benchmarking project. Arch Surg 2006;141:445–9.

[6] Hinojosa MW, Varela JE, Parikh D, et al. National trends in use and outcome of laparoscopic adjustable gastric banding. Surg Obes Relat Dis 2009;5:150–5.

[7] Mognol P, Chosidow D, Marmuse J. Laparoscopic gastric bypass versus Laparoscopic adjustable gastric banding in the super-obese: a comparative study of 290 patients. Obes Surg 2005;15:76–81.

[8] Cottam DR, Atkinson J, Anderson A, et al. A case-controlled matched-pair cohort study of laparoscopic Roux-en-Y gastric bypass and Lap-Band patients in a single US center with three-year follow-up. Obes Surg 2006;16:534–40.

[9] Bowne WB, Julliard K, Castro AE, et al. Laparoscopic gastric bypass is superior to adjustable gastric band in super morbidly obese patients. Arch Surg 2006;141:683–9.

[10] Kim TH, Daud A, Ude AO, et al. Early U.S. outcomes of laparoscopic gastric bypass versus laparoscopic adjustable silicone gastric banding for morbid obesity. Surg Endosc 2006;20:202–9.

[11] Jan JC, Hong D, Bardaro SJ, et al. Comparative study between laparoscopic adjustable gastric banding and laparoscopic gastric bypass: single-institution, 5-year experience in bariatric surgery. Surg Obes Relat Dis 2007;3:42–51.

[12] Puzziferri N, Nakonezny PA, Livingston EH, et al. Variations of weight loss following gastric bypass and gastric banding. Ann Surg 2008;248:233–42.

[13] Riele WW, Vogten JM, Boerma D, et al. Comparison of weight loss and mortality after gastric bypass and gastric banding: a single center European experience. Obes Surg 2008;18:11–6.

[14] Angrisani L, Lorenzo M, Borelli V. Laparoscopic adjustable gastric banding versus Roux-en-Y gastric bypass: 5-year results of a prospective randomized trial. Surg Obes Relat Dis 2007;3:127–33.

[15] Nguyen NT, Sloan JA, Nguyen XT, et al. A prospective randomized trial of laparoscopic gastric bypass versus laparoscopic adjustable gastric banding for the

treatment of morbid obesity; outcomes, quality of life, and costs. Ann Surg 2009;250:631–41.
[16] Tice JA, Karliner L, Walsh J, et al. Gastric banding or bypass? A systematic review comparing the two most popular bariatric procedures. Am J Med 2008;121:885–93.
[17] Bueter M, Thalheimer A, Lager C, et al. Who benefits from gastric banding? Obes Surg 2007;17:1608–13.
[18] Buchwald H, Estok R, Fahrbach K, et al. Weight and type 2 diabetes after bariatric surgery: systematic review and meta-analysis. Am J Med 2009;122:248–56.
[19] Parikh M, Ayoung-Chee P, Romanos E, et al. Comparison of rates of resolution of diabetes mellitus after gastric banding, gastric bypass, and biliopancreatic diverion. J Am Coll Surg 2007;205:631–5.

Advances in Surgery 44 (2010) 59–72

ADVANCES IN SURGERY

Prevention, Detection, and Management of Leaks Following Gastric Bypass for Obesity

Ashish Agarwala, DO, John M. Kellum, MD*

Department of Surgery, Virginia Commonwealth University School of Medicine, 1200 East Broad Street, Richmond, VA 23298, USA

The disease of obesity has reached epidemic proportions, affecting more than 100 million adults in the United States and more than 300 million worldwide. It has adversely affected public health and poses a major burden to society in terms of chronic disease, disability, and associated economic costs. Diet, exercise, and medical weight loss regimens have failed to show significant effectiveness in achieving long-term weight loss in the severely obese adult population [1–5]. However, in contrast with this failure, the surgical treatment of severe obesity has resulted in sustainable long-term results in weight control and resolution of associated comorbid conditions [6–17].

Bariatric surgery was developed slightly more than 50 years ago, representing a post–World War II phenomenon of the late twentieth century [18]. With reports of life-threatening complications of the jejunoileal bypass [19], the gastric bypass of Mason and Ito [20] became the gold standard in the United States for the surgical treatment of morbid obesity. This operation arose from Mason's observation of frequent weight loss after a high subtotal gastrectomy for ulcer disease; he reported the original procedure in 1967 to include a horizontal division of the stomach and the subsequent creation of a loop gastrojejunostomy (Fig. 1) [20].

This operation has since undergone several refinements. In 1977, to prevent bile reflux gastritis and esophagitis, Griffen and colleagues [21] modified the drainage of the proximal gastric pouch to the Roux-en-Y gastrojejunostomy from the original loop gastrojejunostomy. To some extent this may have inadvertently contributed to the leak problem caused by decreased blood flow to the Roux limb. In 1983, Torres and colleagues [22] further altered the procedure by switching from horizontal to a vertical stapling of the stomach. They also reported the creation of a longer alimentary limb, a technique later

*Corresponding author. VCU, PO Box 980519, Richmond, VA 23298-0519. *E-mail address:* jmkellum@vcu.edu.

0065-3411/10/$ – see front matter
doi:10.1016/j.yasu.2010.05.009

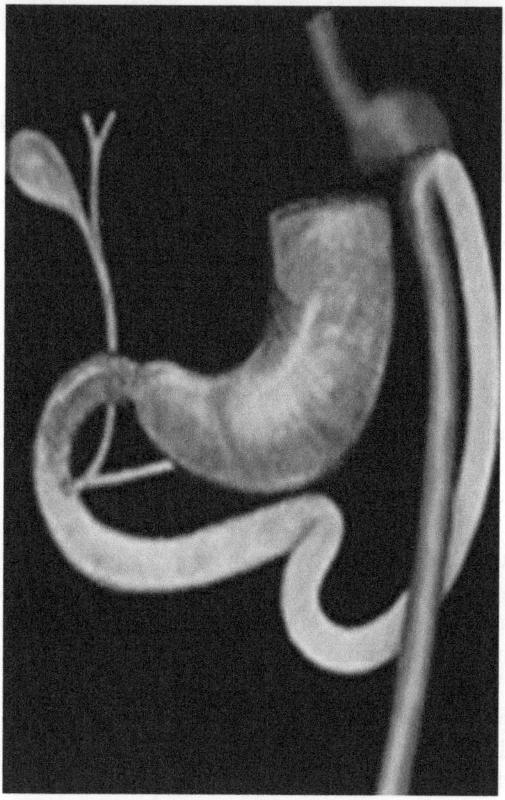

Fig. 1. Gastric bypass; gastric transection with loop gastrojejunostomy. (*From* Buchwald H, Buchwald JN. Evolution of surgery for morbid obesity. In: Pitombo C, Jones KB, Higa KD, et al, editors. Obesity surgery: principles and practice. China: McGraw-Hill; 2008. p. 7; with permission.)

popularized by Brolin and colleagues [23] (150-cm alimentary limb and 75-cm biliopancreatic limb) in the treatment of the super obese (body mass index [BMI, calculated as weight in kilograms divided by the square of height in meters] >50 kg/m^2). In 1994, Wittgrove and Clark [24] introduced the laparoscopic Roux-en-Y gastric bypass and used a circular stapler passed per orum for construction of the gastrojejunostomy. Their laparoscopic approach underwent various modifications including the use of the intra-abdominal linear stapler by Schauer and colleagues [25] to the hand-sewn gastrojejunostomy first described by Higa and colleagues [26]. The laparoscopic procedure also involved the division of the proximal gastric pouch from the gastric remnant, greatly reducing the risk of gastrogastric fistula from a disrupted staple line.

The laparoscopic Roux-en-Y gastric bypass (L-RYGB) has become the preferred operation for morbid obesity; however, it is not free of risk and complications, the gravest of which is a leak. A leak is defined as an anastomotic disruption at the gastrojejunostomy, the jejunojejunostomy, an intestinal perforation, or a blowout of the gastric remnant (excluded stomach). It has proven to be a major source of morbidity and mortality. Patients who suffer a leak often require longer hospitalizations, prolonged ventilatory support, subsequent reoperations, and, in some cases, they die. Mortality as high as 20% has been reported as a result of leaks [27].

The causes of a leak are multifactorial. Early leaks (those occurring within the first 48 hours) are usually attributable to technical factors such as improperly placed sutures or stapler malfunction. Late leaks (those occurring after the first 48 hours) are more likely to result from tissue ischemia and impaired wound healing. Ischemic injury in this setting is often explained by excessive dissection leading to division or interruption of blood supply, dissection injury, or tension on the anastomosis and staple lines. Impaired wound healing is a common phenomenon seen in conditions such as diabetes mellitus, renal failure, peripheral arterial occlusive disease, and advanced age. Age, male gender, sleep apnea, and revisional surgery have been identified as independent risk factors for the development of a leak [27].

The incidence of anastomotic leaks is 0% to 5.6% [25,27–31]. Tables 1 and 2 list the occurrence of leaks in open and L-RYGB in selected series.

The incidence of leaks in the laparoscopic era, although once reported to be higher, has now proven to be comparable with the open gastric bypass [27]. This improvement can be attributed to refinement in operative techniques, improving technology, and accumulated experience in laparoscopy.

The most common site for an anastomotic leak is the gastrojejunostomy [47]. Other commonly affected sites include the jejunojejunostomy, the excluded stomach, and staple line leaks from the gastric pouch or blind end of the alimentary limb. A multi-institutional study by Gonzalez and colleagues [48] described the incidence of leaks at different locations, as illustrated in Fig. 2.

The diagnosis of a leak following gastric bypass can be challenging. The symptoms are often vague and nonspecific. There is no single test or modality to reliably detect leaks in these patients. Therefore, it is prudent for the treating surgeon to maintain a high index of suspicion, because an unrecognized leak can be fatal.

Leaks often present with overt signs of clinical sepsis, peritonitis, or hemodynamic instability early in the postoperative period. These patients require immediate operative exploration. A recent report by Al-Sabah and colleagues [49] from McGill University suggests that it is not the infectious process (leak) but the host's aggressive systemic inflammatory response to the infectious process that leads to poor outcomes in these patients. This may be related to each patient's innate ability to isolate the contamination from the leak. It should be the goal of the surgeon to detect the leak early in its initial phase in the hope of preventing the development of severe sepsis. Early detection in conjunction with benign clinical parameters may allow for nonoperative management in many cases. In patients with free or poorly localized leaks or septic clinical parameters, urgent operation is indicated.

Table 1
Incidence of leak during L-RYGB as reported in selected large series from English literature

Source	Year	Number of patients	Leak rate (%)
Schauer et al [25]	2000	275	3.3
Wittgrove and Clark [24]	2000	500	2.2
Nguyen et al [32]	2001	79	1.3
Higa et al [26]	2001	1500	0.9
Oliak et al [33]	2002	300	1.3
Champion et al [34]	2002	743	0.4
Gonzalez et al [31]	2003	108	0
Hamilton et al [35]	2003	210	4.3
Papasavas et al [36]	2003	246	1.6
Gould et al [37]	2004	100	3
Dresel et al [38]	2004	120	0.8
Fernandez et al [27]	2004	554	4.3
Carrasquilla et al [39]	2004	1000	0.1

From Gonzalez R, Nelson LG, Gallagher SF, et al. Anastomotic leaks after laparoscopic gastric bypass. Obes Surg 2004;14:1300; with permission.

CLINICAL SIGNS AND SYMPTOMS

Any change in patients' clinical status should raise the suspicion for a leak and warrants a thorough workup. Tachycardia, tachypnea, and fever are often the earliest markers in patients with leaks, and usually precede the more perilous signs of sepsis, hemodynamic instability, and vascular collapse. In a study by Hamilton and colleagues [35] patients who had severe tachycardia (sustained heart rate >120) and respiratory distress (SaO_2 <92% on room air, or respiratory rate ≥24) were found to have a 20% chance of harboring a leak (Fig. 3).

Other notable findings include abdominal pain, fever, persistent leukocytosis, or oliguria. In a study by Ballesta and colleagues [50] the most frequent clinical manifestations found in patients with leaks were abdominal pain,

Table 2
Outcomes for open gastric bypass: selected series

Source	Year	Number of patients	Leak rate (%)
Mason and Ito [40]	1969	26	0
Griffen et al [41]	1981	402	5.47
Linner [42]	1982	174	0.57
Sugerman et al [43]	1989	182	1.6
Hall et al [12]	1990	99	0
Brolin et al [23]	1992	90	0
MacLean et al [44]	1993	106	5.6
Capella and Capella [45]	1996	560	0
Fobi et al [46]	1998	944	3.1

From Schauer PR, Ikramuddin S, Gourash W, et al. Outcomes after laparoscopic Roux-en-Y gastric bypass for morbid obesity. Ann Surg 2000;232:525; with permission.

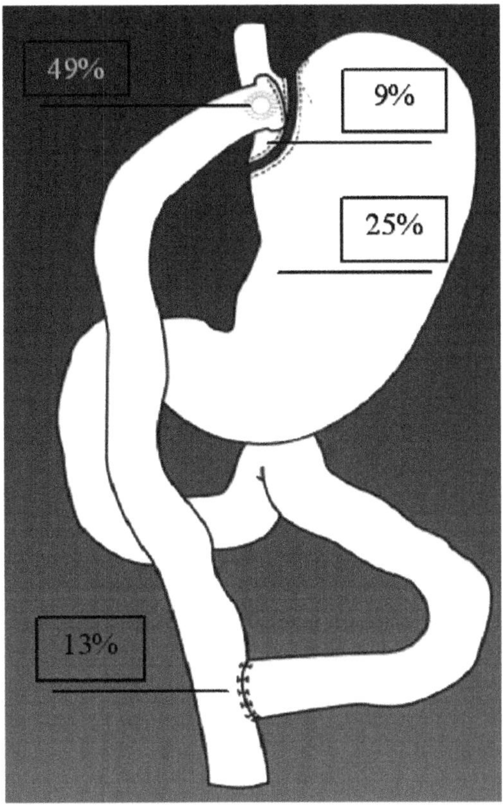

Fig. 2. Incidence of leak at various locations. (*From* Gonzalez R, Sarr MG, Smith CD, et al. Diagnosis and contemporary management of anastomotic leaks after gastric bypass for obesity. J Am Coll Surg 2007;204(1):49; with permission.)

followed by fever and then tachycardia. Another study by Kolakowski and colleagues [51] found that the combination of fever, tachycardia, and tachypnea was a significant predictor of leak (Fig. 4).

As mentioned earlier, these signs are nonspecific and vague, and many of these symptoms can also be found in the normal hypermetabolic postoperative state. Therefore, in the absence of overt sepsis, any clinical suspicion raised by these signs must be confirmed by further workup in the hemodynamically stable patient.

BIOCHEMICAL MARKERS

Amylase is a digestive enzyme found in low concentrations in blood (<150 IU/L) but high concentrations in saliva (70,000 IU/L). In our institution, we routinely measure amylase postoperatively from a juxta-anastomotic drain as a marker of early leak. Studies conducted at this institution [52], involving more than

Clinical sign	Group 1: leak ($n = 9$) n (%)	Group 2: no leak ($n = 201$) n (%)	Odds ratio	95% Confindence interval	p
Severe tachycardia	8/9 (89)	32/201 (15.9)	23.2	2.57–208.5	<0.01
Respiratory distress	6/9 (67)	21/201 (10.5)	6.0	1.2–29.4	<0.05

Fig. 3. Multivariate logistic regression model showing severe tachycardia (heart rate>120) and respiratory distress as independent clinical indicators of leak. (*From* Hamilton EC, Sims TL, Hamilton TT, et al. Clinical predictors of leak after laparoscopic Roux-en-Y gastric bypass for morbid obesity. Surg Endosc 2003;17:682; with permission.)

400 patients, showed that an amylase level of less than 400 IU/L is 90% specific in excluding leaks and has a negative predictive value of 99.6% (Fig. 5). An amylase value greater than 400 IU/L was 94.1% sensitive in detecting a leak with a positive predictive value (PPV) of 33.3%. We believe that an amylase level greater than 400 IU/L is a sensitive and specific adjunct in the detection of postoperative leak. It has a high negative predictive value, but a low PPV.

At the Medical College of Virginia Hospitals, we use the information obtained from the drain amylase along with the patients' clinical status to dictate further management. The presence of an increased amylase level in an otherwise clinically stable patient (afebrile, pulse rate <100), would simply require the drain amylase to be rechecked later the same day and our postoperative feeding regimen would be delayed until the drain amylase value showed a downward trajectory. In contrast, patients with increased drain amylase who exhibit the clinical signs of leak mentioned earlier would be further studied with an upper gastrointestinal water-soluble contrast radiographic

Clinical Indicator	Present[a]	Absent[a]	Odds Ratio (95% Confidence Limits)	*P* Value
		Leaks		
Nausea	1 (8.3)	19 (4.7)	1.85 (0.23 15.06)	.56
Fever and tachycardia	1 (8.3)	6 (1.5)	6.04 (0.67, 54.60)	.50
Fever, tachycardia. nausea. and vomiting	1 (8.3)	0	105.78 (4.08, 2740.80)	.005
Fever.tachycardia and tachypnea	**7 (58.3)**	**1(0.2)**	**565.60 (58.21. 5496.00)**	**<.001**

Fig. 4. Multivariate logistic regression model showing combination of fever, tachycardia, and tachypnea to be a significant predictor of leak. Data are given as number (percentage) of each group. For leaks, n = 12 for the present group and n = 405 for the absent group. (*Adapted from* Kolakowski S, Kirkland ML, Schuricht AL, et al. Routine postoperative upper gastrointestinal series after Roux-en-Y gastric bypass: determination of whether it is necessary. Arch Surg 2007;142(10):932; with permission.)

Variable	≤400 IU/L	>400 IU/L
No leak, n	302	32
Leak, n	1	16
Specificity, %	90	
Negative predictive value, %	99.6	
Sensitivity, %		94.1
Positive predictive value, %		33.3

Fig. 5. Leak rate, sensitivity, and specificity using drain amylase value of 400 IU/L as peak normal value. (*From* Maher JW, Hawver LM, Pucci A, et al. Four hundred and fifty consecutive laparoscopic Roux-en-Y gastric bypasses with no mortality and declining leak rates and lengths of stay in a bariatric training program. J Am Coll Surg 2008;206(5):883; with permission.)

series (UGIS) or possibly a computed tomography (CT) scan of the abdomen with intravenous and oral contrast.

Another study by Salgado and colleagues [53] measured peritoneal cytokines as a marker of leak. This study showed high interleukin-6 levels at 24 hours and interleukin-1b levels at 48 hours postoperatively in the group of patients with leak. They advocated the routine measurement of these cytokine levels as an adjunct for the detection of leak. These tests are less practical because they are cumbersome, more expensive, and not routinely available. The usefulness of peritoneal cytokine levels in clinical practice has yet to be determined.

RADIOLOGIC STUDIES

An UGIS with Gastrografin (diatrizoate meglumine and diatrizoate sodium; Bracco Diagnostics, Princeton, NJ, USA) under fluoroscopy has traditionally been the most commonly used postoperative test to evaluate for leaks. The method used in performing this study is a standard protocol for postoperative swallow studies [54]. Approximately 60 mL of a Gastrografin is administered orally. Next, fluoroscopy is obtained as the patient swallows the contrast, and images of the esophagus, gastric pouch, and jejunum are obtained. Fifteen minutes later images are obtained to assess for emptying of the pouch, passage of contrast through the jejunum, reflux into the duodenum, and possible delayed leaks (Fig. 6).

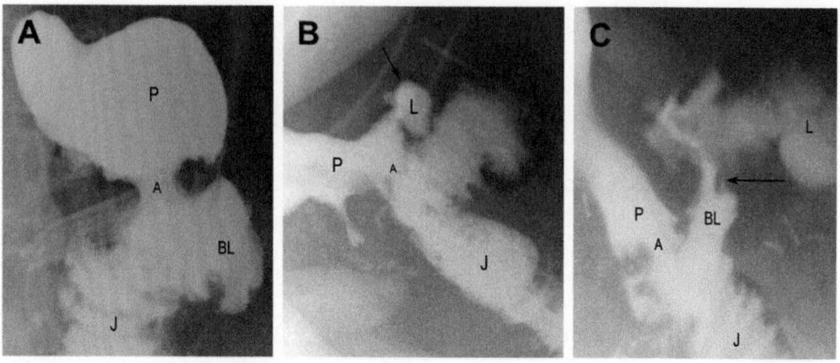

Fig. 6. (*A*) Normal postoperative anatomy after Roux-en-Y gastric bypass surgery. (*B*) Supine left posterior oblique spot image from upper gastrointestinal examination shows a small leak (*L*) and a 1.5-cm collection of contrast material (*arrow*). (*C*) Leak from blind-ending jejunal limb. (*From* Carucci LR, Turner MA, Conklin RC. Roux-en-Y gastric bypass surgery for morbid obesity: evaluation of postoperative extraluminal leaks with upper gastrointestinal series. Radiology 2006;238(1):120, 122, 125; with permission.)

We formerly used routine UGIS within 48 hours after open or laparoscopic gastric bypass to rule out leaks. Although they are still used routinely in some centers, others advocate their selective use based on clinical parameters. This topic is still heavily debated. Proponents of the former strategy argue that routine use of UGIS allows for early detection and management of leaks in an otherwise clinically stable patient, in this sense reducing the morbidity and mortality associated with leaks [28,30,55,56]. Opponents argue that the usefulness of routine UGIS is limited by many factors. First, it has a limited ability to diagnose leaks other than at the gastrojejunostomy site (eg, jejunojejunal leak, excluded stomach), and second, the overall sensitivity and PPV of the study is low. In a study by Carter and colleagues [57] of 654 patients, the overall sensitivity was 43% and overall PPV was 60%. Another study by Doraiswamy and colleagues [58] of 516 patients showed sensitivity of 33.3% and PPV of 11.1%. Singh and Fisher [59] reported PPV of only 27%. They argue that its routine use leads to false-positive results often prolonging hospitalizations, cost, unnecessary interventions, and patient discomfort. Third, the routine use of UGIS has risks. Aspiration of Gastrografin, although rare, can result in fatal pneumonitis. As stated earlier, we do not routinely use the UGIS; the discontinuation of its routine use has resulted in a significantly shorter length of stay for our patients having L-RYGB [60]. Multiple studies have shown that the selective approach to UGIS is safe and effective [51,57,58,60,61]. Furthermore, the selective approach also leads to increased sensitivity of the study. In summary, the routine use of UGIS in postoperative management of patients is still debatable. It may have a role in the initial learning process of the surgeon or the institution, and it may also be of aid in patients undergoing revisional surgery or a newer technique.

Because of the limitations of UGIS, as mentioned earlier, the CT scan is considered by many to be a better initial diagnostic test [62–64]. It provides better assessment of the distal gastric bypass anatomy as well as of the excluded stomach. It also serves as a useful follow-up study in patients with clinical signs of leak but equivocal UGIS findings. When used in conjunction with UGIS, the CT scan increases the overall sensitivity of both. Findings suggestive of an anastomotic leak include contrast extravasation from the gastrojejunostomy or the jejunojejunostomy, collections adjacent to the gastric pouch or remnant, diffuse abdominal fluid, and the presence of free intraperitoneal gas (Figs. 7 and 8).

However, there are inherent limitations in the use of CT, one being that many CT scanners have a weight limit of around 160 kg and may not accommodate larger patients. Also, because of the higher BMI of these patients, the

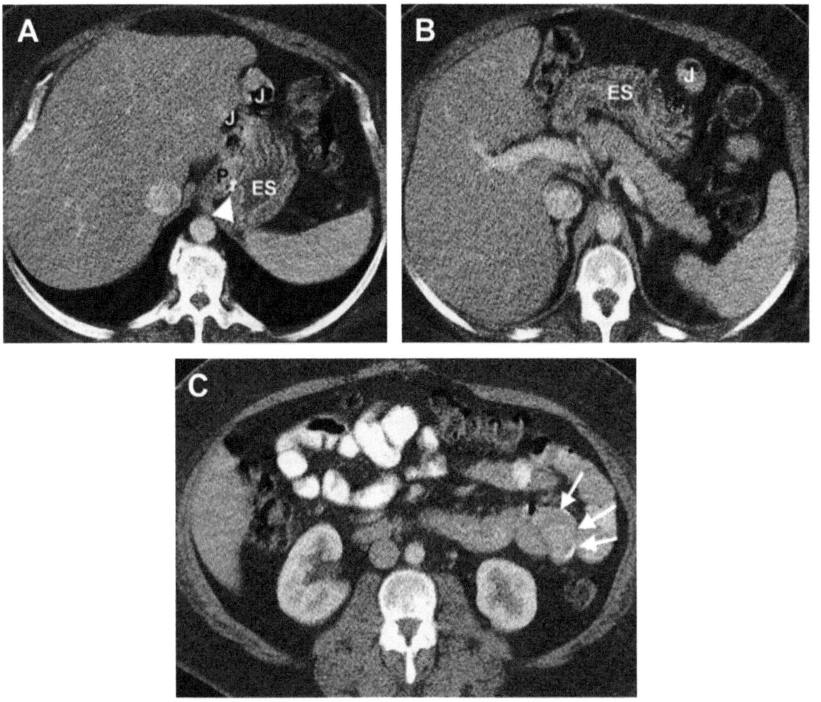

Fig. 7. Expected postoperative anatomy on CT after Roux-en-Y gastric bypass surgery. (*A*) Axial contrast-enhanced CT shows the expected postoperative anatomy including the gastric pouch (P), the gastric staple line (*arrowhead*), the 2 jejunal limbs (J), and the excluded stomach (ES). (*B*) Axial contrast-enhanced CT image slightly more caudally shows the decompressed, unopacified excluded stomach (ES). The Roux jejunal limb (J) is anterior and to the left of the excluded stomach (ES). (*C*) Axial contrast-enhanced CT image through the midabdomen shows the distal jejunojejunal anastomosis (*arrows*). (*From* Carucci LR, Turner MA, Yu J. Imaging evaluation following Roux-en-Y gastric bypass surgery for morbid obesity. Radiol Clin North Am 2007;45(2):249; with permission.)

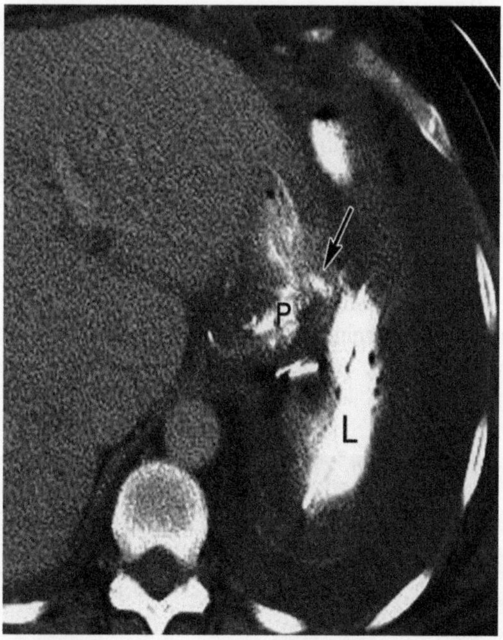

Fig. 8. Leak from gastrojejunal anastomosis extending to the left with resultant left upper quadrant collection (*arrow*). (*From* Carucci LR, Turner MA, Conklin RC. Roux-en-Y gastric bypass surgery for morbid obesity: evaluation of postoperative extraluminal leaks with upper gastrointestinal series. Radiology 2006;238(1):123; with permission.)

images are often of poor quality secondary to poor enhancement of the contrast. Furthermore, leaks may present with subtle signs radiographically and can easily be missed by an inexperienced radiologist. Even together, the CT and UGIS are not foolproof in detecting leaks. In a study by Gonzalez [48] of more than 3000 patients from 4 different institutions, UGIS and CT were negative in one-third of the patients with leaks. Therefore, the final diagnostic test remains operative exploration. In a patient with clinical suspicion of leak with equivocal biochemical and radiographic findings but signs of lack of improvement or deterioration, operative exploration should be undertaken. It has the highest sensitivity and specificity compared with any other diagnostic modality. Laparoscopic or open exploration is appropriate, and multiple studies have shown its safety and efficacy compared with the consequences of a missed leak [28,48,65]. A position statement from the American Society of Metabolic and Bariatric Surgery in January 2009 states "Surgical reexploration is an acceptable strategy to diagnose and treat patients who are highly suspected of having a postoperative leak after gastric bypass. A surgical reexploration that reveals no explanation for a postoperative patients' worrisome clinical findings or deterioration after gastric bypass should be considered an appropriate and indicated intervention and not a complication."

INTRAOPERATIVE DETECTION

Intraoperative leak tests are routinely performed by many surgeons to evaluate the gastrojejunostomy anastomosis using a variety of different methods. One of the most common techniques involves clamping of the Roux limb and insufflation of air through intraoperative endoscopy or nasogastric tube with the anastomosis submerged under saline [34]. The presence of bubbles indicates a leak. Another method involves instillation of methylene blue and evaluating for extravasation at the anastomosis. Some centers have reported on the use of intraoperative UGIS performed by instillation of Gastrografin under fluoroscopy [66].

Although these tests require additional equipment and increase the operative time and cost, they do allow for earlier detection and intraoperative repair of leaks from the gastrojejunostomy, including stapler malfunction in the proximal gastric pouch. At our institution, we routinely perform intraoperative endoscopy and use the bubble test on every gastric bypass procedure. We believe that its routine use has enabled us to decrease our postoperative leak rate. All patients, regardless of their bubble tests, have a suction drain placed posterior to the gastrojejunostomy.

PREVENTION

Comprehensive patient care in the perioperative period, as well as good operative techniques, are the keys to preventing leaks. Every attempt should be made to optimize the patients' medical conditions. Perioperative glycemic control should be attempted in diabetics. All of our patients are required to be on a two-week low-carbohydrate liquid diet before surgery. In the superobese patient, whose BMI exceeds 55 kg/m^2, we require a 10% weight loss before surgery. Alami and colleagues [67] reported that preoperative weight loss shortens operative time and that a low-carbohydrate liquid diet may result in lessening of liver mass, making laparoscopic gastric bypass less technically challenging. Although no improvement in complications or improvement in comorbidities could be documented in their small series, we believe that its routine use has contributed to our declining leak rates.

Excessive dissection should be avoided and adequate blood supply to the gastric pouch should be preserved. Any tension on the staple line should be avoided by ensuring adequate mobility of the alimentary limb. We routinely imbricate the staple line of the gastric pouch as well as of the excluded stomach by a running nonabsorbable suture. Others have reported on the use fibrin sealant, treated bovine pericardial strips, and other agents to reinforce the staple line. There are no randomized clinical trials to support the use of these techniques in reducing or preventing leak rates in the gastric bypass population. However, we believe that, by imbricating staples lines of the proximal and excluded gastric pouches, we have been able to substantially reduce our leak rate [68].

References

[1] Perri MG, Fuller PR. Success and failure in the treatment of obesity: where do we go from here? Med Exerc Nutr Health 1995;4:255–72.

[2] National task force on the prevention and treatment of obesity: very low calorie diets. JAMA 1993;270:967–74.
[3] Safer DJ. Diet, behaviour modification and exercise. A review of obesity treatments from a long term perspective. South Med J 1991;84(12):1470–4.
[4] Weintraub M, Sundaresan PR, Schuster B, et al. Long-term weight control study. IV (weeks 156–190). The second double-blind phase. Clin Pharmacol Ther 1992;51: 608–14.
[5] Powers PS. Conservative treatments for morbid obesity. In: Deitel M, editor. Surgery for the morbidly obese patient. Philadelphia: Lea & Febiger; 1989. p. 27–37.
[6] Pories WJ, Swanson MS, Macdonald KG, et al. Who would have thought it? An operation proves to be the most effective therapy for adult-onset diabetes mellitus. Ann Surg 1995;222(3):339–50 [discussion: 350–2].
[7] Sugerman HJ, Kellum JM, Engle KM, et al. Gastric bypass for treating severe obesity. Am J Clin Nutr 1992;55(Suppl 2):560S–6S.
[8] Linner JH, Drew RL. Why the operation we prefer is the Roux-Y gastric bypass. Obes Surg 1991;1(3):305–6.
[9] Mason EE. Gastric surgery for morbid obesity. Surg Clin North Am 1992;72(2):501–13.
[10] Yale CE. Gastric surgery for morbid obesity. Complications and long-term weight control. Arch Surg 1989;124(8):941–6.
[11] MacLean LD, Rhode BM, Forse RA. Late results of vertical banded gastroplasty for morbid and super obesity. Surgery 1990;107(1):20–7.
[12] Hall JC, Watts JM, O'Brien PE, et al. Gastric surgery for morbid obesity. The Adelaide Study. Ann Surg 1990;211(4):419–27.
[13] Charuzi I, Lavie P, Peiser J, et al. Bariatric surgery in morbidly obese sleep-apnea patients: short- and long-term follow-up. Am J Clin Nutr 1992;55(Suppl 2):594S–6S.
[14] Sugerman HJ, Fairman RP, Sood RK, et al. Long-term effects of gastric surgery for treating respiratory insufficiency of obesity. Am J Clin Nutr 1992;55(Suppl 2):597S–601S.
[15] Benotti PN, Bistrain B, Benotti JR, et al. Heart disease and hypertension in severe obesity: the benefits of weight reduction. Am J Clin Nutr 1992;55(Suppl 2):586S–90S.
[16] Brolin RE. Results of obesity surgery. Gastroenterol Clin North Am 1987;16(2):317–38.
[17] Gleysteen JJ. Results of surgery: long-term effects on hyperlipidemia. Am J Clin Nutr 1992;55(Suppl 2):591S–3S.
[18] Buchwald H, Buchwald JN. Evolution of surgery for morbid obesity. In: Pitombo C, Jones KB, Higa KD, et al, editors. Obesity surgery: principles and practice. China: McGraw-Hill; 2008. p. 1.
[19] Griffen WJ, Bivins B, Bell R. The decline and fall of the jejunoileal bypass. Surg Gynecol Obstet 1983;157:301–8.
[20] Mason EE, Ito C. Gastric bypass in obesity. Surg Clin North Am 1967;47:1345–52.
[21] Griffen WJ, Young V, Stevenson C. A prospective comparison of gastric and jejunoileal bypass procedures for morbid obesity. Ann Surg 1977;186:500–9.
[22] Torres J, Oca C, Garrison R. Gastric bypass: Roux-en-Y gastrojejunostomy from the lesser curvature. South Med J 1983;76:1217–21.
[23] Brolin RE, Kenler HA, Gorman JH, et al. Long-limb gastric bypass in the superobese: a prospective randomized trial. Ann Surg 1991;215:387–95.
[24] Wittgrove AC, Clark WG. Laparoscopic gastric bypass, Roux-en-Y: 500 patients: technique and results, with 3–60 month follow-up. Obes Surg 2000;10:233–8.
[25] Schauer PR, Ikramuddin S, Gourash W, et al. Outcomes after laparoscopic Roux-en-Y gastric bypass for morbid obesity. Ann Surg 2000;232:515–29.
[26] Higa KD, Ho T, Boone KB. Laparoscopic Roux-en-Y gastric bypass: technique and 3-year follow-up. J Laparoendosc Adv Surg Tech A 2001;11:377–82.
[27] Fernandez AZ Jr, DeMaria EJ, Tichansky DS, et al. Experience with over 3,000 open and laparoscopic bariatric procedures: multivariate analysis of factors related to leak and resultant mortality. Surg Endosc 2004;18:193–7.

[28] Marshall JS, Srivastava A, Gupta SK, et al. Roux-en-Y gastric bypass leak complications. Arch Surg 2003;138:520–3.
[29] Arteaga JR, Huerta S, Livingston EH. Management of gastrojejunal anastomotic leaks after Roux-en-Y gastric bypass. Am Surg 2002;68:1061–5.
[30] Gonzalez R, Nelson LG, Gallagher SF, et al. Anastomotic leaks after laparoscopic gastric bypass. Obes Surg 2004;14:1299–307.
[31] Gonzalez R, Lin E, Venkatesh KR, et al. Gastrojejunostomy during laparoscopic gastric bypass. Analysis of 3 techniques. Arch Surg 2003;138:181–4.
[32] Nguyen NT, Goldman C, Rosenquist CJ, et al. Laparoscopic versus open gastric bypass: a randomized study of outcomes, quality of life, and costs. Ann Surg 2001;234:279–91.
[33] Oliak D, Ballantyne GH, Davies RJ, et al. Short-term results of laparoscopic gastric bypass in patients with BMI $\geq$ 60. Obes Surg 2002;12:643–7.
[34] Champion JK, Hunt T, DeLisle N. Role of intraoperative endoscopy in laparoscopic bariatric surgery. Surg Endosc 2002;16:1663–5.
[35] Hamilton EC, Sims TL, Hamilton TT, et al. Clinical predictors of leak after laparoscopic Roux-en-Y gastric bypass for morbid obesity. Surg Endosc 2003;17:679–84.
[36] Papasavas PK, Caushaj PF, McCormick JT, et al. Laparoscopic management of complications following laparoscopic Roux-en-Y gastric bypass for morbid obesity. Surg Endosc 2003;17:610–4.
[37] Gould JC, Garren MJ, Starling JR. Lessons learned from the first 100 cases in a new minimally invasive bariatric surgery program. Obes Surg 2004;14:618–25.
[38] Dresel A, Kuhn JA, McCarty TM. Laparoscopic Roux en-Y gastric bypass in morbidly obese and super morbidly obese patients. Am J Surg 2004;187:230–2.
[39] Carrasquilla C, English WJ, Esposito P, et al. Total stapled, total intra-abdominal (TSTI) laparoscopic Roux en-Y gastric bypass: one leak in 1,000 cases. Obes Surg 2004;14:613–7.
[40] Mason EE, Ito C. Gastric bypass. Ann Surg 1969;170:329–39.
[41] Griffen WO, Bivins BA, Bell RM, et al. Gastric bypass for morbid obesity. World J Surg 1981;5:817–22.
[42] Linner JH. Comparative effectiveness of gastric bypass and gastroplasty. Arch Surg 1982;117:695–700.
[43] Sugerman HJ, Londrey GL, Kellum JM, et al. Weight loss with vertical banded gastroplasty and Roux-Y gastric bypass for morbid obesity with selective versus random assignment. Am J Surg 1989;157:93–102.
[44] MacLean LD, Rhode BM, Sampalis J, et al. Results of the surgical treatment of obesity. Am J Surg 1993;165:155–62.
[45] Capella JF, Capella RF. The weight reduction operation of choice: vertical banded gastroplasty or gastric bypass. Am J Surg 1996;171:74–9.
[46] Fobi MA, Lee H, Holness R, et al. Gastric bypass operation for obesity. World J Surg 1998;22:925–35.
[47] MacLean LD, Rhode B, Nohr CW. Late outcome of isolated gastric bypass. Ann Surg 2000;231:524–8.
[48] Gonzalez R, Sarr MG, Smith CD, et al. Diagnosis and contemporary management of anastomotic leaks after gastric bypass for obesity. J Am Coll Surg 2007;204(1):47–55.
[49] Al-Sabah S, Ladouceur M, Christou N. Anastomotic leaks after bariatric surgery: it is the host response that matters. Surg Obes Relat Dis 2008;4:152–8.
[50] Ballesta C, Berindoague R, Cabrera M, et al. Management of anastomotic leaks after laparoscopic Roux-en-Y gastric bypass. Obes Surg 2008;18:623–30.
[51] Kolakowski S, Kirkland ML, Schuricht AL, et al. Routine postoperative upper gastrointestinal series after Roux-en-Y gastric bypass: determination of whether it is necessary. Arch Surg 2007;142(10):930–4.
[52] Maher JW, Bakhos W, Nahmias N, et al. Drain amylase levels are an adjunct in detection of gastrojejunostomy leaks after Roux-en-Y gastric bypass. J Am Coll Surg 2009;208(5): 881–4.

[53] Salgado W, de Queiroz Cunha F, dos Santos JS, et al. Early identification of infectious complication in bariatric surgery by the determination of peritoneal and systemic cytokines. Obes Surg 2009;19:867–72.
[54] Carucci LR, Turner MA, Conklin RC, et al. Roux-en-Y gastric bypass surgery for morbid obesity: evaluation of postoperative extraluminal leaks with upper gastrointestinal series. Radiology 2006;238(1):119–27.
[55] Sims TL, Mullican MA, Hamilton EC, et al. Routine upper gastrointestinal Gastrografin swallow after laparoscopic Roux-en-Y gastric bypass. Obes Surg 2003;13:66–72.
[56] Madan AK, Stoecklein HH, Ternovits CA, et al. Predictive value of upper gastrointestinal studies versus clinical signs for gastrointestinal leaks after laparoscopic gastric bypass. Surg Endosc 2007;21(2):194–6.
[57] Carter JT, Tafreshian S, Campos GM, et al. Routine upper GI series after gastric bypass does not reliably identify anastomotic leaks or predict stricture formation. Surg Endosc 2007;21: 2172–7.
[58] Doraiswamy A, Rasmussen JJ, Pierce J, et al. The utility of routine postoperative upper GI series following laparoscopic gastric bypass. Surg Endosc 2007;21(12):2159–62.
[59] Singh R, Fisher BL. Sensitivity and specificity of postoperative upper GI series following gastric bypass. Obes Surg 2003;1:73–5.
[60] Lee SD, Khouzam MN, Kellum JM, et al. Selective, versus routine, upper gastrointestinal series leads to equal morbidity and reduced hospital stay in laparoscopic gastric bypass patients. Surg Obes Relat Dis 2007;3(4):413–6.
[61] White S, Han SH, Lewis C, et al. Selective approach to use of upper gastroesophageal imaging study after laparoscopic Roux-en-Y gastric bypass. Surg Obes Relat Dis 2008;4(2):122–5.
[62] Esmailzadeh H, Powell W, Lourie D. Use of computed tomography in diagnosis of major postoperative gastrointestinal complications of laparoscopic Roux-en-Y gastric bypass surgery. Am Surg 2004;70(11):964–6.
[63] Lyass S, Khalili TM, Cunneen S, et al. Radiological studies after laparoscopic Roux-en-Y gastric bypass: routine or selective? Am Surg 2004;70:918–21.
[64] Perugini RA, Mason R, Czerniach DR, et al. Predictors of complication and suboptimal weight loss after laparoscopic Roux-en-Y gastric bypass: a series of 188 patients. Arch Surg 2003;138(5):541–5 [discussion: 545–6].
[65] Durak E, Inabnet WB, Schrope B, et al. Incidence and management of enteric leaks after gastric bypass for morbid obesity during a 10-year period. Surg Obes Relat Dis 2008;4(3):389–93.
[66] Nami F, Fletcher S, Nusbaum MJ. Intra-operative upper gastrointestinal fluoroscopy to detect and repair leaks in laparoscopic gastric bypass surgery. Surg Endosc 2004;18: S201 [abstract].
[67] Alami RS, Morton JM, Schuster R, et al. Is there a benefit to preoperative weight loss in gastric bypass patients? A prospective randomized trial. Surg Obes Relat Dis 2007;3: 141–5.
[68] Maher JW, Hawver LM, Pucci A, et al. Four hundred and fifty consecutive laparoscopic Roux-en-Y gastric bypasses with no mortality and declining leak rates and lengths of stay in a bariatric training program. J Am Coll Surg 2008;206(5):940–4 [discussion: 944–5].

ELSEVIER
MOSBY

Advances in Surgery 44 (2010) 73–85

ADVANCES IN SURGERY

Distinguishing Acute from Ruptured Appendicitis Preoperatively in the Pediatric Patient

Ankush Gosain, MD, PhD, Regan F. Williams, MD, Martin L. Blakely, MD, MS*

Division of Pediatric Surgery, Department of Surgery, University of Tennessee Health Sciences Center, 777 Washington Avenue, Suite P220, Memphis, TN 38105, USA

Appendicitis is the most common intra-abdominal condition requiring urgent operation in pediatric patients. Annually, more than 100,000 children are treated for appendicitis in the United States [1]. The spectrum of presentation ranges from acute nonruptured appendicitis to ruptured appendicitis (RA) with abscess formation. Although the management of acute appendicitis (AA) is rarely debated, the optimal treatment for ruptured appendicitis remains controversial. It is clear from the literature that patients with ruptured appendicitis undergo more diagnostic studies and invasive procedures and these patients have longer hospitalizations than those with nonruptured appendicitis. For these reasons, preoperatively diagnosing ruptured appendicitis may allow for triage of limited resources and informed discussions of expected clinical course. The distinction between nonruptured and ruptured appendicitis is also important because the optimal treatment of each condition may differ. Additionally, the design of prospective studies to compare early versus interval appendectomy for ruptured appendicitis will rely on the accurate preoperative diagnosis of ruptured appendicitis.

DIAGNOSIS OF APPENDICITIS VERSUS NONAPPENDICITIS CAUSES OF ABDOMINAL PAIN

Historically, there has been a great deal of focus in the primary care, emergency medicine, and surgical literature on the preoperative diagnosis of appendicitis in patients presenting with abdominal pain [2]. These studies have been motivated by the desire to accurately make the diagnosis of appendicitis while avoiding or reducing the incidence of negative appendectomy (appendectomy for a histologically normal appendix). Traditionally, a false-positive rate as high as 25% has been accepted to avoid high perforation rates [3,4]. However, an

*Corresponding author. *E-mail address*: mblakely@uthsc.edu.

0065-3411/10/$ – see front matter
doi:10.1016/j.yasu.2010.05.021

improved understanding of the morbidity associated with a negative appendectomy, including abscess formation, wound infection, and bowel obstruction, has lowered the acceptance level of negative appendectomies [5].

Because infants and children will often present with atypical symptoms, clinical scoring systems focusing on differentiating appendicitis from nonappendicitis conditions in adults and children are plentiful in the literature [6–9]. The Alvarado and Samuel scoring systems have received the most attention [8,10]. These systems have been based on elements of the history, physical examination, and laboratory findings. The MANTRELS score, described by Alvarado, includes migration of pain, anorexia, nausea/vomiting, tenderness in the right lower quadrant, rebound tenderness, elevation of temperature, leukocytosis, and shift to the left on the cell count differential. Since its publication, the MANTRELS score has been prospectively evaluated and shown to have a sensitivity of 76% to 90% and specificity of 50% to 81% [11]. The reported accuracy of these scoring systems has varied, depending on the study cohort involved [12].

Additionally, various groups have evaluated the value of imaging modalities, namely ultrasound or CT, for the diagnosis of appendicitis. Broadly speaking, ultrasound appears to be most helpful in nonobese patients and may provide alternative diagnoses to appendicitis [13,14]. Additionally, ultrasound has the benefit of avoiding exposing children to ionizing radiation [15]. Limitations of ultrasound include its operator-dependant nature, lack of sensitivity in early appendicitis when only a portion of the appendix is involved, and inability to visualize the appendix in obese individuals. Because of these limitations, the reported sensitivity varies from 78% to 94% and specificity from 89% to 98% in the pediatric literature [16–19].

CT is not subject to the limitations of operator dependence and is useful for identifying alternative diagnoses or sequelae of ruptured appendicitis. Additionally, CT is able to demonstrate a normal appendix in 66% to 100% of cases [20]. CT is highly sensitive for acute appendicitis, with most studies reporting 95% to 99%, and specificity widely reported as greater than 95% [21,22]. Limitations of CT in the diagnosis of appendicitis include the inability to evaluate the compressibility of the appendix and the administration of ionizing radiation and the subsequent risk of malignancy [2,23]. Additionally, the specific protocols for CT scan vary from institution to institution, with debate over the superiority of noncontrast enhanced studies versus intravenous contrast alone versus rectal contrast in addition to intravenous contrast [24,25].

Although imaging for possible appendicitis has become routine in many centers, there continue to be those that advocate a diagnostic strategy based on the clinical acumen of an experienced surgeon [26]. In their study, Kosloske and colleagues demonstrated 99% sensitivity, 93% specificity, and 97% diagnostic accuracy for appendicitis by surgeon-directed history and physical examination followed by diagnostic imaging. In their series, one-third of subjects had undergone ultrasound or CT imaging before surgical consultation, with another 17% of the subjects receiving imaging after evaluation by the surgeon.

There was no difference in the diagnostic accuracy for those subjects that received imaging before pediatric surgical evaluation as compared with those that received it postreferral. Additionally, the negative appendectomy rate of 5% in their series compares favorably to other published series.

Recently, the authors have demonstrated that pediatric surgeons are quite good at differentiating appendicitis and nonappendicitis causes of abdominal pain, and have focused our attention on the distinction between acute nonruptured and ruptured appendicitis [27].

DEFINITION OF RUPTURED APPENDICITIS

The pathogenesis of appendicitis is well established [28,29]. The initiating event is luminal obstruction, typically caused by lymphoid hyperplasia or an obstructing fecalith. Additional etiologies of luminal obstruction have been described and include foreign bodies, malignancy, and parasitic infections. Luminal obstruction results in bacterial stasis and overgrowth, with resultant distention of the blind-ending appendix (acute appendicitis). With sufficient luminal distention, the intraluminal pressure of the appendix exceeds that of its arterial inflow, resulting in ischemia of the wall (gangrenous appendicitis). Finally, perforation occurs at the site of ischemia, resulting in free spillage of pus (ruptured appendicitis). Numerous investigators have postulated that perforation is more likely at the site of, and in the presence of, an obstructing fecalith [30]. Abscess formation may ensue as part of the normal host response to perforation. Intraoperatively, the distinction between gangrenous and ruptured appendicitis may be difficult to make. Accordingly, the incidence of RA in children varies greatly in multiple large series, from 20% to 76% [31]. Recently, multiple groups have advocated a strict definition of ruptured appendicitis to include the intraoperative or pathologic identification of either a hole in the appendix or the presence of a fecalith in the abdomen [32]. St Peter and colleagues argue that by adopting a strict definition of perforation, cases of suppurative and gangrenous appendicitis that may have been included in the ruptured category in prior studies will be eliminated from analysis and thereby reduce some of the variability in results that are reported in the literature and allow for direct comparisons between studies.

IMPORTANCE OF DISTINGUISHING ACUTE AND RUPTURED APPENDICITIS

Ruptured appendicitis comprises a larger percentage of appendicitis in children than in adults, ranging from 30% to 74% depending on the study population [33]. Although the optimal treatment for AA is rarely debated, the approach to RA varies greatly between pediatric surgeons and medical centers [31,34,35]. Some surgeons advocate early appendectomy, preceded by a brief period of antibiotic administration and fluid resuscitation. Others advocate for interval appendectomy, with antibiotic administration until the child has been afebrile for a variable period of time (typically 24–48 hours). These patients return 6 to 8 weeks after their initial presentation for elective removal of their appendix, often as an outpatient procedure [36]. Finally, there are those that advocate for total nonoperative treatment, with antibiotic therapy and no appendectomy [37]. There exists little consensus among pediatric surgeons as to the optimal treatment of ruptured appendicitis [38].

Initial nonoperative management of appendicitis presenting as appendiceal abscess or phlegmon has been shown to be safe and effective [39–41]. Following nonoperative management, interval appendectomy is employed to avoid a 5% to 37% risk of recurrent appendicitis [39,42,43]. Recently, a few groups have argued against this paradigm, citing low rates of recurrent appendicitis in patients treated nonoperatively. However, the follow-up period in these series is short, and there is some evidence that recurrent appendicitis results in larger resections (eg, cecectomy or hemicolectomy) than would otherwise have been necessary [37].

Retrospective reviews have demonstrated that those patients with a longer duration of symptoms tend to be the ones chosen for nonoperative management [44,45]. Additionally, these studies demonstrate that the patient subset undergoing immediate appendectomy has a higher incidence of complications [46,47], although this is possibly because sicker patients are chosen to undergo immediate appendectomy.

The goals of therapy in the treatment of ruptured appendicitis are minimizing morbidity, costs, hospital length of stay, and readmissions. Following appendectomy, patients with ruptured appendicitis are at higher risk for development of intra-abdominal abscess. A recent trial used a case-control methodology to identify risk factors for abscess formation in patients undergoing appendectomy for ruptured appendicitis [48]. In this study, several demographic and perioperative factors that had previously been identified in the literature as predictive of abscess formation were studied in three-quarters of the subject population and a model to predict abscess formation was developed and tested in the remaining quarter of subjects. The investigators noted that diarrhea at the time of presentation substantially increased the odds of developing an intra-abdominal abscess or other infectious complications postoperatively. However, the predictive model generated based on their data set did not fit their remaining subjects well, decreasing the utility of their findings.

One group has evaluated the incidence of abscess formation in their subject cohort before and after the application of a strict definition of ruptured appendicitis [32]. They have observed an increased incidence of intra-abdominal abscess in the ruptured subject cohort and a decreased incidence in the nonruptured cohort, reinforcing the concept that the risk of postoperative complications increases as one progresses further along the spectrum from acute to ruptured appendicitis.

WHY DO PATIENTS FAIL NONOPERATIVE TREATMENT?

The failure rate for nonoperative management varies in the literature from 9% to 40% [44–46,49]. Bufo and colleagues [50] reviewed 87 cases of ruptured appendicitis of which 41 were treated nonoperatively. In their cohort, 7 subjects

(17%) failed nonoperative management almost exclusively because of the presence of bowel obstruction. Although the nonoperative group had a decreased hospital stay and fewer complications than the operative group, this benefit was not seen when the subjects were analyzed in an intent-to-treat fashion. Other groups have published data indicating that failure of nonoperative management results from persistent or increasing abdominal pain, increasing fevers, and worsening abdominal tenderness [51,52]. Additionally, multiple groups have also reported a higher incidence of complications in those patients that fail nonoperative management [44,53]. These complications include wound infections and abscess formation, resulting in longer hospital stay [54].

PREOPERATIVE DIAGNOSIS OF RUPTURED APPENDICITIS

If treatment recommendations for ruptured and acute appendicitis differ and clinical trials are to be conducted in patients with ruptured appendicitis, it becomes critically important to distinguish between the two preoperatively [27]. In a recent study, the authors proposed to determine the accuracy of pediatric surgeons' preoperative diagnosis of acute and ruptured appendicitis, to prospectively identify and rank patient characteristics that increase the likelihood of having ruptured appendicitis, and to investigate potential methods of improving our ability to distinguish acute from ruptured appendicitis preoperatively.

Data were prospectively collected over a period of 9 months on all subjects younger than 18 years of age referred for surgical consultation for abdominal pain at a regional children's hospital. Subject demographics, elements of the history and physical examination, laboratory values, and diagnostic imaging reports were collected. The pediatric surgical team, including an attending pediatric surgeon, a fellow in pediatric surgery, and a general surgery resident, recorded an agreed initial (preoperative) diagnosis using all data available. Establishing the preoperative diagnosis was a dedicated part of this study and typically involved repeated history and physical examinations by multiple team members (over a brief period, usually in the emergency department), independent reviews of the available data, and consultation with pediatric radiologists when needed for detailed review of the imaging studies. The use of advanced imaging (CT or ultrasonography) was decided by emergency department physicians, referral physicians, or pediatric surgeons. When there was disagreement between team members about the initial diagnosis, the attending pediatric surgeon made the final decision. Final diagnosis was determined using operative findings, pathology reports, or discharge diagnosis in those not undergoing operation.

A total of 247 subjects were evaluated over a 9-month study period. Ninety-eight had AA, 53 had RA, and 96 did not have appendicitis. The median age was 10 years (range 1 to 17 years), 39% were girls, and the median duration of symptoms at the time of surgery consultation was 2.8 days. The majority of the subjects were Caucasian (52%); smaller percentages were African American (34%) or Hispanic (9%). Fifty-five percent of the subjects had localized right lower quadrant pain and 9% presented with generalized peritonitis. Most subjects underwent some form of diagnostic imaging, with 79% of subjects having a CT scan, 21% receiving an abdominal ultrasound, and 15% undergoing both. The perforation rate among all subjects with appendicitis was 35%.

The 98 children with a discharge diagnosis of AA based on intraoperative findings were older and had a shorter duration of symptoms than subjects with ruptured or no appendicitis. These children had a median duration of symptoms of 24 hours, with 73% presenting with emesis and 75% complaining of anorexia. Ninety-one percent of subjects with AA had localized right lower quadrant pain and only 30% had rebound tenderness. The median white blood cell (WBC) count was lower in subjects with AA, although there was no difference in the percentage of bands among the 3 diagnostic groups. Seventy-two percent of these subjects had a CT scan performed and 10% underwent abdominal ultrasonography. All subjects with a preoperative diagnosis of AA underwent an operation, with a negative appendectomy rate of 4.4%.

The RA group consisted of 53 subjects, with a median age of 9.2 years; 34% were girls. Subjects with RA had symptoms for a median of 86.7 hours, similar to the not appendicitis (NA) group, and had a higher WBC count (median 17,900 cells/μL). The majority of subjects with RA had diffuse abdominal pain (62%) and CT scans performed (94%). Of the 53 subjects, 35 underwent immediate appendectomy, 17 had an interval appendectomy 7 to 21 weeks after initial presentation with RA, and 1 subject was managed with intravenous antibiotics but did not return for interval appendectomy.

Ninety-six subjects in the study cohort did not have appendicitis. These subjects were similar to subjects in the RA group in age and duration of symptoms. But the NA group had a larger percentage of girls and a lower median WBC count than the AA or RA groups. There were 8 subjects with diagnoses other than appendicitis that underwent exploratory laparotomy. Two of these subjects had RA identified at the time of exploration. Follow-up was conducted on all subjects who did not undergo an operation (11 to 20 months after discharge) either by telephone follow-up questionnaire (76%), review of the hospital medical record system, or both. No subject reported a subsequent diagnosis of appendicitis during this follow-up period.

Pediatric surgeons at the authors' institution diagnosed acute, ruptured, and not appendicitis with an accuracy of 93.5%, 93.5%, and 96.8%, respectively. Although pediatric surgeons were able to diagnose AA with high sensitivity (92.6%) and specificity (94.9%), these figures for the diagnosis of RA were mixed. RA was correctly diagnosed preoperatively with a sensitivity of 96.4% and a specificity of 83%. Appendicitis was excluded with high sensitivity (98.7%) and specificity (93.8%). Although the overall surgeon's preoperative diagnostic accuracy was 92%, there was variability among the 5 attending pediatric surgeons participating in the study. Accuracy rates varied from 97% (36 subjects) to 83% (30 subjects) among the pediatric surgeons, for an absolute difference of approximately 14%.

Univariate analysis was also performed on all preoperative variables comparing subjects with a discharge diagnosis of RA to those with AA (Table 1). Continuous variables were converted to categorical variables by using a cut point that maximized the Youden's index. The Youden's index is the value that maximizes the sensitivity and specificity of any continuous variable, helping to choose an appropriate cut point for dichotomization. No single variable accurately predicted the final diagnosis. Decreased age and African American race were significantly more common in subjects with RA. Gender had no association with final diagnosis. Elements of the history significantly associated with RA included anorexia, emesis, and duration of symptoms greater than 48 hours. Signs of ruptured appendicitis included fever (temperature >38°C), right lower quadrant tenderness to palpation, diffuse abdominal tenderness, generalized peritonitis, and high white blood cell count (WBC >19,400 cells/μL), although the presence of diffuse abdominal pain and generalized peritonitis was positively correlated with each other and negatively correlated with right lower quadrant tenderness to palpation. Extra-luminal air, fecalith and abscess on CT scan were also associated with RA. All variables from the univariate analysis with a *P* value less than or equal to .2 were placed into the multivariable analysis.

Table 1
Univariate analysis for ruptured appendicitis

Variable	Odds ratio	95% CI	*P* value
Patient demographics			
Age >6 y	0.848	0.386–1.864	.6812
Female gender	0.945	0.465–1.919	.8748
African American	2.357	1.109–5.007	.0258
Hispanic	1.8	0.580–5.58	.3088
Symptoms			
Anorexia	3.810	1.243–11.676	.0192
Diarrhea	1.583	0.754–3.323	.2244
Emesis	3.268	1.176–9.082	.0231
Duration >48 h	11.511	4.991–26.547	<.0001
Signs			
Temperature >38°C	4.514	2.205–9.241	<.0001
Localized RLQ ttp	0.078	0.034–0.176	<.0001
Rebound RLQ ttp	0.725	0.335–1.567	.4131
Diffuse ttp	12.912	5.647–29.526	<.0001
Generalized peritonitis	18.364	5.086–66.303	<.0001
WBC >19,400 cells/μL	4.049	1.926–8.509	.0002
CT findings			
Extraluminal air	8.654	1.782–42.025	.0074
Fecalith	4.070	1.893–8.752	.0003
Free fluid	1.703	0.822–3.528	.1520
Abscess	14.194	4.464–45.131	<.0001
Dilated appendix	0.767	0.372–1.579	.4710

Abbreviations: CI, confidence interval; RLQ, right lower quadrant.

Table 2
Multivariate analysis for ruptured appendicitis and scoring system

Variable	Odds ratio	95% CI	*P* value	Beta coefficient	Score
Generalized tenderness	7.4	2.2–24.5	<.01	2.00	4
Abscess on CT	6.7	1.6–27.1	<.01	1.90	3
Duration >48 h	6.4	1.9–21.7	<.01	1.86	3
WBC >19,400 cells/μL	5.6	1.6–19.6	<.01	1.75	2
Fecalith on CT	4.5	1.4–14.7	.01	1.51	1

Abbreviation: CI, confidence interval.

The final multivariable model of RA was completed in a manual, backward, stepwise fashion to determine preoperative variables independently associated with RA (Table 2). Based on this analysis, 5 preoperative variables were independently associated with the diagnosis of RA: duration of symptoms greater than 48 hours, pain not localized to the right lower quadrant, WBC greater than 19,400 cells/μL, and fecalith and abscess on CT scan.

Using the predictors identified with multivariable analysis, a scoring system was constructed to evaluate whether an objective score based on available data might improve the ability to accurately diagnose RA (see Table 2). Points were assigned to each preoperative variable based on the beta coefficients from the multivariable final model. Pain not localized to the right lower quadrant had a beta coefficient of 2.00 and was assigned 4 points. Abscess on CT scan and duration of symptoms greater than 48 hours had similar coefficients (1.90 and 1.86, respectively) and were assigned 3 points each. WBC count greater than 19,400 cells/μL had a beta coefficient of 1.75 and was assigned 2 points, and fecalith on CT scan had the lowest significant correlation with ruptured appendicitis, with a beta coefficient of 1.51 (1 point). The subject's

Table 3
Accuracy of ruptured appendicitis scoring system

Score	Sensitivity	Specificity	PDLR	NDLR
1	98	46	1.8	0.04
2	96	56	2.1	0.07
3	92	65	2.6	0.12
4	92	81	4.9	0.1
5	82	90	7.9	0.19
6	78	92	9.1	0.24
7	68	94	11.3	0.33
8	62	97	24.3	0.38
9	47	98	27.0	0.53
10	35	99	41.0	0.65
11	18	1	—	0.82
12	7	1	—	0.92
13	6	1	—	0.94

Abbreviations: NDLR, negative diagnostic likelihood ratio; PDLR, positive diagnostic likelihood ratio.

score was calculated by adding the appropriate points based on the number of significant preoperative variables present. Positive and negative likelihood ratios (LR) were calculated for the pediatric surgeon's preoperative diagnosis and the score according to the scoring system (Table 3).

SUMMARY

There have been several retrospective studies addressing which patient characteristics are associated with an increased risk for RA rather than AA. The most common variables reported to increase the risk of RA from these studies include longer duration of symptoms (>2 to 3 days), signs of diffuse peritoneal irritation on abdominal examination, age younger than 8 to 9 years, higher temperature elevation, and multiple CT findings [55–60]. Laboratory data reported to be associated with ruptured appendicitis include elevated C-reactive protein, erythrocyte sedimentation rate greater than 25 mm/h, increased band neutrophils, and increased total white blood cell count [55,58–60]. The authors' data provide a ranking of variables that are routinely available preoperatively in patients referred for surgical consultation to rule out appendicitis in order of strength of association with a final diagnosis of RA. The most important preoperative risk factors identified in the authors' study cohort, in rank order, were duration of symptoms greater than 48 hours, diffuse abdominal pain, WBC greater than 19,400 cells/μL, abscess identified on CT, and fecalith identified on CT. Age was not an independent significant risk factor for RA.

The derivation of a novel scoring system, based on the variables found to be significant in the multivariable regression analyses, is an attempt to improve the diagnostic accuracy of RA in the future. As mentioned earlier, the pediatric surgeon's preoperative diagnosis was somewhat variable between the 5 attending surgeons participating in this study. Because the distinction between AA and RA was a major part of this prospective study, it is possible that this distinction in routine clinical practice could be somewhat lower. Also, the accuracy of other pediatric surgeon groups and other medical centers is largely unknown. An objective scoring system, if validated, could decrease the variability of this diagnostic process and potentially improve overall distinction between AA and RA. Depending on the cut point chosen, the sensitivity and specificity of the scoring system vary considerably. The authors propose that a cut point that achieves a high specificity (at the expense of sensitivity) would potentially be most valuable. The authors' data indicate that the pediatric surgeons accurately distinguish appendicitis from nonappendicitis abdominal pain with high sensitivity, specificity, and accuracy. Distinguishing AA from RA is more difficult. Once a diagnosis of appendicitis has been made, the scoring system might be used to assist in distinguishing the acute from the ruptured form. Deciding where the cut point should be in this scoring system significantly influences its performance. As the cut-point value increases, specificity and the positive likelihood ratio increase, and the sensitivity decreases markedly. Using a cut point of 9, the scoring system outperforms the surgeon's preoperative diagnosis in terms of positive LR and specificity by a degree that, if reproducible, would likely help practicing pediatric surgeons make clinically relevant decisions. Confirmation of this scoring system in a different subject cohort will be necessary to validate its clinical utility. To this end, plans are underway to test this scoring system in a multicenter, prospective cohort study.

FUTURE DIRECTIONS

The diagnosis of appendicitis has shifted from one made purely on the basis of history and physical examination to a sophisticated evaluation of elements of the presentation and imaging. This evolution has resulted from an improved understanding of the differing natural history of acute and ruptured appendicitis and the ongoing debate as to optimal treatment of these conditions (eg, initial nonoperative vs immediate operation). Additionally, as imaging techniques improve, the diagnosis of appendicitis is more frequently being made before consultation with a surgeon. As more data are published about potential harmful effects of ionizing radiation from abdominal and pelvic CT scans, heavy reliance on these studies is problematic. Limitations of the authors' recent study, and those of others, include single-center design, low numbers of subjects, and frequent use of advanced imaging (especially abdominal CT). Many scoring systems appear accurate when applied to the study populations from which they are derived, but then are less accurate when one attempts to validate them in other studies. It remains unknown how accurate pediatric surgeons' preoperative diagnoses are across multiple centers or how the authors' recently developed scoring system might perform in larger and more diverse study populations.

References

[1] Addiss DG, Shaffer N, Fowler BS, et al. The epidemiology of appendicitis and appendectomy in the United States. Am J Epidemiol 1990;132(5):910–25.
[2] Brennan GD. Pediatric appendicitis: pathophysiology and appropriate use of diagnostic imaging. CJEM 2006;8(6):425–32.
[3] Larsson PG, Henriksson G, Olsson M, et al. Laparoscopy reduces unnecessary appendectomies and improves diagnosis in fertile women. A randomized study. Surg Endosc 2001;15(2):200–2.
[4] Wilson EB. Surgical evaluation of appendicitis in the new era of radiographic imaging. Semin Ultrasound CT MR 2003;24(2):65–8.
[5] Colson M, Skinner KA, Dunnington G. High negative appendectomy rates are no longer acceptable. Am J Surg 1997;174(6):723–6 [discussion: 726–7].
[6] Bundy DG, Byerley JS, Liles EA, et al. Does this child have appendicitis? JAMA 2007;298(4):438–51.
[7] Kharbanda AB, Taylor GA, Fishman SJ, et al. A clinical decision rule to identify children at low risk for appendicitis. Pediatrics 2005;116(3):709–16.
[8] Alvarado A. A practical score for the early diagnosis of acute appendicitis. Ann Emerg Med 1986;15(5):557–64.
[9] Enochsson L, Gudbjartsson T, Hellberg A, et al. The Fenyo-Lindberg scoring system for appendicitis increases positive predictive value in fertile women–a prospective study in 455 patients randomized to either laparoscopic or open appendectomy. Surg Endosc 2004;18(10):1509–13.
[10] Samuel M. Pediatric appendicitis score. J Pediatr Surg 2002;37(6):877–81.

[11] Kwok MY, Kim MK, Gorelick MH. Evidence-based approach to the diagnosis of appendicitis in children. Pediatr Emerg Care 2004;20(10):690–8 [quiz: 699–701].
[12] Schneider C, Kharbanda A, Bachur R. Evaluating appendicitis scoring systems using a prospective pediatric cohort. Ann Emerg Med 2007;49(6):778–84, 784, e771.
[13] Blebea JS, Meilstrup JW, Wise SW. Appendiceal imaging: which test is best? Semin Ultrasound CT MR 2003;24(2):91–5.
[14] Even-Bendahan G, Lazar I, Erez I, et al. Role of imaging in the diagnosis of acute appendicitis in children. Clin Pediatr (Phila) 2003;42(1):23–7.
[15] Taylor GA. Suspected appendicitis in children: in search of the single best diagnostic test. Radiology 2004;231(2):293–5.
[16] Hayden CK Jr, Kuchelmeister J, Lipscomb TS. Sonography of acute appendicitis in childhood: perforation versus nonperforation. J Ultrasound Med 1992;11(5):209–16.
[17] Rubin SZ, Martin DJ. Ultrasonography in the management of possible appendicitis in childhood. J Pediatr Surg 1990;25(7):737–40.
[18] Sivit CJ, Newman KD, Boenning DA, et al. Appendicitis: usefulness of US in diagnosis in a pediatric population. Radiology 1992;185(2):549–52.
[19] Vignault F, Filiatrault D, Brandt ML, et al. Acute appendicitis in children: evaluation with US. Radiology 1990;176(2):501–4.
[20] Sivit CJ, Applegate KE. Imaging of acute appendicitis in children. Semin Ultrasound CT MR 2003;24(2):74–82.
[21] Rao PM, Rhea JT, Rattner DW, et al. Introduction of appendiceal CT: impact on negative appendectomy and appendiceal perforation rates. Ann Surg 1999;229(3):344–9.
[22] Stroman DL, Bayouth CV, Kuhn JA, et al. The role of computed tomography in the diagnosis of acute appendicitis. Am J Surg 1999;178(6):485–9.
[23] Hall EJ. Lessons we have learned from our children: cancer risks from diagnostic radiology. Pediatr Radiol 2002;32(10):700–6.
[24] Kaiser S, Finnbogason T, Jorulf HK, et al. Suspected appendicitis in children: diagnosis with contrast-enhanced versus nonenhanced Helical CT. Radiology 2004;231(2):427–33.
[25] Kharbanda AB, Taylor GA, Bachur RG. Suspected appendicitis in children: rectal and intravenous contrast-enhanced versus intravenous contrast-enhanced CT. Radiology 2007;243(2):520–6.
[26] Kosloske AM, Love CL, Rohrer JE, et al. The diagnosis of appendicitis in children: outcomes of a strategy based on pediatric surgical evaluation. Pediatrics 2004;113(1 Pt 1):29–34.
[27] Williams RF, Blakely ML, Fischer PE, et al. Diagnosing ruptured appendicitis preoperatively in pediatric patients. J Am Coll Surg 2009;208(5):819–25 [discussion: 826–8].
[28] Fitz R. Perforating inflammation of the vermiform appendix with special reference to its early diagnosis and treatment. Trans Assoc Am Physicians 1886;1:107–44.
[29] Wangensteen OH, Dennis C. Experimental proof of the obstructive origin of appendicitis in man. Ann Surg 1939;110(4):629–47.
[30] Ein SH, Langer JC, Daneman A. Nonoperative management of pediatric ruptured appendix with inflammatory mass or abscess: presence of an appendicolith predicts recurrent appendicitis. J Pediatr Surg 2005;40(10):1612–5.
[31] Newman K, Ponsky T, Kittle K, et al. Appendicitis 2000: variability in practice, outcomes, and resource utilization at thirty pediatric hospitals. J Pediatr Surg 2003;38(3):372–9 [discussion: 372–9].
[32] St Peter SD, Sharp SW, Holcomb GW 3rd, et al. An evidence-based definition for perforated appendicitis derived from a prospective randomized trial. J Pediatr Surg 2008;43(12):2242–5.
[33] Ponsky TA, Huang ZJ, Kittle K, et al. Hospital- and patient-level characteristics and the risk of appendiceal rupture and negative appendectomy in children. JAMA 2004;292(16):1977–82.
[34] Morrow SE, Newman KD. Current management of appendicitis. Semin Pediatr Surg 2007;16(1):34–40.

[35] Muehlstedt SG, Pham TQ, Schmeling DJ. The management of pediatric appendicitis: a survey of North American Pediatric Surgeons. J Pediatr Surg 2004;39(6):875–9 [discussion: 875–9].
[36] Whyte C, Tran E, Lopez ME, et al. Outpatient interval appendectomy after perforated appendicitis. J Pediatr Surg 2008;43(11):1970–2.
[37] Kaminski A, Liu IL, Applebaum H, et al. Routine interval appendectomy is not justified after initial nonoperative treatment of acute appendicitis. Arch Surg 2005;140(9): 897–901.
[38] Chen C, Botelho C, Cooper A, et al. Current practice patterns in the treatment of perforated appendicitis in children. J Am Coll Surg 2003;196(2):212–21.
[39] Brown CV, Abrishami M, Muller M, et al. Appendiceal abscess: immediate operation or percutaneous drainage? Am Surg 2003;69(10):829–32.
[40] Oliak D, Yamini D, Udani VM, et al. Initial nonoperative management for periappendiceal abscess. Dis Colon Rectum 2001;44(7):936–41.
[41] Janik JS, Ein SH, Shandling B, et al. Nonsurgical management of appendiceal mass in late presenting children. J Pediatr Surg 1980;15(4):574–6.
[42] Friedell ML, Perez-Izquierdo M. Is there a role for interval appendectomy in the management of acute appendicitis? Am Surg 2000;66(12):1158–62.
[43] Yamini D, Vargas H, Bongard F, et al. Perforated appendicitis: is it truly a surgical urgency? Am Surg 1998;64(10):970–5.
[44] Henry MC, Gollin G, Islam S, et al. Matched analysis of nonoperative management vs immediate appendectomy for perforated appendicitis. J Pediatr Surg 2007;42(1):19–23 [discussion: 23–4].
[45] Weber TR, Keller MA, Bower RJ, et al. Is delayed operative treatment worth the trouble with perforated appendicitis is children? Am J Surg 2003;186(6):685–8 [discussion: 688–9].
[46] Vane DW, Fernandez N. Role of interval appendectomy in the management of complicated appendicitis in children. World J Surg 2006;30(1):51–4.
[47] Roach JP, Partrick DA, Bruny JL, et al. Complicated appendicitis in children: a clear role for drainage and delayed appendectomy. Am J Surg 2007;194(6):769–72 [discussion: 772–3].
[48] Henry MC, Walker A, Silverman BL, et al. Risk factors for the development of abdominal abscess following operation for perforated appendicitis in children: a multicenter case-control study. Arch Surg 2007;142(3):236–41 [discussion: 241].
[49] Samuel M, Hosie G, Holmes K. Prospective evaluation of nonsurgical versus surgical management of appendiceal mass. J Pediatr Surg 2002;37(6):882–6.
[50] Bufo AJ, Shah RS, Li MH, et al. Interval appendectomy for perforated appendicitis in children. J Laparoendosc Adv Surg Tech A 1998;8(4):209–14.
[51] Aprahamian CJ, Barnhart DC, Bledsoe SE, et al. Failure in the nonoperative management of pediatric ruptured appendicitis: predictors and consequences. J Pediatr Surg 2007;42(6): 934–8 [discussion: 938].
[52] Whyte C, Levin T, Harris BH. Early decisions in perforated appendicitis in children: lessons from a study of nonoperative management. J Pediatr Surg 2008;43(8):1459–63.
[53] Kogut KA, Blakely ML, Schropp KP, et al. The association of elevated percent bands on admission with failure and complications of interval appendectomy. J Pediatr Surg 2001;36(1):165–8.
[54] Gillick J, Mohanan N, Das L, et al. Laparoscopic appendectomy after conservative management of appendix mass. Pediatr Surg Int 2008;24(3):299–301.
[55] Beltran MA, Almonacid J, Vicencio A, et al. Predictive value of white blood cell count and C-reactive protein in children with appendicitis. J Pediatr Surg 2007;42(7):1208–14.
[56] Bickell NA, Aufses AH Jr, Rojas M, et al. How time affects the risk of rupture in appendicitis. J Am Coll Surg 2006;202(3):401–6.
[57] Brender JD, Marcuse EK, Koepsell TD, et al. Childhood appendicitis: factors associated with perforation. Pediatrics 1985;76(2):301–6.

[58] Lin CJ, Chen JD, Tiu CM, et al. Can ruptured appendicitis be detected preoperatively in the ED? Am J Emerg Med 2005;23(1):60–6.
[59] Nelson DS, Bateman B, Bolte RG. Appendiceal perforation in children diagnosed in a pediatric emergency department. Pediatr Emerg Care 2000;16(4):233–7.
[60] Peng YS, Lee HC, Yeung CY, et al. Clinical criteria for diagnosing perforated appendix in pediatric patients. Pediatr Emerg Care 2006;22(7):475–9.

Advances in Surgery 44 (2010) 87–100
ADVANCES IN SURGERY

Screening Criteria for Breast Cancer

Subhasis Misra, MD, Naveenraj L. Solomon, MD, Frederick L. Moffat, MD, Leonidas G. Koniaris, MD*
Division of Surgical Oncology, Department of Surgery, Sylvester Comprehensive Cancer Center, University of Miami Miller School of Medicine, 3550 SCCC (310T), 1475 NW 12th Avenue, Miami, FL 33136, USA

Breast cancer remains the most common malignancy and the second most common cause of cancer death among women in the United States. Overall, more than 99% of all breast cancers occur in women [1]. The lifetime risk for a woman developing breast cancer surviving at least until age 85 years in the United States has reportedly increased over the past 5 years to 1 in 7. In 2006, more than 200,000 new cases of breast cancer were diagnosed and there were more than 40,000 breast cancer mortalities in that same year [1].

Current breast cancer screening modalities and their strengths and limitations are discussed in this article. Identification of high-risk patients and screening recommendations for these individuals are also discussed, as are various screening approaches, established and new. The clinician involved in the screening of women for breast cancer is encouraged to develop a logical approach that may use many or select tests to better screen women for breast cancer. Awareness of patients' risk factors as well as their personal preferences and cultural values should also always be considered in approaching screening and therapy.

GENERAL CONSIDERATIONS IN INITIATING CANCER SCREENING

Overall, population-based screening and early detection are important public health measures in cancer control. Screening is particularly beneficial when the cancer affects a large portion of the population and when current therapies may leverage earlier diagnosis into improved patient cure or palliation rates. Screening implementation must strike a balance between the reduction in cancer mortality and the costs associated with screening and false-positive screening tests [2]. False-positive screening subjects patients to needless procedures and expenses, significant anxiety, and potential morbidity and mortality [3,4]. Furthermore, screening approaches are evolving as new and often more

*Corresponding author. *E-mail address:* lkoniaris@med.miami.edu.

0065-3411/10/$ – see front matter
doi:10.1016/j.yasu.2010.05.008

expensive screening modalities are introduced. The clinician may be further challenged in trying to integrate such newer screening tests into clinical practice when incompletely validated and conflicting reports exist for such newer procedures. Finally, the treating physician must also discuss the relative benefits and limitations of various approaches for patients in terms that they understand for them to be able to make an informed choice [5].

GENERAL SCREENING MODALITIES FOR BREAST CANCER AND THEIR LIMITATIONS

Effective screening methods for breast cancer have been developed and implemented, which increase the chances for patient cure and palliation [3,4]. The relatively high incidence of breast cancer makes this disease an ideal target for widespread screening. Current breast cancer screening protocols aim to optimize sensitivity and specificity while limiting overall costs and false-positive results. The rationales for breast cancer screening are that breast cancers so identified are smaller and earlier in their course, and potentially require less aggressive and deforming treatments, while prognosis improves commensurately [6–8]. Available data support the hypothesis that breast cancer screening saves lives, in contrast to lung cancer, for which the efficacy of screening remains highly controversial [9].

SCREENING APPROACHES

Breast awareness

Also known as breast self-examination (BSE), breast awareness is a long-advocated approach, although not currently recommended for screening as per National Comprehensive Cancer Network guidelines [2]. Recent data have failed to demonstrate that instructing BSE has any population-based effect on breast cancer mortality [2]. Recently the United States Preventive Services Task Force (USPSTF) recommended that clinicians should not teach women how to perform BSE [10]. Nonetheless, for individual patients breast cancer self-screening may result in earlier diagnosis that may affect individual patient outcomes. This earlier diagnosis particularly may apply in the detection of interval cancers that may arise between routine screenings. Unlike other modalities, there is no economic cost associated with BSE, and education of individuals through weekly BSE of what their breasts normally feel like and how they change with the menstrual cycle may increase the likelihood of interval detection of cancer between screenings. Frequency of BSE may be important; examining once a month may be too infrequent for negotiation of the learning curve, whereas daily examination may be inappropriate for psychological reasons. Beginning in their 20s, women should be informed of the benefits and limitations of BSE. The importance of prompt reporting of any new breast symptoms to a health care professional should be emphasized. Women who choose to do BSE should receive proper instruction and have their technique reviewed during a periodic health examination. For menstruating women, weekly BSE is a salutary compromise.

It is acceptable for women to choose whether not to do BSE or to do BSE irregularly. Women should have an opportunity to become informed about the benefits, limitations, and potential harms associated with regular screening [6]. In general most clinicians, although recognizing the difficulty of demonstrating a population-based benefit for BSE, still encourage patients to undergo BSE and to arrange an appointment should worrisome changes develop.

Clinical breast examination

Screening mammography may miss at least 10% of breast cancers [8,11]. Some of these may be detected by clinical breast examination (CBE), and this potential increase in cancer detection is the rationale for the technique's inclusion by many clinicians in breast cancer screening protocols. Nonetheless, the benefit of CBE without radiological screening remains unproven. All suspicious palpable lesions identified should be evaluated with ultrasonography (US) and biopsy, irrespective of mammographic findings [2]. US prior to biopsy is indicated to rule out simple breast cysts which, in the absence of complexity or a solid tissue component, may generally be observed.

It should be stressed that CBE with or without US, in the absence of mammography, is insufficient for screening [12]. Sensitivity of CBE in particular was estimated to be only 54% in a recent meta-analysis [13]. The USPSTF under the auspices of the Agency for Health Care Research and Quality, in fact, recommends mammography with or without CBE. There is insufficient evidence to recommend for or against CBE in breast cancer screening, and evidence of additional benefit of CBEs beyond mammography is inadequate [7,10].

However, inclusion of CBE is nonetheless recommended because it may benefit individual patients in providing earlier diagnosis of their breast cancer [7]. CBE also provides an important clinical opportunity to raise breast cancer awareness and educate patients on breast cancer–related matters, such as breast cancer symptomatology, genetic considerations, risk factors, and new cancer detection technologies [6]. For patients after mastectomy for either ductal carcinoma in situ (DCIS) or invasive breast cancer, CBE remains the main technique to determine potential recurrences [14].

Mammography: X-Ray and digital

Screening mammography is performed in asymptomatic women with the goal of detecting breast cancer that is not yet clinically evident. Screening mammography remains the main breast cancer screening tool for women. The tool has been demonstrated to reduce breast cancer mortality by 20% to 35% in women aged 50 to 69 years and slightly less in women aged 40 to 49 years, at 14 years of follow-up [15]. A recent USPSTF report recommends against routine screening mammography in women aged 40 to 49 years [10]. This report also mentions that starting regular biennial screening instead of annual screening for the age group of 50 to 75 years is more cost-effective and preserves most of the benefits of annual screening while reducing the associated harms by half [10]. These recommendations have been highly controversial, and currently are not considered by most physicians who treat breast cancer to represent the best standard of care. The American Cancer Society along with other public forums has similarly voiced significant concerns over this report.

Widespread adoption of screening mammography has also dramatically increased the number of patients diagnosed with DCIS in the past 20 years [16]. Many of these patients with DCIS represent women in their 40s diagnosed by screening mammography. It remains unclear whether DCIS detected by screening mammography follows the same natural history as DCIS presenting with a mass; exactly which patients actually benefit from the earlier diagnosis and treatment of DCIS remains uncertain [17]. Screening mammography also is somewhat limited in the detection of inflammatory breast cancer (IBC). Failure of screening mammography to determine breast cancer in the dermis may be a factor in the dire prognosis of IBC [18]. The risk from radiation exposure due to mammography in young women with an inherited cancer predisposition is unknown, and there is concern about whether this genetic factor may increase sensitivity to irradiation. The cumulative risk of breast cancer due to repeated radiation and genetic predisposition, however, may be as high as 19% by age 40 years in women with *BRCA1* mutations [19].

Mediolateral oblique and craniocaudal mammographic views of each breast are obtained. In women with augmentation mammoplasties, additional Eklund views are taken. Abnormalities or changes as compared with prior studies are pursued with additional magnification and compression views of the relevant part of the breast. US is also increasingly being used to further image potential areas of concern. Mammographic sensitivity is limited by breast density, with as many as 10% to 15% of clinically evident breast cancers having no associated mammographic abnormality [20–22].

Digital mammography is an improved imaging modality for breast screening relative to standard film-screen mammography. Digital mammography acquires images and stores them electronically, thereby allowing manipulation and enhancement to facilitate interpretation and increase sensitivity [23]. Digital mammography seems to be particularly superior to traditional film-screen mammography for detecting cancer in younger women and those with dense breasts [23].

The Breast Cancer Detection Demonstration Project (BCDDP) explicitly addressed several questions, including the effectiveness of applying research-based screening to a general population and whether identification of nonpalpable breast cancer would save lives otherwise lost to breast cancer. The BCDDP also addressed the question of whether groups of women at high risk for developing breast cancer could be defined. Mammographic screening in the BCDDP conferred an equal survival advantage to younger and older women [24]. Patients diagnosed with cancer by mammography had significantly improved survival rates compared with those diagnosed by BSE/CBE across the early stages of breast cancer. Mean survival for those undergoing BSE/CBE screening versus BSE/CBE plus mammography was 43 and 57 months, respectively [25].

Ultrasonography

The diagnostic acuity of breast US is greatest when used as an adjunct to mammography in women with significant breast density. Prevalence screening studies in women with radiographically dense breasts have reported 3 to 4 cases of breast cancer per 1000 women who were detected by US only [26–31]. US is less sensitive than magnetic resonance imaging (MRI) but has the advantage of being more widely available, considerably less expensive, and without the complications of contrast agent injection. US is useful as a secondary diagnostic tool rather than as a screening technique in that it provides additional information on whether a lesion detected by other modalities is solid or cystic. US also has the ability to determine contour and internal echogenicities of a lesion as well as its vascularity [20–22]. Recent improvements in breast ultrasound technology have aided in the distinction of benign from malignant abnormalities using this modality [27].

Breast US has numerous limitations as a screening tool. It is an operator-dependent imaging modality that requires specialty training for technologists and radiologists to interpret the results, which varies greatly between professionals and institutions. Other concerns include the lack of standardized examination techniques and interpretation criteria. There are further limitations regarding the inability of breast US to detect microcalcifications, variability in available equipment with respect to clarity and resolution, and preliminary data suggesting a substantially higher false-positive rate than mammography [26,29,30]. Nonetheless, there are several studies supporting the use of US for breast cancer screening as an adjunct to mammography for high-risk women or women with dense breast tissue [32].

Magnetic resonance imaging

MRI is increasingly being used to evaluate breast abnormalities, but its application, more than any other imaging modality in breast cancer, remains controversial for its high false-positive rate and high costs. Breast MRI breast imaging does appear to be of clear value in identifying primary breast cancer in patients with malignant axillary nodes but with no palpable or mammographic evidence of a breast neoplasm. MRI may also be more accurate than mammography in assessing the extent of the primary tumor, particularly in young women with dense breast tissue. The technique may be helpful in diagnosing invasive lobular cancer and may elucidate patient eligibility for breast conservation [33]. MRI has a role in early detection of malignancy in younger patients with *BRCA* gene mutations who choose not to have prophylactic bilateral mastectomy. The sensitivity of MRI for invasive cancer is more than 90% but only 60% or less for DCIS. Because of the high false-positive rate, the specificity of MRI is commensurately low [33].

The use of MRI for breast cancer screening remains highly controversial and, in any case, is not recommended as a breast cancer screening tool for the general population [2]. Numerous breast cancer–specific algorithms for interpretation of MRI have been instituted, which may provide better sensitivity and specificity. Examples of such improved protocols include the Rotating Delivery of Excitation Off-Resonance Protocol. The current consensus is that current evidence does not support the routine use of breast MRI as a screening procedure in average-risk women. Furthermore, a recent study emphasized that there is little evidence for routine preoperative use of MRI in women who already have a diagnosis of breast cancer on one side to effectively screen for the presence of cancer in the contralateral side [34].

Nonetheless, MRI may be beneficial in select patients. There is a demonstrated role for the use of breast MRI screening as an adjunct to mammography for high-risk women if any of these criteria are met (Table 1):

- Have a *BRCA1* or *BRCA2* mutation
- Have a first-degree relative with a *BRCA1* or *BRCA2* mutation and are untested
- Have a lifetime risk of breast cancer of 20% to 25% or more as defined by models that are largely dependent on family history
- Have received radiation treatment to the chest between 10 and 30 years of age
- Carry or have a first-degree relative who carries a genetic mutation in the *TP53* or *PTEN* genes (Li-Fraumeni, Cowden, and Bannayan-Riley-Ruvalcaba syndromes) [35].

The use of MRI in breast screening is also constrained by its cost. At present, the average cost for bilateral screening mammography is $50, whereas the cost for bilateral MRI is $965 [36]. Although breast MRI may provide benefits

Table 1
Recommendations for breast MRI screening as an adjunct to mammography

Recommend Annual MRI Screening (Based on Evidence[a])
BRCA mutation
First-degree relative of *BRCA* carrier, but untested
Lifetime risk of ~20%–25% or greater, as defined by BRCAPRO or other models that are largely dependent on family history
Recommend Annual MRI Screening (Based on Expert Consensus Opinion[b])
Irradiation to chest between 10 and 30 years of age
Li-Fraumeni syndrome and first-degree relatives
Cowden and Bannayan-Riley-Ruvalcaba syndromes and first-degree relatives
Insufficient evidence to recommend for or against MRI screening[c]
Lifetime risk of 15%–20%, as defined by BRCAPRO or other models that are largely dependent on family history
Lobular carcinoma in situ or atypical lobular hyperplasia
Atypical ductal hyperplasia
Heterogeneously or extremely dense breast on mammography
Women with a personal history of breast cancer, including DCIS
Recommend Against MRI Screening (Based on Expert Consensus Opinion)
Women at <15% lifetime risk

[a]Evidence from nonrandomized screening trials and observational studies.
[b]Based on evidence of lifetime risk for breast cancer.
[c]Payment should not be a barrier. Screening decisions should be made on a case-by-case basis, as there may be particular factors to support MRI.
Data from caonline.amcancersoc.org. Accessed July 8, 2009, © American Cancer Society, Inc.

compared with screening mammography in certain high-risk individuals, it does not appear to be cost-effective even at willingness-to-pay thresholds of more than $120,000 per quality-adjusted life-year [36].

Role of Positron Emission Tomography

Positron emission tomography (PET) scans create computerized images of glucose uptake in tissue and are increasingly applied in the staging for various malignancies [37]. PET scans are better at detecting large and more aggressive tumors than at locating tumors that are smaller than 8 mm and/or more indolent. Nonetheless, PET may be falsely positive in a large number of patients and thus is not considered a screening test. PET scans may play a role in determining whether a breast mass is cancerous when other imaging techniques show normal results. The high rate of false-positive results with PET is clinically problematic. PET scans certainly are helpful in staging patients after the initial diagnosis of cancer and in the setting of potential recurrent disease [37]. A National Cancer Institute–sponsored clinical trial is evaluating the usefulness of PET scan results in women who have breast cancer as compared with the findings from other imaging and diagnostic techniques [37]. Current evidence does not support the routine use of PET scans as a screening procedure to detect breast cancer.

Computer-Aided Detection

Computer-aided detection (CAD) involves the use of computers to bring suspicious areas on a mammogram to the radiologist's attention. The technique is used after the radiologist has done the initial review of the mammogram.

In 1998, the Food and Drug Administration (FDA) approved the first breast-imaging device that used CAD technology. An example of a breast-imaging device that uses CAD technology is the ImageChecker (R2 Technology, Sunnyvale, CA, USA) This device scans the mammogram with a laser beam and converts it into a digital signal that is processed by a computer. The image is then displayed on a video monitor, with suspicious areas highlighted for the radiologist to review. The radiologist can compare the digital image with the conventional mammogram to see if any of the highlighted areas were missed on the initial review and require further evaluation. CAD technology may improve the accuracy of screening mammography. The incorporation of CAD technology into digital mammography continues to be under evaluation and remains unproven [37].

Electrical impedance scanning

Electrical impedance is a measurement of how fast electricity travels through a given material. Different types of tissue have different electrical impedance levels. Some types of tissue have high electrical impedance whereas others have low electrical impedance. Breast tissue that is cancerous has a lower electrical impedance (conducts electricity much better) than normal breast tissue; hence, breast tumors may appear as bright white spots on the computer screen [37]. Electrical impedance scanning devices are used along with conventional mammography to detect breast cancer. The T-Scan 2000 (TransScan, Ramsey, NJ, USA), also known as the T-Scan, is an example of such a device that was approved by the FDA in 1999. These devices do not emit any radiation, and may improve the specificity of breast cancer detection by reducing the number of biopsies needed to determine whether a mass is cancerous [37].

Electrical impedance scanning is not approved as a screening device for breast cancer and is not used when mammography or other findings clearly indicate the need for a biopsy. This device has not been studied with patients who have implanted electronic devices, such as pacemakers, and is not recommended for use on such patients [37].

Miscellaneous

Current evidence does not support the routine use of breast scintigraphy (eg, sestamibi scan) or ductal lavage as a screening procedure [2].

RISK ASSESSMENT

Overall, the lifetime risk for the development of breast cancer in women may vary considerably. As the risk for the development of breast cancer increases, additional screening tests may be beneficial for a specific patient. To better determine the breast cancer risk in individual patients, several risk models have been developed. The 2 most frequently used models for breast cancer risk assessment are the Gail model and the Claus model. The Gail model was developed from case-control data in the BCDDP by Gail and colleagues [38]. These investigators determined that age, race, age at menarche, age at first live birth, number of previous breast biopsies, presence of proliferative disease with atypia, and number of first-degree female relatives with breast cancer influence the risk for breast cancer [38]. This model is available for clinical use at http://cancer.gov/bcrisktool or at http://brca.nci.nih.gov/brc. The Gail model does not include detailed information about genetic factors, and may underestimate the risk for a *BRCA1* or *BRCA2* mutation carrier and overestimate the risk in a noncarrier [33]. Furthermore, because the Gail model was derived from studies of upper middle class white women in Chicago, there are real limitations with respect to generalizability beyond this demographic [39].

Another risk-adjustment model developed by Claus and colleagues [40] is based on assumptions about the prevalence of high-penetrance breast cancer susceptibility genes. This model provides individual estimates of breast cancer risk by the decade of life, based on the knowledge of first- and second-degree relatives with breast cancer and their age at diagnosis. The Claus model includes more information about family history than the Gail model, but excludes other risk factors mentioned earlier [39,40].

RISK CLASSIFICATION

Women are classified into 2 basic groups for screening recommendations: those at normal risk and those at increased risk. The increased risk category currently consists of 5 groups: (1) women who have previously received therapeutic thoracic irradiation or mantle irradiation, (2) women aged 35 years or older with a 5-year risk of invasive breast carcinoma greater than or equal to 1.7% (Gail model), (3) women with a strong family history or genetic predisposition, (4) women with high-risk breast histologies (lobular carcinoma in situ or atypical ductal hyperplasia, atypical lobular hyperplasia, sclerosing papillary lesions, radial scars), and (5) women with a prior history of breast cancer [2].

SCREENING RECOMMENDATIONS BASED ON PATIENT BREAST CANCER RISK

For women at average risk, current recommendations are to begin mammography between 40 and 50 years of age. For women before that age, it is generally recommended that CBE be part of a periodic health examination, preferably at least every 3 years. Asymptomatic women aged 40 years and older should continue to receive a CBE as part of a periodic health examination, preferably annually [2].

With the exception of women with a strong family history/genetic predisposition, the current recommendations for all high-risk groups include CBE every 6 to 12 months, annual mammography, and periodic BSE beginning at age 25 years. Patients with prior thoracic irradiation should start this process 10 years after irradiation or at 40 years of age, whichever is earlier [2]. Strong family history includes breast cancer before 40 years of age, multiple cases of breast cancer in the same individual or close maternal and paternal relatives, a family member with a known mutation in a breast cancer susceptibility gene, or a cluster of breast cancer with other cancers indicating Li-Fraumeni syndrome or Cowden syndrome [41].

SCREENING FOR PATIENTS WITH A STRONG FAMILY HISTORY OR GENETIC PREDISPOSITION FOR BREAST CANCER

Genetic predisposition for hereditary breast and ovarian cancer

Obtain CBEs every 6 to 12 months and annual mammograms beginning at age 25 years.

Strong family history or other genetic predisposition for breast cancer

For women 25 years or older, (1) performing CBE every 6 to 12 months and annual mammograms starting 5 to 10 years prior to the youngest breast cancer case in the family is required, (2) periodic BSE is encouraged, and (3) annual MRI may also be recommended as an adjunct to mammogram and CBE, as mentioned earlier.

For women younger than 25 years, obtaining annual CBE and periodic BSE is recommended, and risk reduction strategies, including genetic counseling, regular exercise, limitation of alcohol consumption, and proper weight control are also advisable [42].

INTERPRETATION OF SCREENING MAMMOGRAPHY

In 1993, The American College of Radiology [43] developed the Breast Imaging Reporting and Data System (BI-RADS) to standardize mammographic reporting, improve communication, reduce confusion regarding mammographic findings, aid research, and facilitate outcomes monitoring. Ninety-five percent of all breast calcifications seen on mammography, whether macro or micro, are benign. Although there are 7 assessment categories in BI-RADS, only 4 outcomes are possible: (1) routine interval mammography, (2) additional imaging studies, (3) short-term follow-up, and (4) biopsy (Table 2) [44]. The positive predictive value for malignancy increases from 2% for BI-RADS category 3 mammograms to 23% to 30% for category 4 mammograms, and as high as 95% for category 5 mammograms [45,46].

CONDITIONS THAT MAY MIMIC BREAST CANCER

There are groups of benign breast pathology that can mimic cancer on clinical examination. These conditions include, but are not limited to, fat necrosis, sclerosing adenosis, and mammary duct ectasia/plasma cell mastitis. Fat necrosis of the breast is a benign inflammatory process that is common in obese, usually middle-aged women with fatty, pendulous breasts, and frequently occurs in a superficial or periareolar portion of the breast. The most common causes of fat necrosis are surgery (biopsy, lumpectomy, reduction mammoplasty, implant removal, breast reconstruction), radiation therapy, and trauma [47]. Sclerosing adenosis also is frequently confused with cancer. Both fat necrosis and sclerosing adenosis can be definitively diagnosed by core needle biopsy. Mammary duct ectasia/plasma cell mastitis is associated with obstruction of the lactiferous duct and can manifest as nipple retraction, inversion, bloody discharge, and pain. On histologic examination, dilation of the mammary ducts and periductal fibrosis are seen.

SCREENING IN THE POSTSURGICAL BREAST

Women who have had total, modified radical, or radical mastectomy for breast cancer need no further routine screening mammograms of the affected side. However, a subcutaneous mastectomy does require follow-up with

Table 2
BI-RADS classification of breast imaging

BI-RADS class	Findings	Action	Risk of malignancy
0	Incomplete examination	Additional imaging	
1	Normal	Routine screening	
2	Benign finding	Routine screening	
3	Probably benign finding	Repeat imaging in 6 months	<2%
4	Suspicious abnormality	Biopsy recommended	Widely variable
5	Highly suggestive of malignancy	Biopsy recommended	>95%
6	Known biopsy-proven malignancy		

mammography [48]. Post mastectomy, if the breast was reconstructed with silicon or saline implants, mammography is not needed. With tissue reconstruction, such as transverse rectus abdominis myocutaneous flap reconstruction, further imaging may be necessary if there is concern after physical examination [48].

The presence of radio-opaque implants interferes with the sensitivity of screening mammography [14,49]. Techniques that displace the implants posteriorly (Eklund views) improve the sensitivity, but at least a third of the breast is still not visualized, leading to an increase in the rate of false-negative mammograms [49]. New radiolucent implants have been developed to increase the sensitivity of mammography, but these are still under evaluation [50]. Physical examination continues to be crucial in the detection of palpable masses in the reconstructed breast [14]. As compared with the nonaugmented breast, tumors of equivalent size are more easily palpated in the augmented breast, and this tends to offset to some degree the decreased sensitivity of mammography [51]. US may be useful in screening augmented women without risk of rupturing the implant. In appropriate cases, MRI should be considered as an adjunct to mammography and US [14].

SCREENING IN ELDERLY WOMEN

Screening decisions in older women should be individualized by the potential benefits and risks of mammography in the context of current health status and estimated life expectancy. One should also consider severe comorbid conditions limiting life expectancy and whether therapeutic interventions are planned. As long as a woman is in reasonably good health and would be a candidate for treatment, she should continue to be screened with mammography. An upper age limit for screening is not yet established [2]. The USPSTF reports that there is insufficient evidence to assess additional benefits or harms of screening mammography in women 75 years or older [10].

DISPARITIES AND SCREENING

There has been renewed interest in the disparity of outcomes in breast cancer with race and socioeconomic status. It is well documented in the literature that African American patients present with breast cancer at younger ages and with more aggressive tumors [52–55]. Although breast cancer is more common in white than in African American women, among patients younger than 45 years, breast cancer is more common in African Americans. In addition, 12.5% of African American women diagnosed with breast cancer are 40 years or younger, and 24.1% of breast cancers in African American patients present before 45 years of age. Earlier breast cancer presentation among African American patients is accompanied by more aggressive tumor characteristics and advanced stage.

One possible target for improvement of breast cancer outcomes in African American women would be to revise current screening guidelines by lowering the age of initial screening in African American women to 33 years if initial screening for the general population remains at 40 years of age. It is at age 33 that the incidence of breast cancer among African American women is similar to the incidence of breast cancer in white women at 40 years of age. How a cost-effective screening program should be implemented needs to be examined, but the program might include digital mammography and/or US [56].

SUMMARY

Breast cancer screening constitutes an integral part of surgical practice for many surgeons and is an important tool in the war against breast cancer. Among many modalities, mammography plays a central role, with MRI now being increasingly used for women with high risk for breast cancer. Current guidelines for screening are in the process of evolution as more scientific knowledge is gained. The challenge lies in developing cost-effective methods to reach the maximum number of the population at risk.

References

[1] Jemal A, Siegel R, Ward E, et al. Cancer statistics, 2006. CA Cancer J Clin 2006;56(2): 106–30.

[2] Bevers TB, Anderson BO, Bonaccio E, et al. Breast cancer screening and diagnosis. NCCN clinical practice guidelines in oncology. V.1.2009.

[3] Berry DA, Cronin KA, Plevritis SK, et al. Effect of screening and adjuvant therapy on mortality from breast cancer. N Engl J Med 2005;353(17):1784–92.

[4] Tabar L, Vitak B, Chen HH, et al. Beyond randomized controlled trials: organized mammographic screening substantially reduces breast carcinoma mortality. Cancer 2001;91(9): 1724–31.

[5] Housri N, Weil RJ, Shalowitz DI, et al. Should informed consent for cancer treatment include a discussion about hospital outcome disparities? PLoS Med 2008;5(10):e214.

[6] Smith RA, Saslow D, Sawyer KA, et al. American Cancer Society guidelines for breast cancer screening: update 2003. CA Cancer J Clin 2003;53(3):141–69.

[7] Humphrey LL, Helfand M, Chan BK, et al. Breast cancer screening: a summary of the evidence for the U.S. Preventive Services Task Force. Ann Intern Med 2002; 137(5 Part 1):347–60.

[8] Seidman H, Gelb SK, Silverberg E, et al. Survival experience in the Breast Cancer Detection Demonstration Project. CA Cancer J Clin 1987;37(5):258–90.

[9] Calonge N, Berg AO, Allan JD, et al. Lung cancer screening: recommendation statement. Ann Intern Med 2004;140(9):738–9.

[10] US Preventive Services Task Force. Screening for breast cancer: U.S. preventive services task force recommendation statement. Ann Intern Med 2009;151(10): 716–26, W-236.

[11] Shapiro S, Venet W, Strax P, et al. Periodic screening for breast cancer the Health Insurance Plan Project and its sequelae, 1963–86. Baltimore (MD): The Johns Hopkins University Press; 1988.

[12] USPST Force. Screening for breast cancer: recommendations and rationale. Ann Intern Med 2002;137(5):3.

[13] Barton MB, Harris R, Fletcher SW. The rational clinical examination. Does this patient have breast cancer? The screening clinical breast examination: should it be done? How? JAMA 1999;282(13):1270–80.

[14] Uematsu T. Screening and diagnosis of breast cancer in augmented women. Breast Cancer 2008;15(2):159–64.

[15] Elmore JG, Armstrong K, Lehman CD, et al. Screening for breast cancer. JAMA 2005;293(10):1245–56.
[16] Sumner WE 3rd, Koniaris LG, Snell SE, et al. Results of 23,810 cases of ductal carcinoma-in-situ. Ann Surg Oncol 2007;14(5):1638–43.
[17] Nakhlis F, Morrow M. Ductal carcinoma in situ. Surg Clin North Am 2003;83(4):821–39.
[18] Yang R, Cheung MC, Hurley J, et al. A comprehensive evaluation of outcomes for inflammatory breast cancer. Breast Cancer Res Treat 2009;117(3):631–41.
[19] Burke W, Daly M, Garber J, et al. Recommendations for follow-up care of individuals with an inherited predisposition to cancer. II. BRCA1 and BRCA2. Cancer Genetics Studies Consortium. JAMA 1997;277(12):997–1003.
[20] Stefanick ML, Anderson GL, Margolis KL, et al. Effects of conjugated equine estrogens on breast cancer and mammography screening in postmenopausal women with hysterectomy. JAMA 2006;295(14):1647–57.
[21] Powles TJ. Anti-oestrogenic prevention of breast cancer—the make or break point. Nat Rev Cancer 2002;2:787–94.
[22] Hartmann LC, Schaid DJ, Woods JE, et al. Efficacy of bilateral prophylactic mastectomy in women with a family history of breast cancer. N Engl J Med 1999;340(2):77–84.
[23] Pisano ED, Gatsonis CA, Yaffe MJ, et al. American College of Radiology Imaging Network digital mammographic imaging screening trial: objectives and methodology. Radiology 2005;236(2):404–12.
[24] Cunningham MP. The Breast Cancer Detection Demonstration Project 25 years later. CA Cancer J Clin 1997;47(3):131–3.
[25] Misra S, Tarr S, Pratt D. Comparison of various breast cancer detection methods with survival rates. J Clin Oncol 2007;25(18S):17033.
[26] Gordon PB. Ultrasound for breast cancer screening and staging. Radiol Clin North Am 2002;40(3):431–41.
[27] Stavros AT, Thickman D, Rapp CL, et al. Solid breast nodules: use of sonography to distinguish between benign and malignant lesions. Radiology 1995;196(1):123–34.
[28] Gordon PB, Goldenberg SL. Malignant breast masses detected only by ultrasound. A retrospective review. Cancer 1995;76(4):626–30.
[29] Kolb TM, Lichy J, Newhouse JH. Occult cancer in women with dense breasts: detection with screening US—diagnostic yield and tumor characteristics. Radiology 1998;207(1):191–9.
[30] Buchberger W, DeKoekkoek-Doll P, Springer P, et al. Incidental findings on sonography of the breast: clinical significance and diagnostic workup. AJR Am J Roentgenol 1999;173(4):921–7.
[31] Kolb TM, Lichy J, Newhouse JH. Comparison of the performance of screening mammography, physical examination, and breast US and evaluation of factors that influence them: an analysis of 27,825 patient evaluations. Radiology 2002;225(1):165–75.
[32] Berg WA, Blume JD, Cormack JB, et al. Combined screening with ultrasound and mammography vs mammography alone in women at elevated risk of breast cancer. JAMA 2008;299(18):2151–63.
[33] Townsend CM Jr, Beauchamp RD, Evers BM, et al. Diseases of the breast. Sabiston textbook of surgery. Philadelphia: Saunders Elsevier; 2007.
[34] Houssami N, Hayes DF. Review of preoperative magnetic resonance imaging (MRI) in breast cancer: should MRI be performed on all women with newly diagnosed, early stage breast cancer? CA Cancer J Clin 2009;59(5):290–302.
[35] Saslow D, Boetes C, Burke W, et al. American Cancer Society guidelines for breast screening with MRI as an adjunct to mammography. CA Cancer J Clin 2007;57(2):75–89.
[36] Moore SG, Shenoy PJ, Fanucchi L, et al. Cost-effectiveness of MRI compared to mammography for breast cancer screening in a high risk population. BMC Health Serv Res 2009;9:9.
[37] Institute NC. Improving methods for breast cancer detection and diagnosis. 2002.

[38] Gail MH, Brinton LA, Byar DP, et al. Projecting individualized probabilities of developing breast cancer for white females who are being examined annually. J Natl Cancer Inst 1989;81(24):1879–86.
[39] Domchek SM, Eisen A, Calzone K, et al. Application of breast cancer risk prediction models in clinical practice. J Clin Oncol 2003;21(4):593–601.
[40] Claus EB, Risch N, Thompson WD. Autosomal dominant inheritance of early-onset breast cancer. Implications for risk prediction. Cancer 1994;73(3):643–51.
[41] Daly MB, Axilbund JE, Bryant E, et al. Genetic/familial high-risk assessment: breast and ovarian. NCCN clinical practice guidelines in oncology. V.1.2009.
[42] Bevers TB, Armstrong D, Arun B, et al. Breast cancer risk reduction. NCCN clinical practice guidelines in oncology. V.2.2009.
[43] American College of Radiology. The ACR breast imaging reporting and data system (BI-RADS) [web source]. Available at: http://www.acr.org/departments/stand_accred/birads/contents.html; November 11, 2003; Accessed September 9, 2009.
[44] Liberman L, Menell JH. Breast imaging reporting and data system (BI-RADS). Radiol Clin North Am 2002;40(3):409–30, v.
[45] Lacquement MA, Mitchell D, Hollingsworth AB. Positive predictive value of the breast imaging reporting and data system. J Am Coll Surg 1999;189(1):34–40.
[46] Orel SG, Kay N, Reynolds C, et al. BI-RADS categorization as a predictor of malignancy. Radiology 1999;211(3):845–50.
[47] Cyrlak D, Carpenter PM. Breast imaging case of the day. Fat necrosis of the breast. Radiographics 1999;19(Spec No):S80–3.
[48] American Cancer Society. Mammograms and other breast imaging procedures [web source]. September 30, 2009. Available at: http://www.cancer.org/docroot/cri/content/cri_2_6x_mammography_and_other_breast_imaging_procedures_5.asp. 2009 Accessed October 20, 2009.
[49] Handel N, Silverstein MJ, Gamagami P, et al. Factors affecting mammographic visualization of the breast after augmentation mammaplasty. JAMA 1992;268(14):1913–7.
[50] Monstrey S, Christophe A, Delanghe J, et al. What exactly was wrong with the Trilucent breast implants? A unifying hypothesis. Plast Reconstr Surg 2004;113(3):847–56.
[51] Handel N, Gutierrez J. Long-term safety and efficacy of polyurethane foam-covered breast implants. Aesthet Surg J 2006;26(3):265–74.
[52] Joslyn SA. Racial differences in treatment and survival from early-stage breast carcinoma. Cancer 2002;95(8):1759–66.
[53] Eley JW, Hill HA, Chen VW, et al. Racial differences in survival from breast cancer. Results of the National Cancer Institute Black/White Cancer Survival Study. JAMA 1994;272(12):947–54.
[54] Elmore JG, Moceri VM, Carter D, et al. Breast carcinoma tumor characteristics in black and white women. Cancer 1998;83(12):2509–15.
[55] Furberg H, Millikan R, Dressler L, et al. Tumor characteristics in African American and white women. Breast Cancer Res Treat 2001;68(1):33–43.
[56] Yang R, Cheung MC, Franceschi D, et al. African-American and low-socioeconomic status patients have a worse prognosis for invasive ductal and lobular breast carcinoma: do screening criteria need to change? J Am Coll Surg 2009;208(5):853–68 [discussion: 869–70].

Advances in Surgery 44 (2010) 101–116

ADVANCES IN SURGERY

Laparoscopic and Thoracoscopic Esophagectomy

Ryan M. Levy, MD, Joseph Wizorek, MD, Manisha Shende, MD, James D. Luketich, MD*

Department of Surgery, Division of Thoracic and Foregut Surgery, Heart, Lung and Esophageal Surgery Institute, University of Pittsburgh, 200 Lothrop Street Suite C-800, Pittsburgh, PA 15213, USA

During the past decade, minimally invasive approaches to esophagectomy have emerged as safe, technically feasible alternatives to open esophageal resection. There has been a significant evolution in technique since the initial descriptions of hybrid approaches using thoracoscopic esophageal mobilization with a laparotomy [1–4]. Although technically demanding and associated with a significant operator learning curve, totally minimally invasive esophagectomy (MIE) has been shown to be a viable option for esophageal resection while reducing blood loss, length of hospital stay, and narcotic requirements [5–9]. In our experience, a minimally invasive approach reduces postoperative pain and pulmonary complications while comparing favorably with the best published open series with regard to morbidity, mortality, and oncologic outcomes [10]. At present, minimally invasive techniques include laparoscopic transhiatal, laparoscopic-thoracoscopic 3-hole (McKeown), and laparoscopic-thoracoscopic (Ivor Lewis) esophagectomy. Each of these can be performed with lymph node sampling or a more complete lymph node dissection. Although the choice between approaches is, to a large degree, based on surgeon preference, the operative approach is at times dictated by anatomic location of the tumor margins. For example, a midthoracic esophageal tumor or long segment of Barrett's esophagus may require a more proximal resection margin and mandate a cervical anastomosis, whereas a gastroesophageal (GE) junction tumor extending onto the gastric cardia might limit conduit length and thus require an intrathoracic anastomosis. The choice of operative approach also impacts postoperative morbidity depending on which body cavities are entered. Specifically, approaches that include a cervical anastomosis have been shown to have a higher incidence of anastomotic stricture, leak, recurrent nerve injury, and pharyngoesophageal swallowing dysfunction [6,11–13]. In comparison, transthoracic approaches

*Corresponding author. *E-mail address:* luketichjd@upmc.edu.

0065-3411/10/$ – see front matter
doi:10.1016/j.yasu.2010.05.002

have an increased incidence of cardiopulmonary complications and more morbid consequences when an anastomotic leak does occur [14].

Emerging data suggest that the number of lymph nodes sampled at operation has important prognostic and treatment implications. It is also clear that to obtain a more aggressive resection with complete 2-field lymph node dissection, the operation must include thoracic exposure via an Ivor Lewis or McKeown modification [15–18]. A trend toward improved 5-year survival has been observed in specific subsets of patients with more locally advanced cancers treated with an Ivor Lewis approach [19,20]. In addition, local recurrence rates have been reported in the low single digit numbers with complete lymph node dissections using a thoracic approach compared with local recurrence rates upwards of 40% with transhiatal operations [21–23]. However, it should be emphasized that no randomized trial has shown significant survival or mortality differences between transhiatal and transthoracic esophageal resection.

We have previously reported on our extensive experience with MIE using a 3-field technique [10,24]. In those publications, we demonstrated that MIE could be performed safely with stage-specific survival that was equivalent to previously published open series [25,26]. However, in light of the concerns delineated previously regarding cervical dissection and anastomosis, our preferred approach is now a completely laparoscopic-thoracoscopic (Ivor Lewis) esophagectomy with complete lymph node dissection for typical GE junction tumors. The minimally invasive Ivor Lewis approach works well for most distal esophageal cancers, short-to-moderate length Barrett's with high-grade dysplasia, and gastroesophageal junction tumors extending onto the gastric cardia. In addition, in situations in which there exists concern for the length of the gastric conduit, an intrathoracic anastomosis is preferable. In more extreme cases of cardia extension, we prefer a total gastrectomy and roux Y reconstruction. Total laparoscopic and thoracoscopic Ivor Lewis resections should not be performed for upper third or mid-esophageal cancers with significant proximal extension because of concern for adequate margins of resection. Herein, we describe our current operative technique and present some early results and insights we have attained.

SURGICAL TECHNIQUE

Our initial step in performing total laparoscopic and thoracoscopic esophagectomy is an on-table esophagogastroduodenoscopy (EGD) following intubation with a double-lumen endotracheal tube. EGD is important to confirm the anatomic location and extent of pathology, as well as ensuring suitability of the gastric conduit.

Laparoscopic phase

We perform the laparoscopic portion of the procedure first. The patient is positioned supine in a steep reverse Trendelenburg position with a footboard in place. The surgeon stands on the patient's right, the assistant on the left. Five abdominal trocars (four 5 mm and one 10 mm) are then placed as depicted in Fig. 1. Initially, we place the 10-mm port via a cut-down technique approximately 3 cm to the right of the junction between the lower and middle third of a line connecting the xiphoid and umbilicus. Carbon dioxide insufflation is used for pneumoperitoneum to a pressure of 15 mm Hg. The remaining four 5-mm ports are then placed: 5 cm to the left of the operating port (30° camera port), subcostally on the right and left midclavicular lines (tissue grasper ports), and in the right flank (liver retractor port).

A thorough staging procedure is then performed to evaluate for occult metastatic disease. If satisfactory, we then proceed with gastric mobilization. The gastrohepatic ligament (lesser omentum) is first divided and the right and left crura of the diaphragm are dissected. Care is taken not to divide the phrenoesophageal membrane at this point so as to prevent loss of pneumoperitoneum into the chest cavity. The greater curvature of the stomach is then mobilized by first dividing the short gastric vessels, followed by division of the gastrocolic omentum while carefully preserving the right gastroepiploic arcade (Fig. 2). Recently, on the basis of published data and personal communication (Dr Earle Wilkins, personal communication, 2008), we have started using an omental pedicle wrap of the intrathoracic esophagogastric anastamosis [27]. It is at this point in the operation that

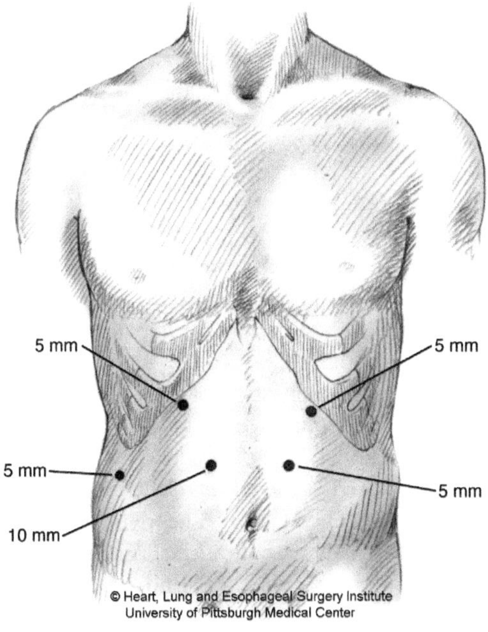

Fig. 1. Laparoscopic port placement for MIE.

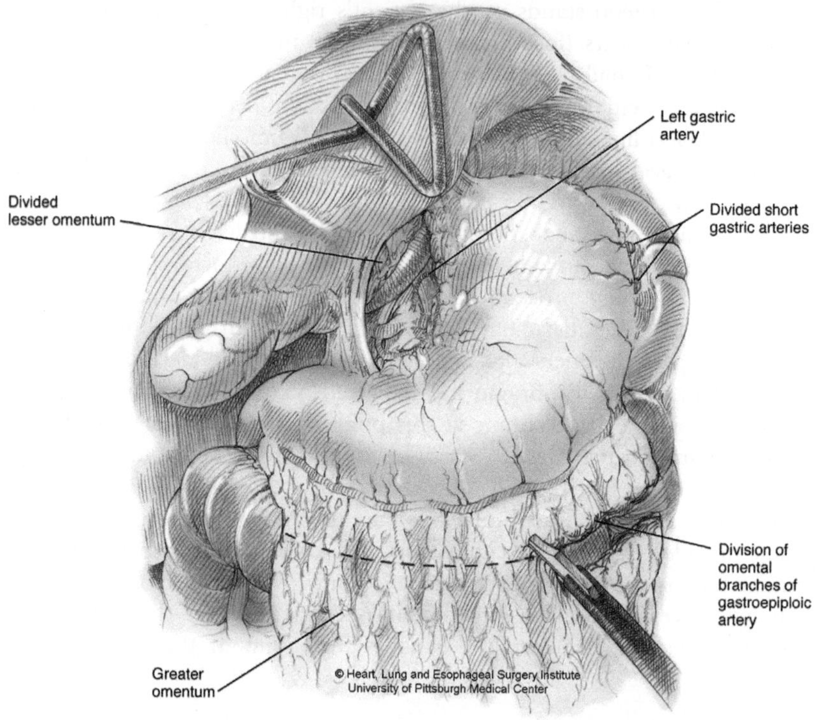

Fig. 2. Gastric mobilization.

we mobilize a long, narrow tongue of omentum from the mid-to-upper third of the greater curvature. We attempt to base this omental pedicle off of 2 feeding vessels to ensure viability (Fig. 3). The mobilized stomach is retracted superiorly, and any remaining adhesions between the posterior wall of the stomach and the pancreas are divided as well. The left gastric vessels are then identified, dissected, and divided with a vascular load of the stapler. Before division, a complete celiac lymph node dissection is performed, continuing along the superior border of the splenic artery and pancreas toward the splenic hilum.

Attention is then turned to mobilization of the pyloric-antral area and subsequent pyloroplasty (Fig. 4). Adequate mobilization is evident when the pylorus can be gently lifted up to the level of the right crus in a tension-free manner. Two traction sutures are placed at the edges of the pylorus with the Endostitch (2-0, US Surgical, Norwalk, CT, USA). The pyloroplasty is performed by incising the pylorus longitudinally with the ultrasonic shears, and closing it transversely with interrupted sutures using the Endostitch device in a Heineke-Mikulicz fashion. A 4-cm diameter gastric conduit is then constructed using multiple fires of the stapler (4.8 mm) beginning from the lesser curve antral area, just proximal to the pylorus and heading toward the angle of His (Fig. 5).

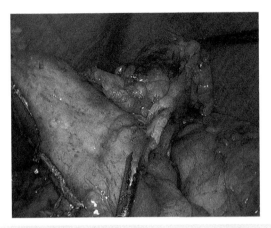

Fig. 3. Creation of omental pedicle flap.

It is essential to avoid excessive manipulation and resulting trauma to the gastric conduit during all steps. To facilitate exposure, staple alignment, and adequate conduit length during this step, we have found it helpful to have the assistant grasp the greater curve of the stomach, along the line of the proximal short gastric arteries and retract gently toward the spleen, while simultaneously another assistant grasps the antrum and retract inferiorly. This essentially elongates the entire stomach and provides the alignment necessary to construct a consistent diameter gastric conduit. The tip of the gastric conduit is then secured to the specimen with 2 Endostitches (Fig. 6). During this step, care is taken to maintain alignment so that subsequent retrieval of the specimen through the hiatus into the chest does not lead to any rotation and maintains perfect anatomic alignment of the gastric

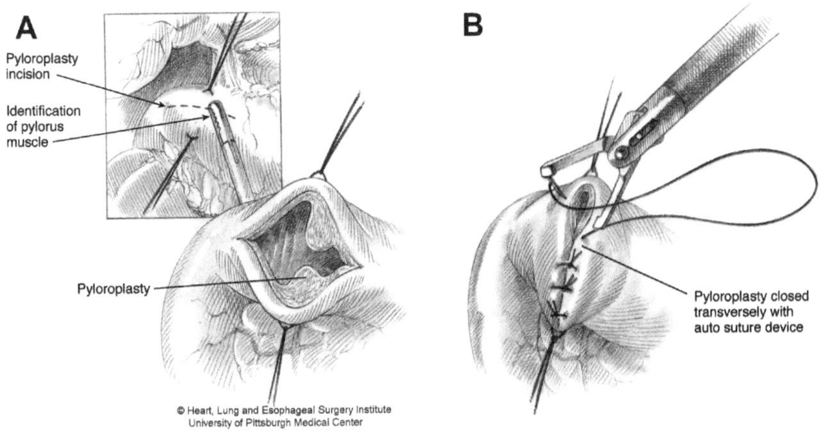

Fig. 4. (*A, B*) Laparoscopic pyloroplasty.

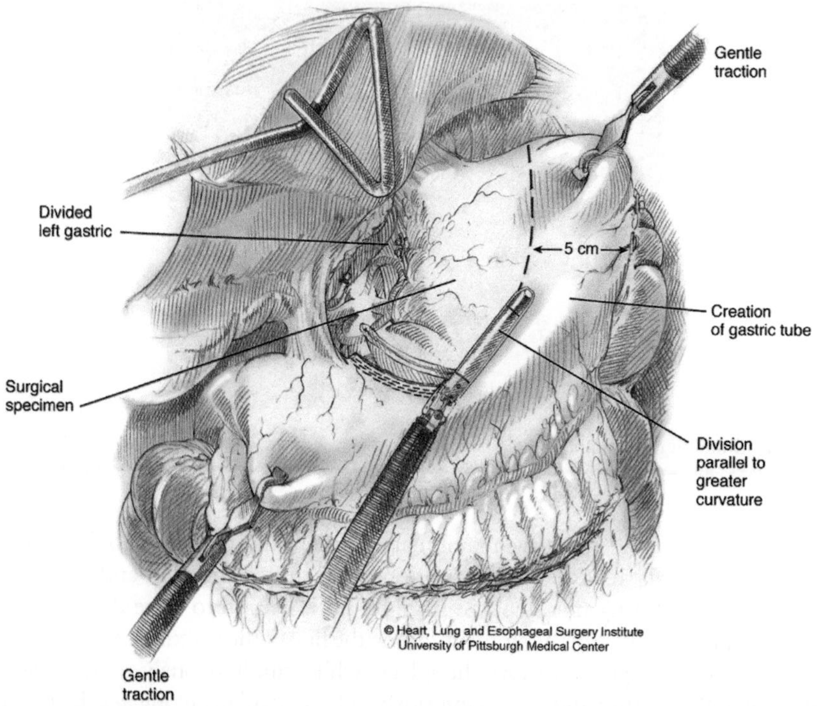

Fig. 5. Creation of gastric conduit.

conduit, with the short gastrics facing the direction of the spleen and the lesser curve staple line facing the right chest. With our recent use of omental pedicles, we have also started tacking the omental pedicle wrap to the proximal end of the conduit so as to facilitate bringing it through the hiatus without trauma to the omentum or the supplying vasculature.

A feeding jejunostomy is placed next, as depicted in Fig. 7. The patient is placed in the Trendelenburg position with the transverse colon and greater omentum retracted cranially. The ligament of Treitz is identified and approximately 30-cm distal to this point, a suitable limb of proximal jejunum is tacked to the lateral, anterior abdominal wall in the left mid-quadrant with a single 2-0 Endostitch. We often place an additional 10-mm port in the right lower quadrant to facilitate this maneuver. Under direct visualization, a needle jejunostomy catheter (Compat Biosystems, Minneapolis MN, USA) is then placed, with intraluminal position confirmed by distending the jejunum with 10 mL air insufflated via the catheter. The jejunum is then securely tacked to the abdominal wall at the catheter entry site over a distance of a few centimeters with interrupted 2-0 Endostitches. One of these sutures should be at least 3 cm distal to the catheter insertion site so as to prevent torsion and possible strangulation around a single fixed point (Fig. 8). The

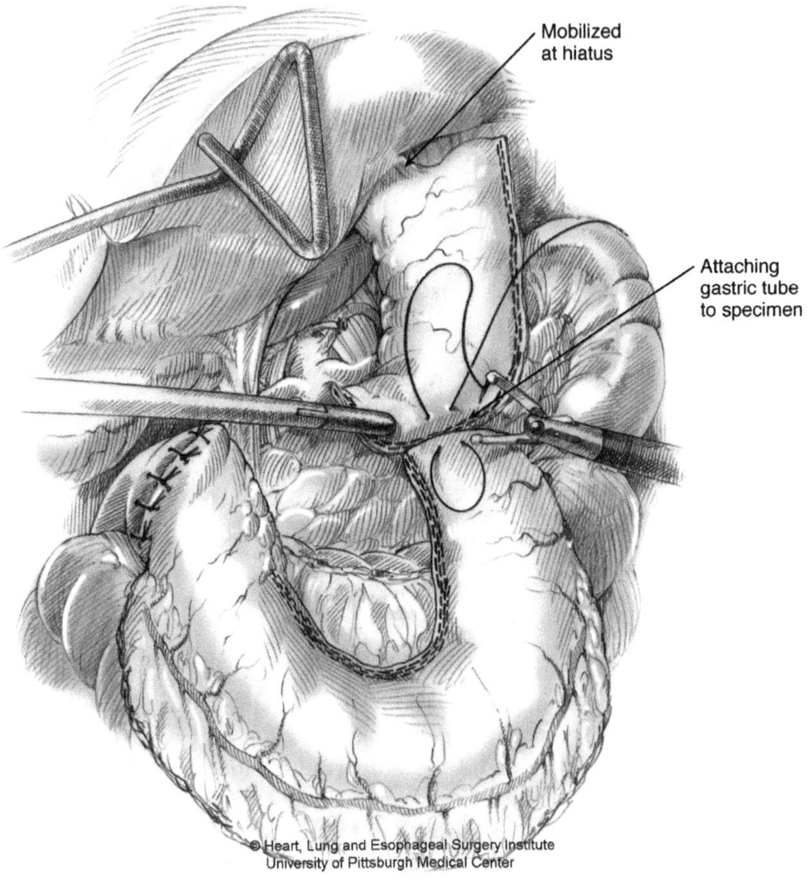

Fig. 6. Completed schematic of gastric conduit sutured to specimen.

final step in the laparoscopic stage of the operation is division of the phrenoesophageal membrane with partial division of the right and left crura. This allows for circumferential mobilization of the distal esophagus. A Penrose drain may be passed around the distal esophagus to aid in retraction during the thoracic portion of the procedure. Before leaving the abdomen, we add an omental patch to the pyloroplasty. Also in most cases of GE junction tumors, there is a hiatal hernia, so we add one or two 0-Surgidac sutures to approximate the right and left crus to minimize the size of the hiatal defect to approximate the size of the relatively narrow gastric conduit, and minimize the likelihood of a delayed hiatal hernia [28].

Thoracoscopic phase

After completion of the laparoscopic abdominal stage, the patient is repositioned in a left lateral decubitus position. Four thoracoscopic ports are then

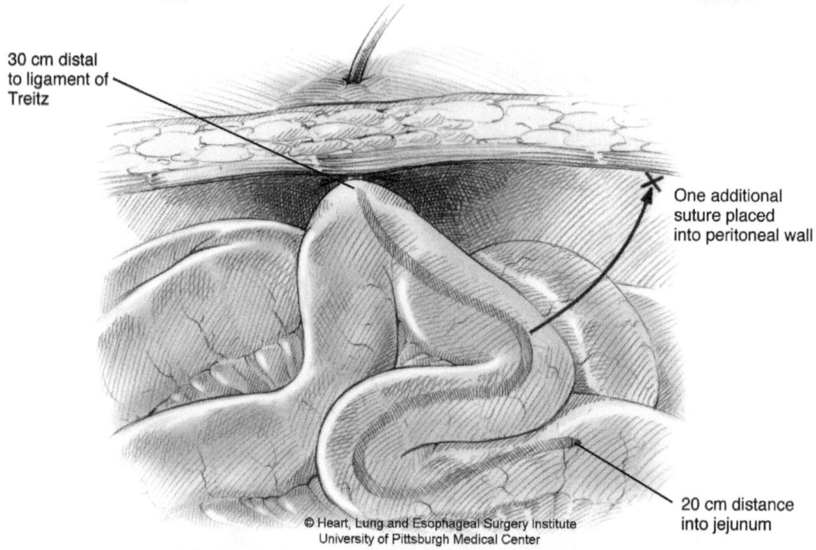

Fig. 7. Needle jejunostomy feeding tube.

introduced as follows: 10-mm port in the seventh intercostal space, mid-axillary line (camera port); a 10-mm port in the eighth intercostal space 2 cm posterior to the posterior axillary line (ultrasonic shears working port); a 5-mm port posterior to the scapular tip; and a 10-mm port in the fourth intercostal space at the anterior axillary line for retraction during the esophageal dissection (Fig. 9). Generally, we add a small 5-mm port anteriorly to allow a second assistant to pass a suction-irrigator to maintain a clean operating field. Ultimately, the

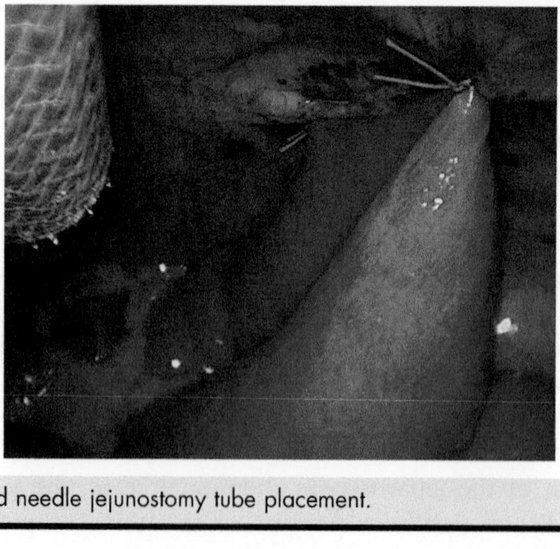

Fig. 8. Completed needle jejunostomy tube placement.

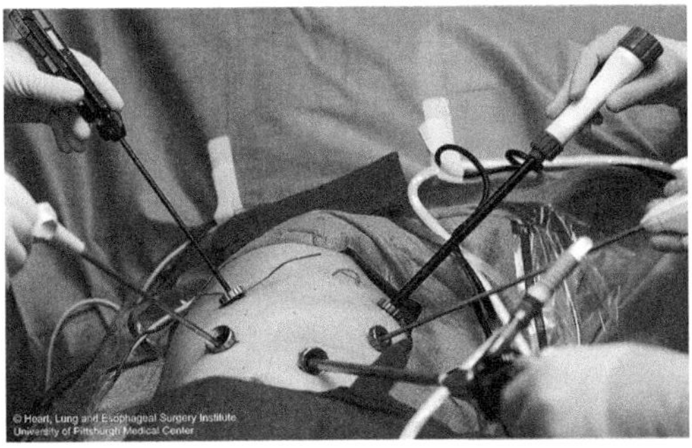

Fig. 9. Thoracoscopic port placement for MIE.

eighth posterior interspace port will be enlarged to 5 cm to enable passage of the end-to-end stapler (EEA, US Surgical, Norwalk, CT, USA) and removal of the specimen. An important maneuver at the beginning of the thoracoscopic phase is placement of an 0-silk stitch into the central tendon of the diaphragm using the Endostitch. The suture is brought out through a 2-mm stab incision in the skin at the lowest anterior part of the costophrenic angle. Traction on this suture pulls the diaphragm inferiorly and improves visualization of the esophageal hiatus.

Mobilization of the esophagus is begun by dividing the inferior pulmonary ligament and retracting the lung anterolaterally. This facilitates incision of the mediastinal pleura over the esophagus. Dissection moves in a cranial direction from this point posterior to the inferior pulmonary vein, and along the line of the mediastinal pleura connection to the lung. The esophagus and accompanying periesophageal tissue and lymph nodes are mobilized circumferentially en bloc toward the right mainstem bronchus and carina. We use the ultrasonic shears for much of the dissection, as the sharp blade of this instrument is ideal for a precise dissection plane. Endoscopic clips are used for hemostasis on larger vessels. Because of the extensive lymphatics in this area and fragile vessels attached to the subcarinal nodes, careful use of endoclips also aids in minimizing oozing of chyle and blood. The azygous vein is mobilized and divided as it overlies the esophagus posteriorly with a vascular staple load. The esophagus is then mobilized circumferentially from the hiatus to near the thoracic inlet, the ultimate cephalad extent depends on the proximal extent of the tumor or Barrett's and the length and condition of the gastric conduit. It should be noted that the plane of dissection should stay directly on the esophagus above the azygous vein so as to prevent injury to the posterior membranous trachea and recurrent laryngeal nerve. We do not perform an aggressive lymph node dissection in the area of the recurrent nerves. The distal esophagus and previously constructed gastric conduit are then brought up through the hiatus into the chest (Fig. 10). The proximal esophagus is then transected above the azygous vein with an Endo GIA stapler (US Surgical). Again, the precise

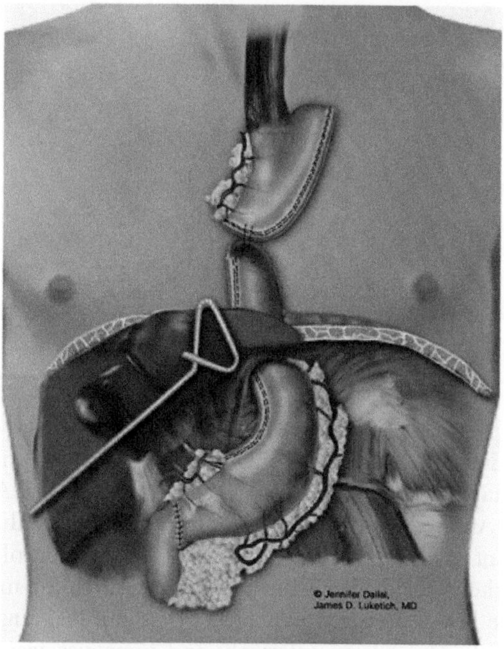

Fig. 10. Delivery of specimen and gastric conduit into the chest.

location of this division and ultimate location of the anastomosis tends to be high, near the thoracic inlet; however, cutting the esophagus too proximal may make the anastomosis technically difficult and should be avoided. In the case of concern over tumor margin, we may rescope at this point to precisely determine where to transect the esophagus. The specimen is then sent for frozen section analysis of the esophageal and gastric margins. The eighth interspace port site is enlarged and a wound protector (Applied Medical, Rancho Santa Margarita, CA, USA) placed for specimen removal after cutting the previously placed sutures that secured the conduit to the specimen.

Attention is then directed to the intrathoracic esophagogastric anastomosis. A 28-mm EEA anvil is placed into the proximal divided esophagus through the eighth interspace incision and secured in a purse string fashion using the 2.0 Endostitch. It is technically difficult to make the first stitch perfect, as the anvil wants to migrate out of the open esophagus during suturing. Thus, a second stitch is always added to ensure perfect subsequent complete rings following EEA firing. The EEA stapler is then introduced through the eighth interspace incision into the tip of the gastric conduit via a gastrotomy at the apex of the conduit. This is technically challenging for most trainees, and care must be taken to carefully angle the gastric tube facing straight up to accept the tip of the EEA device aimed straight down, much the same way one angles the tip of your foot as you pull on your sock. A circular anastomosis is then created in an end- (proximal esophagus) to-side (gastric conduit) fashion above the level of the azygous vein (Fig. 11). Gastrotomy closure and the redundant portion of the gastric conduit is removed with a reticulating Endo GIA stapler (Fig. 12). We have recently starting wrapping a tongue of omentum mobilized from the greater curve of the stomach around the anastamosis, securing in place with several 2-0 Surgidac Endostitches (Fig. 13). It is important to ensure that the conduit is not twisted in the process of wrapping the omentum around the anastamosis. The chest is drained with a 28-F chest tube placed posteriorly but not on the anastomosis and a number 10 Jackson Pratt drain placed directly posteriorly to the anastomosis and tracked behind the gastric conduit, down to the diaphragmatic hiatus, across the dome of the diaphragm and out through a small stab incision near the costrophrenic angle. A nasogastric tube is placed across the anastomosis under direct vision. To prevent herniation, the conduit is tacked to the right crus with several interrupted 2.0 Endostitches.

RESULTS

Outside of case reports, there are currently few series reporting experience with laparoscopic/thoracoscopic Ivor Lewis esophagectomy [29,30]. Kunisaki and colleagues [31] described a small series of laparoscopic and thoracoscopic Ivor Lewis esophagectomies (n = 15), but the anastomotic leak rate was somewhat high (13.3%) and length of stay was prolonged (30 days). We recently reported the largest series of minimally invasive Ivor Lewis esophagectomies (n = 50) published to date [32]. Of these, the first 35 included a hybrid

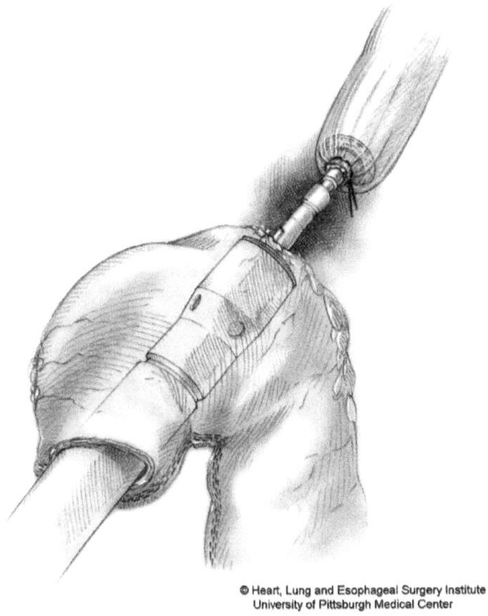
© Heart, Lung and Esophageal Surgery Institute
University of Pittsburgh Medical Center

Fig. 11. Thoracoscopic creation of esophago-gastric anastomosis with EEA stapler.

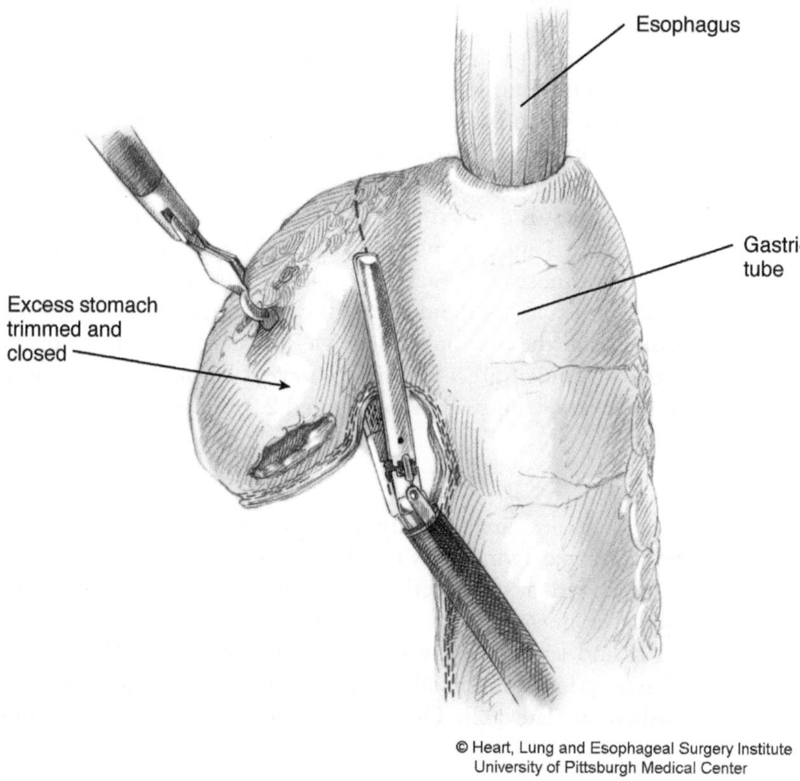

Fig. 12. Resection and closure of gastrotomy.

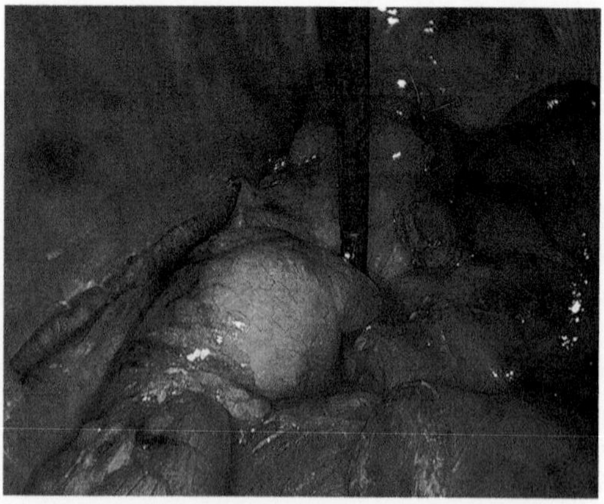

Fig. 13. Completed anastomosis with omental pedicle wrap.

approach with a planned mini-thoracotomy. The last 15 patients in this series were performed with a completely laparoscopic-thoracoscopic method without need for minithoracotomy. The median length of stay was 9 days for the entire group, with the completely minimally invasive group having a significantly shorter hospitalization (7 days vs 9 days). The median ICU stay was 1 day for both groups. Anastomotic leak rate was 6%. All pneumonias (10%) occurred in the hybrid minithoracotomy group. Importantly, there were no recurrent nerve injuries.

SUMMARY

Over the past decade, our technique of MIE has evolved considerably. In the incipient phase of our experience, we used a totally laparoscopic approach similar to that described in the initial reports from DePaula and colleagues [33] and Swanstrom and Hansen [34]. However, it was soon apparent that there were several critical disadvantages to a purely laparoscopic approach. Laparoscopic transhiatal mobilization of the esophagus offers suboptimal visualization of important periesophageal structures, including the inferior pulmonary vein and the left mainstem bronchus. Moreover, decreased visibility hindered hemostatic division of periesophageal vessels and negatively impacted the completeness of the mediastinal lymph node dissection. These problems are further exacerbated in taller patients.

In light of these considerations, we soon transitioned to a laparoscopic-thoracoscopic McKeown approach (thoracoscopic mobilization of the intrathoracic esophagus, laparoscopic gastric tube creation, cervical anastomosis). To this date, the great majority of our minimally invasive esophagectomies (>500 cases) have been performed with this 3-field technique. Indeed, the procedure has been the mainstay of our experience in the past 10 years with reduced perioperative morbidity and mortality compared with many other open series [10]. In our experience, perhaps the most significant technical concern with this operation is the cervical dissection. Recurrent laryngeal nerve injuries, perturbations in pharyngeal transit, and swallowing dysfunction even in the absence of recurrent nerve injury are not infrequent. Moreover, as described in open series using a cervical anastomosis, anastomotic stricture and leak have been shown to occur with increased frequency [35]. In short, there is a significant learning curve with the cervical dissection. Out of these concerns emerged our more recent experience with completely thoracoscopic-laparoscopic Ivor Lewis esophagectomy. However, we did first evolve through a transition phase whereby a mini-thoracotomy (hybrid approach) was performed for creation of the intrathoracic anastomosis.

We believe that the experience with totally thoracoscopic-laparoscopic Ivor Lewis esophagectomy will ultimately reproduce the low morbidity and mortality we have previously published with our established MIE technique. The omission of a cervical dissection has reduced our recurrent nerve injury rate to zero. From a theoretical standpoint, one would presume that pharyngeal transit problems and oropharyngeal swallowing dysfunction should be reduced as well with a chest anastomosis. It should be emphasized that there is a steep operator learning curve associated with this approach. Indeed, thoracoscopic port placement is critical, as poorly positioned trocars can result in difficulty maneuvering instruments through the rigid chest wall. Additionally, both blood and lung can obscure visualization of the esophagus, which lies at the dependent aspect of the operative field. Prone positioning has been described as an alternative approach that may facilitate operative exposure and address such technical concerns. Low rates of anastomotic leak (3%), low mortality (1.5%), and equivalent stage-specific survival compared with open series have been shown with this thoracoscopic prone approach [36].

In conclusion, our technique of MIE has evolved such that laparoscopic-thoracoscopic Ivor Lewis esophagectomy has become our preferred approach. Although somewhat early in our experience, we are convinced that this operative technique is feasible with reproducible results. Perioperative morbidity and mortality are comparable with our previously established MIE with cervical anastomosis while essentially eliminating recurrent nerve injury, limiting the length of the gastric conduit required, and allowing a more aggressive gastric resection margin. Recent data from other publications also suggests that lymph node yields may be improved, although insufficient data exist at this time to comment on oncologic results or outcomes with this technique.

References

[1] McAnena OJ, Rogers J, Williams NS. Right thoracoscopically assisted oesophagectomy for cancer. Br J Surg 1994;81(2):236–8.

[2] Collard JM, Lengele B, Otte JB, et al. En bloc and standard esophagectomies by thoracoscopy. Ann Thorac Surg 1993;56(3):675–9.

[3] Peracchia A, Rosati R, Fumagalli U, et al. Thoracoscopic esophagectomy: are there benefits? Semin Surg Oncol 1997;13(4):259–62.

[4] Cuschieri A. Endoscopic subtotal oesophagectomy for cancer using the right thoracoscopic approach. Surg Oncol 1993;2(Suppl 1):3–11.

[5] Law S, Wong J. Use of minimally invasive oesophagectomy for cancer of the oesophagus. Lancet Oncol 2002;3(4):215–22.

[6] Atkins BZ, Shah AS, Hutcheson KA, et al. Reducing hospital morbidity and mortality following esophagectomy. Ann Thorac Surg 2004;78(4):1170–6 [discussion: 1170–6].

[7] Law S, Wong KH, Kwok KF, et al. Predictive factors for postoperative pulmonary complications and mortality after esophagectomy for cancer. Ann Surg 2004;240(5):791–800.

[8] Bailey SH, Bull DA, Harpole DH, et al. Outcomes after esophagectomy: a ten-year prospective cohort. Ann Thorac Surg 2003;75(1):217–22 [discussion: 222].

[9] Narumiya K, Nakamura T, Ide H, et al. Comparison of extended esophagectomy through mini-thoracotomy/laparotomy with conventional thoracotomy/laparotomy for esophageal cancer. Jpn J Thorac Cardiovasc Surg 2005;53(8):413–9.

[10] Luketich JD, Alvelo-Rivera M, Buenaventura PO, et al. Minimally invasive esophagectomy: outcomes in 222 patients. Ann Surg 2003;238(4):486–94 [discussion: 494–5].

[11] Hulscher JB, Tijssen JG, Obertop H, et al. Transthoracic versus transhiatal resection for carcinoma of the esophagus: a meta-analysis. Ann Thorac Surg Jul 2001;72(1):306–13.

[12] Martin RE, Letsos P, Taves DH, et al. Oropharyngeal dysphagia in esophageal cancer before and after transhiatal esophagectomy. Dysphagia 2001;16(1):23–31.

[13] Easterling CS, Bousamra M 2nd, Lang IM, et al. Pharyngeal dysphagia in postesophagectomy patients: correlation with deglutitive biomechanics. Ann Thorac Surg 2000;69(4): 989–92.
[14] Hulscher JB, van Sandick JW, de Boer AG, et al. Extended transthoracic resection compared with limited transhiatal resection for adenocarcinoma of the esophagus. N Engl J Med 2002;347(21):1662–9.
[15] Greenstein AJ, Litle VR, Swanson SJ, et al. Effect of the number of lymph nodes sampled on postoperative survival of lymph node-negative esophageal cancer. Cancer 2008;112(6): 1239–46.
[16] Altorki NK, Zhou XK, Stiles B, et al. Total number of resected lymph nodes predicts survival in esophageal cancer. Ann Surg 2008;248(2):221–6.
[17] Veeramachaneni NK, Zoole JB, Decker PA, et al. Lymph node analysis in esophageal resection: American College of Surgeons Oncology Group Z0060 trial. Ann Thorac Surg 2008;86(2):418–21 [discussion: 421].
[18] Wolff CS, Castillo SF, Larson DR, et al. Ivor Lewis approach is superior to transhiatal approach in retrieval of lymph nodes at esophagectomy. Dis Esophagus 2008;21(4): 328–33.
[19] Rizzetto C, DeMeester SR, Hagen JA, et al. En bloc esophagectomy reduces local recurrence and improves survival compared with transhiatal resection after neoadjuvant therapy for esophageal adenocarcinoma. J Thorac Cardiovasc Surg 2008;135(6): 1228–36.
[20] Omloo JM, Lagarde SM, Hulscher JB, et al. Extended transthoracic resection compared with limited transhiatal resection for adenocarcinoma of the mid/distal esophagus: five-year survival of a randomized clinical trial. Ann Surg 2007;246(6):992–1000 [discussion: 1000–1].
[21] Lerut T, Coosemans W, Decker G, et al. Extended surgery for cancer of the esophagus and gastroesophageal junction. J Surg Res 2004;117(1):58–63.
[22] Lagarde SM, Reitsma JB, Ten Kate FJ, et al. Predicting individual survival after potentially curative esophagectomy for adenocarcinoma of the esophagus or gastroesophageal junction. Ann Surg 2008;248(6):1006–13.
[23] Schuchert MJ, Luketich JD, Landreneau RJ, et al. Minimally-invasive esophagomyotomy in 200 consecutive patients: factors influencing postoperative outcomes. Ann Thorac Surg 2008;85(5):1729–34.
[24] Luketich JD, Schauer PR, Christie NA, et al. Minimally invasive esophagectomy. Ann Thorac Surg 2000;70(3):906–11 [discussion: 911–2].
[25] Kent MS, Schuchert M, Fernando H, et al. Minimally invasive esophagectomy: state of the art. Dis Esophagus 2006;19(3):137–45.
[26] Nguyen NT, Roberts P, Follette DM, et al. Thoracoscopic and laparoscopic esophagectomy for benign and malignant disease: lessons learned from 46 consecutive procedures. J Am Coll Surg 2003;197(6):902–13.
[27] Bhat MA, Dar MA, Lone GN, et al. Use of pedicled omentum in esophagogastric anastomosis for prevention of anastomotic leak. Ann Thorac Surg 2006;82(5):1857–62.
[28] Kent MS, Luketich JD, Tsai W, et al. Revisional surgery after esophagectomy: an analysis of 43 patients. Ann Thorac Surg 2008;86(3):975–83 [discussion: 967–74].
[29] Watson DI, Davies N, Jamieson GG. Totally endoscopic Ivor Lewis esophagectomy. Surg Endosc 1999;13(3):293–7.
[30] Nguyen NT, Follette DM, Lemoine PH, et al. Minimally invasive Ivor Lewis esophagectomy. Ann Thorac Surg 2001;72(2):593–6.
[31] Kunisaki C, Hatori S, Imada T, et al. Video-assisted thoracoscopic esophagectomy with a voice-controlled robot: the AESOP system. Surg Laparosc Endosc Percutan Tech 2004;14(6):323–7.
[32] Bizekis C, Kent MS, Luketich JD, et al. Initial experience with minimally invasive Ivor Lewis esophagectomy. Ann Thorac Surg 2006;82(2):402–6 [discussion: 406–7].

[33] DePaula AL, Hashiba K, Ferreira EA, et al. Laparoscopic transhiatal esophagectomy with esophagogastroplasty. Surg Laparosc Endosc 1995;5(1):1–5.

[34] Swanstrom LL, Hansen P. Laparoscopic total esophagectomy. Arch Surg 1997;132(9): 943–7 [discussion: 947–9].

[35] Rizk NP, Bach PB, Schrag D, et al. The impact of complications on outcomes after resection for esophageal and gastroesophageal junction carcinoma. J Am Coll Surg 2004;198(1): 42–50.

[36] Palanivelu C, Prakash A, Senthilkumar R, et al. Minimally invasive esophagectomy: thoracoscopic mobilization of the esophagus and mediastinal lymphadenectomy in prone position—experience of 130 patients. J Am Coll Surg 2006;203(1):7–16.

Advances in Surgery 44 (2010) 117–130

ADVANCES IN SURGERY

Biomedical and Health Informatics for Surgery

Genevieve B. Melton, MD, MA

Department of Surgery, Institute for Health Informatics, 420 South East Delaware Street, Mayo Medical Code 450, Minneapolis, MN 55405, USA

Biomedical and health informatics is a growing discipline focused on the science of information and its use for the improvement of health care and biomedicine. Although the largest focus of informatics to date has been the application of electronic health records (EHR) systems and other health information technology (HIT) in clinical care, informatics uses other techniques to effectively use biomedical and health information beyond the computer, including algorithms, devices, system redesign, and other artifacts (ie, items or things) that assist with health care processes. Moreover, technology alone is not the goal; rather, informatics seeks to use information principles to synergize with care providers so that better clinical care can be provided [1].

Because health care and the use of its information is inherently complex, informatics is multidisciplinary and pulls from a wide range of areas, including computer science, sociology, statistics, industrial engineering, biomedical engineering, human factors research, and other fields [2]. It is also important to distinguish biomedical and health informatics from bioinformatics, which applies informatics approaches to information in basic biomedical research. In addition, work in translational informatics has been expanding rapidly; this related discipline seeks to transform discoveries from biomedical research to clinical care or from clinical care to the population level [3]. Table 1 contains some of the common terms and abbreviations used in biomedical and health informatics.

The application of biomedical and health informatics to surgery will be essential to advancing modern surgical practice. In particular, informatics has far-reaching implications with respect to patient care throughout the spectrum of surgical practice, including preoperative, perioperative, and postoperative settings. Additional areas in surgery in which informatics can assist and inform surgeons include operative simulation technologies, surgical education, optimization of scheduling and other operating room resources, intraoperative decision making, and surgical research.

At present, several mandates in the United States have substantially increased resources devoted to HIT and universal adoption of EHR systems,

E-mail address: gmelton@umn.edu.

0065-3411/10/$ – see front matter
doi:10.1016/j.yasu.2010.05.015

Table 1
Common terms used in biomedical and health informatics

Term (Abbreviation)	Definition
Informatics	Science of information encompassing artificial intelligence, cognitive science, computer science, information science, and social science with multiple field applications (eg, health informatics, bioinformatics, legal informatics)
Bioinformatics	Application of informatics to biology. Example research areas include sequence analysis, genome annotation, computational biology, and protein structure
Biomedical and health informatics	Informatics applied to clinical care (including medicine, nursing, dentistry), public health, translational medicine (bringing biomedical discoveries to bedside), and clinical research
Health Information Technology (HIT)	Use of information technology in health care. Commonly includes E and PHRs, alerts and reminders, decision-support systems, and other technologies for clinical, financial, and administrative information in health care
Electronic Health Record (EHR)	A medical record or other information relating to the physical and mental health, or condition of a patient, which resides in computers for the primary purpose of providing health care and health-related services
Personal Health Record (PHR)	An electronic application through which individuals can maintain and manage their health information (and that of others for whom they are authorized) in a private, secure, and confidential environment
Computerized Provider Order Entry (CPOE)	A computer application that allows for orders (such as medication prescribing, laboratory tests, nursing care orders, and other tests) to be entered electronically
Controlled medical vocabularies (CMV)	Standards for accurate data definitions, data representation, and content. Various CMV are commonly used including SNOMED-CT and LOINC. The UMLS is a compendium of biomedical CMV maintained by the NLM
Decision Support Systems (DSS)	A system that assists in applying new information to patient care. Many of these systems include computer-based programs that analyze information entered by the clinician
Health Information Exchange (HIE)	Electronic movement of health-related information among organizations according to nationally recognized standards

Abbreviations: LOINC, Logical Observation Identifier Names and Codes; NLM, National Library of Medicine; SNOMED-CT, Systemized Nomenclature of Medicine—Clinical Terms; UMLS, Unified Medical Language System.

including initiatives through the Institute of Medicine [4], the new Office of the National Coordinator for Health Information Technology within the Department of Health and Human Services [5], and the Stimulus Bill (American Recovery and Reinvestment Act of 2009) which contains the key legislative piece pertaining to health information technology entitled the *Health Information Technology for Economic and Clinical Health* Act (HITECH Act) [6]. These developments have focused efforts on key functionalities of the EHR and the idea of "meaningful use" for EHR systems in the form of incentives and penalties to individual clinicians and institutions. Significant monetary investments in HIT alone, however, will not be enough to allow for positive changes to occur within health care. Substantial progress continues to be needed in standards development, health care delivery redesign, and data interoperability.

Historically there have been a paucity of surgeon stakeholders in informatics. This problem is particularly important because changes within the health care system and HIT are occurring with greater rapidity. A larger emphasis on the unique issues with informatics and surgery can potentially help maximize the benefit of these investments on surgical care.

INFORMATICS PRINCIPLES IN CLINICAL CARE

Biomedical and health informatics focuses on methods for effectively using the large amounts of data and information required to improve clinical practice, research, and quality. As clinical care becomes more complex, the potential for "information overload" and cognitive errors increases (Fig. 1) [7,8]. As illustrated graphically in Fig. 1, when minimal information is available, information improves understanding and comprehension. However, beyond a certain threshold amount of information, overload occurs and confusion increases.

Informatics can help clinicians manage information overload by assisting them in various ways such as giving focus to important pieces of information, adding important functionality such as summarization and attention to new pieces of information, and improving the presentation of data through the use of better HIT system interface design. Systems that provide information and prompt clinicians electronically are termed decision support systems (DSS). One aspect of care in which DSS have been used extensively are inpatient and ambulatory drug-prescribing systems, often referred to as Computerized Provider Order Entry (CPOE) [9], which often have alerting functionality for potential adverse drug events, drug interactions, and other prescribing suggestions for clinicians.

Although the "primary use" of patient information is for direct clinical care, "secondary use" of data for research, administrative, and other functions has

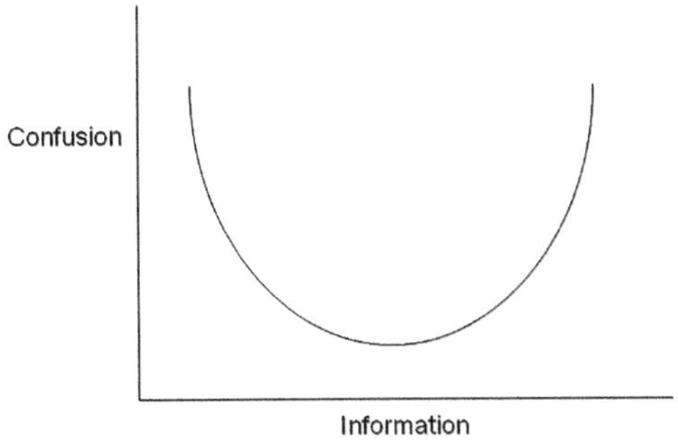

Fig. 1. Relationship of information quantity and confusion. *From* Hagy J. Needles and haystacks and such. Available at: http://thisisindexed.com/2009/10/needles-andhaystacks-and-such/; 2009. With permission.

important implications for quality care improvements. An example of secondary data use would be systems and technologies that use EHR patient data to automatically populate research databases and generate business intelligence metrics for health care administrators. This process allows for tasks to be computerized, thereby decreasing the need for manual extraction and summarization of data, which is typically error-prone and resource intensive. It also can potentially allow for comparative effectiveness research into therapeutic and diagnostic modalities.

INFORMATICS TO SUPPORT SURGEONS

An essential factor in the development of informatics tools to effectively support surgical practice is for HIT developers to create systems that function well within the workflow of surgeons. Surgical practice, whether general surgery or a subspecialty practice, has unique elements. One distinction of surgical care is that unlike primary care, internal medicine, and hospitalist practices, surgical procedures are often the central component of the therapeutic encounter. In addition, surgeons practice in various care settings with ambulatory and inpatient phases of care, including the operating room, clinic, and hospital settings.

Surgery also encompasses multiple organ systems (from general surgery to subspecialty practice), patient groups, practice types (solo, private-practice, academic), and locations (rural, community, tertiary-care, academic). Multiple modalities of information are also commonly used in the care of the surgical patient, not limited to radiological studies, pathologic studies, laboratory investigations, medication therapies, surgical and other interventions (including bedside interventions), and subspecialty consultations. Moreover, the process of operating requires several important and poorly defined skills and information resources, including intraoperative decision making with application of surgical principles, an understanding of anatomy in relation to a procedure and a patient's pathology, and technical skill.

Certain surgical disciplines also conduct a significant amount of ambulatory and medical management. For instance, otolaryngologists manage many medical conditions of the aerodigestive tract, just as colon and rectal surgery practices include medical proctology. Tailoring EHR systems to the information needs of surgical subspecialty care is one of the important challenges that must be met for these systems to have maximal effectiveness when care for a particular condition can be highly protocolized.

Informatics can help surgeons make use of best practices, clinical pathways, and guidelines, and facilitate the acquisition of information "just in time" to support surgeons in practice. The concept of "just-in-time" information is particularly important in a climate of increasing patient complexity and workloads, changes in resident and medical student training and hour restrictions, information resources (which are often not well integrated), and care teams with multiple team members (ie, surgeon, residents and students, nurses, physical therapists, other medical teams, and others).

INFORMATION NEEDS FOR THE SPECTRUM OF SURGICAL CARE

Information needs in the preoperative setting

Diagnosis and treatment in the preoperative care of patients ranges from straightforward, such as a young healthy patient with a symptomatic inguinal hernia, to complex, in the presence of significant comorbidities, diagnostic complexity, or other treatment workup. For instance, the management of morbidly obese patients prior to bariatric surgery requires the involvement of multiple subspecialists, diagnostic tests, and other eligibility requirements. Also, patients with considerable comorbidities, such as significant heart or liver disease, often have increased operative risk. These patients may require multiple diagnostic and therapeutic measures, as well as involvement of specialists, in the preoperative phases of care. Surgical interventions will sometimes need to be tailored, taking into account these comorbidities and other clinical factors.

Analogous systems in primary care have been developed that tailor and coordinate information gaps in the care of elderly patients with multiple comorbidities [10]. These systems aim to improve this complex collaborative care process and assign increased resources to coordinate the care of these patients. Other systems developed allow for monitoring and care of patients with chronic medical diseases, such as diabetes mellitus, hypertension, and heart disease. In a parallel and analogous fashion, the preoperative phase of care could be enhanced with EHR system redesign and coordination of preoperative surgical care processes for patients with more critical needs.

The development of informatics tools that streamline preoperative surgical care to address specific disease-centric, procedure-centric, and patient-centric needs will be the key to effective management in the preoperative setting. For instance, the preoperative phase of care for renal transplant candidates includes certain standard tests for all candidates ("disease-centric"), possible diagnostic studies to assess anatomic issues such as vascular anatomy to determine the correct surgical approach ("procedure-centric"), and individualized preoperative tests for a patient with multiple comorbidities ("patient-centric").

Moreover, as in the case of renal transplantation, surgical care can often require multidisciplinary participation or opinions from large teams with collaborative decision making. In another example, a patient that has a resectable mass in the head of the pancreas with portal vein involvement might require opinions and care from radiation or medical oncologists, interventional or diagnostic radiologists, pathologists, a hepatobiliary surgeon or surgical oncologist (for consideration of performing a pancreaticoduodenectomy), and a vascular surgeon (for portal vein reconstruction). Sophisticated informatics tools in complex scenarios such as this example can help to facilitate, coordinate, and care-model these processes in the preoperative setting. In addition, informatics studies are needed to understand optimal presentation of information for the needs of surgeons, and for methods to improve the ability of teams of practitioners to provide collaborative care for surgical patients.

Information needs in the perioperative setting

Informatics tools and DSS that help surgeons implement current guidelines and make decisions related to perioperative processes are particularly important for improving surgical outcomes. For instance, nationally mandated requirements for quality, such as the Surgical Care Improvement Project, which seek to reduce surgical complications, can be implemented with pathways and electronic order sets to "cue" and encourage compliance by surgeons [11]. Guidelines and automated systems that assist surgeons to implement evidence-based measures for routine patients such as early feeding, optimal pain control, thromboembolic disease prophylaxis, updated guidelines on intravenous fluid administration, glucose control, use of beta-blockers, and other aspects of perioperative care are examples whereby informatics solutions may be able to facilitate best practices with electronic order sets, evidence-based guidelines, and information integration at the point of care.

Perioperative care in the inpatient setting often involves care teams with surgical house staff, nursing, ancillary support staff, and other specialists. Tools to aid in the collaborative process of inpatient care are an important target area to improve patient care. For example, automated tools that assist with inpatient rounding and patient sign-out have been demonstrated to help surgical house staff in filling information gaps in clinical care and in decreasing time devoted to data transcription with "prerounding" [12]. In addition, informatics tools that can aid with information transfer and communication between clinicians in the perioperative period can potentially positively affect the quality and efficiency in inpatient care [13].

An important target area for quality researchers is the development of mechanisms to improve transitions in care [14]. With respect to surgical care, the greatest opportunity for positive change will be improvements in the transition from the inpatient to the outpatient or transitional-care settings. This issue is a particularly difficult one if surgical patients have ongoing care needs including skilled nursing, physical therapy, and occupational therapy. It is at this time that errors in medication and other needs of care can occur; conversely, this is also an opportunity in select cases where patients may have the ability to transition more quickly to the outpatient setting if effective automated systems are in place for care to occur at home in a more rapid and efficient fashion. For instance, patients with moderately high gastrointestinal outputs that require further monitoring (in cases of short intestinal length or an ileostomy) may be candidates for a home program whereby laboratory values, inputs and outputs, and patient status can be monitored remotely with feedback and treatment from a designated clinician. While several recent initiatives are looking at processes at the transition of care, few have specifically focused on opportunities with surgical patients.

Information needs in the operating room

Important advancements in the past decade regarding information access in the operating room have included increased computer access within operating rooms, most prominently to EHR systems and the Picture Archiving and Communication System, which provide patient information and radiology images, respectively, within the operating room. Some operating rooms provide large screens, which have been particularly useful for intraoperative viewing of radiographic images that have largely replaced the need for having hardcopies of these films.

Despite this, most operating rooms and surgeons continue to have substantial information needs that remain unmet. There are complementary efforts ongoing to increase information resources for the operating room by anesthesia, perioperative nursing, and operating room administrators. Within anesthesiology, there have been continued improvements in patient monitoring, electronic recording of vital signs, and accessibility of computers as tools for accessing relevant anesthesia information. Perioperative nursing through the Association of Perioperative Registered Nurses has developed, ratified, and implemented documentation standards for the operating room [15].

Human factors studies can potentially have an important impact on our understanding of the cognitive issues and methods to improve care complexity and quality in operating rooms [16,17]. Although investigators have attributed issues in communication and a systems approach as a possible method to decrease surgical complications, recent studies demonstrate that human factors, including human error, have the greatest influence on complications in surgery [18].

Because the operating room involves large teams and surgery is resource intensive, the development of automated tools to improve the allocation and use of these resources is an important informatics issue that brings together surgeons, anesthesiologists, operating room nurses, and hospital administrators. Some investigators have started to design automated systems to better predict procedure times and to provide improved support to streamline this process [19]. Some of the models being explored to improve resource use in the operating room include the use of parallel-workflow patterns, such as case staggering and multiple room allocations; the use of induction rooms as is done commonly in Europe, blocking rooms for local anesthesia, and epidural rooms; increasing personnel at the beginning and ends of cases; methods to decrease nonoperative times by improving supply efficiency (including separate sterile rooms for instrument counting and pulling); and video feeds to give current, ongoing monitoring of rooms to coordinate subsequent case scheduling and allocation [20–25]. In addition, automated cataloging systems for stocking, sterile supply planning and allocation, and allowing feedback by surgeons that bring about change have important implications for cost containment, effective use of equipment, reduction of waste, and automation of these processes [26]. Integration of operating room information systems, which today typically function on disparate platforms for supply, scheduling, billing, and other hospital operations, is an important unmet challenge in many centers. The development of operating room dashboards for surgical managers with proactive information can provide useful and timely trends that would not be apparent with more traditional information sources [27]. Most hospitals have not embraced and applied these types of interventions to any great extent, and more efficient information models to implement, develop, and link operating room systems are needed.

Important future technologies aim to improve information access for and facilitate the work of surgeons in the operating room in revolutionary ways. With respect to telesurgery, standards are being developed as this technology becomes more mainstream [28]. Future development of innovative interfaces and vigilance systems for surgeons with novel displays and voice recognition, and other new navigation methods designed for use in the operating room will enhance information access for surgeons, with minimal impact on workflow [29]. Finally, future developments at the intersection of surgery, biomedical engineering, informatics, and radiology with intraoperative image-guided technologies allowing more sophisticated image registration, overlay, and anatomic visualization, including 3-dimensional virtual models, could also fundamentally change the way surgeons perform operative procedures [30–32].

Information needs in the postoperative setting

Although most efforts in surgical practice have focused on preoperative, intraoperative, and perioperative settings, the importance of the postoperative period is being increasingly appreciated. Close follow-up of patients postoperatively helps surgeons better measure outcomes from operative interventions. This follow-up includes immediate operative outcomes (like 30-day morbidity and mortality) and long-term operative outcomes, including cancer survival for oncologic resections, long-term morbidities, and other important long-term outcomes (such as excess body weight loss or resolution of comorbidities following bariatric surgery).

In addition, for some disease processes surgeons are responsible for aspects of screening or surveillance, and certain diseases are chronically managed with shared input from surgeons and other practitioners. For example, the management of Crohn's disease is often jointly performed by colon and rectal surgeons and gastroenterologists together, just as a kidney transplant patient may be closely followed and managed by transplant nephrology and surgical teams. Similar to HIT systems that assist surgeons with data integration and management of complex patients in the preoperative setting, development of models and functionalities to manage postoperative patient information that are disease-specific and procedure-specific can aid clinicians in the care of these patients.

ADDITIONAL SURGICAL INFORMATICS CHALLENGES

Because biomedical and health informatics has primarily focused on other medical disciplines, there are several informatics gaps in surgery, many already discussed in the context of different aspects of surgical care. This section does not intend to be a comprehensive recitation of these gaps; rather, it covers important additional informatics areas with particular need or opportunity within surgery.

Terminology development

An important prerequisite for sustainable data sharing for the surgical community is ensuring that current biomedical data standards are used and supplemented to contain surgical terms. Biomedical terminologies allow for concepts to be represented in a computable and standard format. A systematic review of existing terminologies and the creation of a series of task forces to identify gaps that need to be filled with new content will be an important foundational step. The leading and most comprehensive controlled biomedical data terminology is the Systemized Nomenclature of Medicine-Clinical Terms (SNOMED-CT) [33]. SNOMED-CT is owned and administered by the International Health Terminology Standards Development Organization (IHTSDO) [1], and is freely distributed in the United States via the Unified Medical Language System (UMLS) [34] through the National Library of Medicine (NLM). Despite continued expansion, the growth of SNOMED-CT has not been comprehensive in specialized areas of clinical medicine, including most areas of surgery. Further ongoing development of surgical terms in SNOMED-CT will facilitate data sharing and result in a more comprehensive standard that gains greater adoption as it becomes more usable. A number of other medical terminologies with other focuses (such as laboratory values or medications) are widely used.

Clinical research informatics focused on surgery

Clinical research informatics has recently emerged as an important discipline for supporting clinical trials, which are often complex and highly resource intensive. Clinical research informatics seeks to facilitate the multidisciplinary nature of clinical research to allow seamless integration of these workflows, information resources, and processes for facilitating large-scale clinical research capabilities of health care institutions [35]. Greater attention and resources for clinical trials has been leveraged recently particularly with initiatives through the Clinical and Translational Science Awards and the cancer Biomedical Informatics Grid (caBIG), which rely extensively on informatics underpinnings [36,37]. While a great deal of resources with these initiatives have been devoted to trials in cancer and medical management of chronic illnesses, surgeon investigators can take advantage of and expand these resources to answer important surgical questions through the conduct of clinical trials with informatics resources and support.

Informatics technologies for high-throughput surgical research

Traditional clinical research in surgery has involved retrospective reviews requiring manual extraction of clinical data from the patient chart. Although this provides detailed information, retrospective reviews are time consuming, costly, and typically involve single institutional datasets. Prospective clinical trials can provide the greatest level of evidence for interventions and are essential to advancing surgery science, but they are time consuming, expensive, labor intensive and in some cases unethical to perform.

By contrast, health services research uses large administrative claims databases. This research involves "mining" patient data based on insurance claims,

Medicare data, and other required administrative (ie, ICD-9 or ICD-10) coding. Although these studies allow researchers to ask questions about populations on a large scale, they rely on error-prone claims data [38]. Furthermore, these datasets often do not contain outcome measures and variables, which are most clinically significant. Initiatives such as the National Surgical Quality Improvement Program (NSQIP) and the National Cancer Institute's Surveillance Epidemiology and End Results (SEER) provide researchers more detailed patient information for operative and cancer outcomes. However, these programs are costly, require institutional commitment, may not cover all patients (ie, in the case of NSQIP's cyclical data collection), and are not inherently flexible for the addition of further variables on a large scale. Powerful informatics tools and increasing adoption of EHR systems can be leveraged to improve the quality of surgical research data in a "high-throughput" manner.

Consumer health informatics and decision aids to improve the therapeutic experience

Consumer health informatics focuses on the information needs of patients and families, including making information accessible and understandable to patients, models to integrate patient preferences into decision aids, and methods to impart this information in a tailored and effective manner to patient needs (such as literacy or education level, non-English version speakers, or cultural factors) [39]. Consumer health informatics also makes use of various media, such as Web site information, patient testimonials, and video. The development of evidence-based information summarized to lay-person reading levels is a particularly important challenge for imparting complex information to patients. Because information resources on the Internet are unregulated and of variable content, there is also a large need to provide measures of quality to patients of these resources.

Although decision making and education for surgical patients can be complex, little emphasis has been placed on these high-impact therapeutic encounters with patients. Education modules help patients to be better informed about surgical outcomes and to have realistic expectations. In addition, decision aids that help patients model and consider different therapeutic options, particularly for multifaceted decision making, are potentially important tools for surgical patients [40,41].

One particular development that bridges the EHR with consumer health informatics has been the introduction of personal health record (PHR) systems. PHR systems allow individual patients to maintain and manage their health information in a private, secure, and confidential format. Some PHR systems permit patients to add information from disparate health systems; to annotate and modify their own health records; or to receive alerts, reminders, and other forms of communication. Although certain ethical and adoption issues exist [42], PHR system development represents an important opportunity for patient engagement in the surgical therapeutic process.

Informatics technologies to improve surgical education, accreditation, and simulation

There have been significant and rapid changes in surgical education, particularly with work-hour restrictions for residency training in the last decade. In addition, new paradigms for residency training are being developed, which will most likely decrease the overall length of training and increase focus on subspecialty training. These changes have important implications for future training of the surgical workforce. In addition, future surgical training will include more formal evaluation of skill-based assessments, bench model exercises, and simulators to supplement skills [43,44], provide more robust feedback [45], and help trainees be more prepared for teaching and technically performing in the operating room [46,47]. While simulators are an effective paradigm for surgical education, there is an opportunity for informatics to add cognitive exercises to these simulations to facilitate learning [48]. Moreover, informatics methods can help and increase usability of these systems and the process of feedback [49].

Increasing informatician surgeon stakeholders

Despite the need for greater application of informatics techniques in the process of clinical care, biomedical and health informatics workforce training has traditionally been aimed at generating researchers. The American Medical Informatics Association (AMIA) has recognized the importance of increasing the number of health care professionals able to assume operational informatics roles. In particular, the AMIA 10X10 program is a multicenter, online initiative that aims to train 10,000 applied informaticians by the year 2010 [50]. This program and other similar certificate programs represent important opportunities through which surgeons can learn about and subsequently work in informatics. In addition, the National Institutes of Health, through the NLM, continues to fund centers for training academic informaticians through both predoctoral and postdoctoral (fellowship) tracts.

There is also a complementary current initiative from AMIA to make clinical informatics a subspecialty for each of the boards in the American Boards of Medical Specialties [51,52]. Creation of a Clinical Informatics subspecialty by the American Board of Surgery would be a formidable and important step in increasing the number of surgeons in informatics. One of the important challenges will be the presence of a sufficient number of surgeons to lead these training programs and to leverage institutional informatics expertise in this effort from other clinical disciplines.

In addition to formally trained surgeons with informatics expertise, surgeons with an interest in HIT and improving system design, who are engaged in this process, play an invaluable and complementary role. Collaboration between surgeons and academic information researchers who lack the clinical understanding and acumen of surgical care is invaluable in helping advances occur in a manner that best assists surgeons in the process of care, with good and efficient system redesign for the needs of surgeons.

SUMMARY

The application of biomedical and health informatics to surgery holds tremendous opportunities to enhance surgical care. Better use of information in surgical practice has the potential to streamline care, remove inefficiencies, and allow for improvements in surgical research. With greater EHR adoption, health care reform, and direct investment in HIT, an increasing opportunity exists for surgeons to access and use patient information more effectively. For this to happen, greater focus on the specific needs of surgeons is particularly important, alongside increasing the number of surgical informatics stakeholders.

References

[1] Friedman CP. A "fundamental theorem" of biomedical informatics. J Am Med Inform Assoc 2009;16(2):169–70.

[2] Musen MA. Medical informatics: searching for underlying components. Methods Inf Med 2002;41(1):12–9.

[3] Gaughan A. Bridging the divide: the need for translational informatics. Pharmacogenomics 2006;7(1):117–22.

[4] Institute of Medicine Committee on Quality of Health Care in America. Crossing the quality chasm: a new health system for the 21st century. Washington, DC: National Academy Press; 2001.

[5] Available at: http://www.healthit.hhs.gov. Accessed March 1, 2010.

[6] American recovery and reinvestment act. Available at: http://frwebgate.access.gpo.gov/cgi-bin/getdoc.cgi?dbname=111_cong_bills&docid=f:h1enr.pdf; 2009. Accessed March 1, 2010.

[7] Hall A, Walton G. Information overload within the health care system: a literature review. Health Info Libr J 2004;21(2):102–8.

[8] Hagy J. Needles and haystacks and such. Available at: http://thisisindexed.com/2009/10/needles-and-haystacks-and-such/; 2009. Accessed March 1, 2010.

[9] Classen DC, Avery AJ, Bates DW. Evaluation and certification of computerized provider order entry systems. J Am Med Inform Assoc 2007;14(1):48–55.

[10] Dorr DA, Wilcox A, Burns L, et al. Implementing a multidisease chronic care model in primary care using people and technology. Dis Manag 2006;9(1):1–15.

[11] Griffin FA. Reducing surgical complications. Jt Comm J Qual Patient Saf 2007;33(11): 660–5.

[12] Van Eaton EG, Horvath KD, Lober WB, et al. A randomized, controlled trial evaluating the impact of a computerized rounding and sign-out system on continuity of care and resident work hours. J Am Coll Surg 2005;200(4):538–45.

[13] Williams RG, Silverman R, Schwind C, et al. Surgeon information transfer and communication: factors affecting quality and efficiency of inpatient care. Ann Surg 2007;245(2): 159–69.

[14] Phillips CO, Wright SM, Kern DE, et al. Comprehensive discharge planning with postdischarge support for older patients with congestive heart failure: a meta-analysis. JAMA 2004;291(11):1358–67.

[15] Kleinbeck SV, Dopp A. The perioperative nursing data set—a new language for documenting care. AORN J 2005;82(1):51–7 [quiz: 59–62].

[16] Parker SE, Laviana AA, Wadhera RK, et al. Development and evaluation of an observational tool for assessing surgical flow disruptions and their impact on surgical performance. World J Surg 2010;34(2):353–61.

[17] Wiegmann DA, El Bardissi AW, Dearani JA, et al. Disruptions in surgical flow and their relationship to surgical errors: an exploratory investigation. Surgery 2007;142(5):658–65.

[18] Fabri PJ, Zayas-Castro JL. Human error, not communication and systems, underlies surgical complications. Surgery 2008;144(4):557–63 [discussion: 563–5].
[19] Eijkemans MJ, van Houdenhoven M, Nguyen T, et al. Predicting the unpredictable: a new prediction model for operating room times using individual characteristics and the surgeon's estimate. Anesthesiology 2010;112(1):41–9.
[20] Marjamaa RA, Torkki PM, Hirvensalo EJ, et al. What is the best workflow for an operating room? A simulation study of five scenarios. Health Care Manag Sci 2009;12(2):142–6.
[21] Mariano ER, Chu LF, Peinado CR, et al. Anesthesia-controlled time and turnover time for ambulatory upper extremity surgery performed with regional versus general anesthesia. J Clin Anesth 2009;21(4):253–7.
[22] Xiao Y, Dexter F, Hu P, et al. The use of distributed displays of operating room video when real-time occupancy status was available. Anesth Analg 2008;106(2):554–60 [table of contents].
[23] Dalstrom DJ, Venkatarayappa I, Manternach AL, et al. Time-dependent contamination of opened sterile operating-room trays. J Bone Joint Surg Am 2008;90(5):1022–5.
[24] Smith MP, Sandberg WS, Foss J, et al. High-throughput operating room system for joint arthroplasties durably outperforms routine processes. Anesthesiology 2008;109(1):25–35.
[25] Sandberg WS, Daily B, Egan M, et al. Deliberate perioperative systems design improves operating room throughput. Anesthesiology 2005;103(2):406–18.
[26] Park KW, Dickerson C. Can efficient supply management in the operating room save millions? Curr Opin Anaesthesiol 2009;22(2):242–8.
[27] Nagy PG, Konewko R, Warnock M, et al. Novel, web-based, information-exploration approach for improving operating room logistics and system processes. Surg Innov 2008;15(1):7–16.
[28] Natarajan S, Ganz A. SURGNET: an integrated surgical data transmission system for telesurgery. Int J Telemed Appl 2009;2009:435849.
[29] Quint DJ. Voice recognition: ready for prime time? J Am Coll Radiol 2007;4(10):667–9 [discussion: 670–1].
[30] Kocak E, Al-Saif O, Satter M, et al. Image guidance during abdominal exploration for recurrent colorectal cancer. Ann Surg Oncol 2007;14(2):405–10.
[31] San Jose Estepar R, Westin CF, Vosburgh KG. Towards real time 2D to 3D registration for ultrasound-guided endoscopic and laparoscopic procedures. Int J Comput Assist Radiol Surg 2009;4(6):549–60.
[32] Foo JL, Lobe T, Winer E. A virtual reality environment for patient data visualization and endoscopic surgical planning. J Laparoendosc Adv Surg Tech A 2009;19(Suppl 1):S211–7.
[33] Spackman KA. Rates of change in a large clinical terminology: three years experience with SNOMED clinical terms. AMIA Annu Symp Proc 2005;714–8.
[34] Lindberg DA, Humphreys BL, McCray AT. The Unified Medical Language System. Methods Inf Med 1993;32(4):281–91.
[35] Embi PJ, Payne PR. Clinical research informatics: challenges, opportunities and definition for an emerging domain. J Am Med Inform Assoc 2009;16(3):316–27.
[36] Zerhouni EA, Alving B. Clinical and translational science awards: a framework for a national research agenda. Transl Res 2006;148(1):4–5.
[37] Saltz J, Oster S, Hastings S, et al. caGrid: design and implementation of the core architecture of the cancer biomedical informatics grid. Bioinformatics 2006;22(15):1910–6.
[38] Campbell SE, Campbell MK, Grimshaw JM, et al. A systematic review of discharge coding accuracy. J Public Health Med 2001;23(3):205–11.
[39] Eysenbach G. Consumer health informatics. BMJ 2000;320(7251):1713–6.
[40] Neuman HB, Charlson ME, Temple LK. Is there a role for decision aids in cancer-related decisions? Crit Rev Oncol Hematol 2007;62(3):240–50.
[41] O'Connor AM, Bennett CL, Stacey D, et al. Decision aids for people facing health treatment or screening decisions. Cochrane Database Syst Rev 2009;3:CD001431.

[42] Weitzman ER, Kaci L, Mandl KD. Acceptability of a personally controlled health record in a community-based setting: implications for policy and design. J Med Internet Res 2009;11(2):e14.
[43] Chipman JG, Schmitz CC. Using objective structured assessment of technical skills to evaluate a basic skills simulation curriculum for first-year surgical residents. J Am Coll Surg 2009;209(3):364–70, e362.
[44] Scott DJ, Bergen PC, Rege RV, et al. Laparoscopic training on bench models: better and more cost effective than operating room experience? J Am Coll Surg 2000;191(3):272–83.
[45] Roach PB, Roggin KK, Selkov E Jr, et al. Use of a novel, web-based educational platform facilitates intraoperative training in a surgical oncology fellowship program. Ann Surg Oncol 2009;16(5):1100–7.
[46] Burkhart HM, Riley JB, Hendrickson SE, et al. The successful application of simulation-based training in thoracic surgery residency. J Thorac Cardiovasc Surg 2010;139(3):707–12.
[47] Wetzel CM, Black SA, Hanna GB, et al. The effects of stress and coping on surgical performance during simulations. Ann Surg 2010;251(1):171–6.
[48] Kahol K, Vankipuram M, Smith ML. Cognitive simulators for medical education and training. J Biomed Inform 2009;42(4):593–604.
[49] Rissanen MJ, Kuroda Y, Nakao M, et al. A novel approach for training of surgical procedures based on visualization and annotation of behavioural parameters in simulators. Stud Health Technol Inform 2007;125:388–93.
[50] Hersh W, Williamson J. Educating 10,000 informaticians by 2010: the AMIA 10x10 program. Int J Med Inform 2007;76(5-6):377–82.
[51] Detmer DE, Lumpkin JR, Williamson JJ. Defining the medical subspecialty of clinical informatics. J Am Med Inform Assoc 2009;16(2):167–8.
[52] Safran C, Shabot MM, Munger BS, et al. Program requirements for fellowship education in the subspecialty of clinical informatics. J Am Med Inform Assoc 2009;16(2):158–66.

ELSEVIER
MOSBY
Advances in Surgery 44 (2010) 131–148
ADVANCES IN SURGERY

Does the Type of Pancreaticojejunostomy After Whipple Alter the Leak Rate?

Chad G. Ball, MD, MSc, FRCSC, Thomas J. Howard, MD*
Department of Surgery, Indiana University School of Medicine, 545 Barnhill Drive, Indianapolis, IN 46202, USA

Leakage of digestive juices from the pancreas with their unpredictable sequelae continues to pose a challenge to surgeons since Whipple's addition of a pancreaticojejunostomy [1] to the classic Kausch-Whipple pancreatoduodenectomy in 1942 [2,3]. Although the mortality associated with pancreatoduodenectomy has been dramatically reduced over the past 70 years (from 20% to <3%), morbidity rates have remained stubbornly constant at approximately 40% [4–14]. Although the list of complications associated with a Whipple operation is substantial, an uncontrolled pancreatic leak and its associated downstream effectors of sepsis, hemorrhage, and multiorgan failure remain the most dramatic and lethal. Although the mortality rates associated with a pancreatic leak have been substantially reduced by the application of modern critical care, nutritional support and percutaneous catheter drainage techniques, systemic sepsis, and visceral pseudoaneurysms still occur, and when present, result in mortality rates of up to 40% [11,15–19]. Efforts to reduce the 10% to 25% incidence of pancreatic-enteric anastomotic leaks have invigorated surgeons to explore innovative technical modifications to this portion of the operation [7,15,16,20]. More than 1700 publications commenting on pancreatic anastomosis have been listed in PubMed over the past 50 years chronicling the employment of different reconstructive organs, sewing techniques, pancreatic duct stenting methods, pharmacologic manipulation of pancreatic secretion, application of topical adhesives, and methods of external drainage [21]. Whenever one encounters a body of literature this extensive that focuses on one technical aspect of an operation, it generally means: (1) it is viewed as an important problem by surgeons, and (2) no adequate solution to the problem exists.

As alluded to in the preceding discussion, there remains a paucity of rigorously designed large multi-institutional randomized controlled trials (RCT)

*Corresponding author. *E-mail address*: tjhoward@iupui.edu.

0065-3411/10/$ – see front matter
doi:10.1016/j.yasu.2010.05.020

to allow one to draw definitive conclusions regarding the optimal technique to use to reduce the pancreatic leak rate following Whipple operation. Although several valid attempts at achieving level I data have been completed, including several moderately large, randomized multi-institutional clinical trials [22–24], much of our current understanding, or lack thereof, is predicated on single-surgeon case series reports. Although it is true that these reports have been authored by many of the true giants in pancreatic surgery, single-surgeon case series remain prone to significant biases, including volume-outcome covariates, learning curves issues, and difficult to transfer knowledge and skill sets. Furthermore, case series reporting poor outcomes using a new or modified technique are rarely published, providing a substantial publication bias in favor of positive studies. The importance of surgeon experience on the postoperative rate of pancreatic leakage is perhaps *the* most important factor in this challenging technical exercise [6,21,25–28]. Although this particular variable has proven nearly impossible to accurately quantify, it remains a significant covariate in all studies. As a result of this confounding factor, regardless of country or center, high-volume surgeons at busy centers who are able to master a given technique through frequent repetition have better outcomes and lower pancreatic leak rates than surgeons who do not have these characteristics [21]. In addition to these single-surgeon case series, a large number of studies have been done using a retrospective cohort design that limits our ability to draw definitive conclusions. Issues, such as selection bias, temporal bias (began with technique *x* and then switched to technique *y* with improved results), confirmation bias, and poor outcome definitions are some of the troubling methodological limitations in this body of literature. Analogous to single-surgeon case series, these studies rarely control for surgeon experience and are often influenced by variables other than the direct technical factors of interest (anastomotic technique) by not controlling for concomitant stent placement, octreotide treatment, or sealant use. It seems to be an infrequent occurrence for surgeons to limit their technical modifications to a single, well-defined measureable variable. This observation is exemplified in a recent report finding fewer pancreatic leaks using a three-stage procedure incorporating a pancreaticogastrostomy, external continuous suction drainage of pancreatic juice, wrapping the pancreatic anastomosis with the round ligament, and applying fibrin glue sealant [29,30]. Which specific factor contributed to the improved results they cite is of course, a matter of speculation, not science. Although conclusions drawn from an RCT in theory are more transferable, variability in definitions, patient populations, clinical endpoints, and individual surgeon's skill sets significantly limits broad generalizations when applied to technique-based investigations. Nevertheless, it is only through carefully designed, large, multi-institutional RCTs do we have any true hope of eliminating the nearly ubiquitous statement, "future randomized studies are required," found at the conclusion of most papers on this topic. Given these significant limitations, this article reviews the recent literature pertaining to the technical approaches designed to reduce pancreatic leaks following a Whipple operation.

DEFINITIONS

Consistent and reliable terminology has not been applied in the literature with regard to pancreatic leaks following a Whipple operation. As a result of this inconsistency, heterogeneous definitions of pancreatic leaks and fistulae, as well as their clinic sequelae, abound [20]. This article defines a pancreatic *fistula* as an abnormal communication between two epithelialized structures. *Leak* or *leakage* is defined as an abnormal escape of fluid from the pancreas gland itself [25]. Because these terms have been used interchangeably within the literature, as well as the fact that amylase-rich pancreatic juice may drain from either the pancreatico-enteric anastomosis or the transected surface of the gland, both terms are included in this article. This inclusiveness is clearly evident in the International Study Group for Pancreatic Fistula (ISGPF) lexicon, which defines a pancreatic fistula in the broadest sense by including all peripancreatic fluid collections, abscesses, leaks, and fistulas thought to originate from either the anastomosis or pancreatic gland surface: "any measurable volume of fluid on or after postoperative day three, with an amylase content greater than three times the upper limit of normal serum" [20]. Until the recent adoption of a common lexicon and grading system by the ISGPF it was nearly impossible to compare the results from different published series or centers in any meaningful manner.

UNMODIFIABLE ANASTOMOTIC RISK FACTORS

Unmodifiable risk factors associated with the occurrence of a pancreatic leak following a Whipple operation include a laundry list of anatomic and physiologic factors: patient age (>70 years), sex (male), jaundice (duration), coronary artery disease, hemoglobin A1c level (diabetes mellitus), creatinine clearance (<50 mL/min), periampullary neoplasms besides pancreatic cancer (duodenum, terminal bile duct, ampulla of Vater), blood supply to the pancreatic remnant, and the volume of pancreatic juice output [17,31–45]. These variables are, for the most part, related to the general capacity for wound healing and not necessarily specific to a pancreatic anastomosis. Although the specific impact of each of these factors can be debated, the direct consequences of pancreatic gland texture and duct size have been repeatedly highlighted over decades of publications. The higher pancreatic leak rate associated with a soft, fatty, nonfibrotic gland with a small (<4 mm) pancreatic duct is clear to even the most junior pancreatic surgeon [6,21,25,26,45]. It appears that a soft pancreas conveys up to a 10-fold increased risk of subsequent pancreatic leak/fistula [17,31,40,45–50] and this risk appears to be independent of the specific type of pancreatico-enteric anastomosis constructed [22]. These same observations of a higher pancreatic leak rate have consistently been made for the presence of a small pancreatic duct [17,38,45]. Ducts less than 4 mm in diameter are particularly problematic and may confer a greater than 3-fold increased risk of subsequent fistula [17,38]. Magnification of the surgical field using a microscope during pancreaticojejunostomy has been proposed in this setting as a useful adjunct [51]. These risk factors coexist with potentially modifiable factors, such as operative time, excessive intraoperative blood loss (>1500 mL), use of neoadjuvant chemoradiotherapy (protective), and type of anastomosis constructed. The remainder of this article focuses on the technical factors of pancreatic-enteric reconstruction that have been associated with a reduced leak rate following Whipple operation.

TECHNICAL FACTORS

Reconstructive organ

Debate over the best reconstructive organ (stomach vs jejunum) for restoration of pancreatic-enteric continuity can be traced to the initial description of pancreaticogastrostomy by Waugh and Claggett in 1946 [52]. Anastomosing the pancreatic remnant to the posterior stomach has several plausible advantages that include: (1) a rich gastric wall blood supply to improve anastomotic healing, (2) a tension-free anastomosis caused by the close proximity of the stomach to the pancreatic remnant, (3) avoidance of a long traction-prone jejunal loop, and (4) inactivation of troublesome digestive pancreatic enzymes (trypsin) by gastric acid secretion (Fig. 1). Similarly, jejunum also has several theoretical advantages as a reconstructive conduit including: (1) ease of approximation because of the mobility of the jejunal mesentery, and (2) a rich jejunal blood supply for anastomotic healing. A recent single-institution randomized clinical trial compared 53 subjects with gastric partition pancreaticogastrostomy to 55 subjects with conventional pancreaticojejunostomy where they reported a lower pancreatic leak rate (4% vs 18%, $P<.01$) using pancreaticogastrostomy [53]. These investigators speculate that although pancreatic juice continues to drain directly into the stomach using this technique, benefits are derived from the anastomosis resting outside the flow of gastric contents into the jejunum (Fig. 2). One concern in the design of this study is that both anastomoses were done using short (6 cm) silastic internal pancreatic stents, an uncontrolled variable that may have influenced their results.

Many authors have attempted to delineate which of these two procedures is superior [8,29,53–69] and 4 prospective randomized clinical trials comparing pancreaticogastrostomy to pancreaticojejunostomy have been completed [23,38,70,71]. Despite variable definitions of end points and incidences (0% to 14%) of pancreatic leak/fistula rates between trials, no significant differences between these two techniques were identified. Further evidence of this clinical equipoise is found in a recent meta-analysis that concluded that the two techniques of anastomosis were not different in terms of pancreatic fistula rate or overall postoperative morbidity rates [66]. Despite the equivalence of these two techniques in the early postoperative period, troubling long-term functional deficits, including both anastomotic stenosis and pancreatic endocrine insufficiency, have been reported with pancreaticogastrostomy [72–75]. To date, jejunum remains the favored conduit for pancreatic enteric anastomosis and its use has provided surgeons with a consistent and predictable pancreatic leak rate in the 2% to 19% range [76]. Use of the stomach for reconstruction remains firmly entrenched in the practice of several high-volume surgical

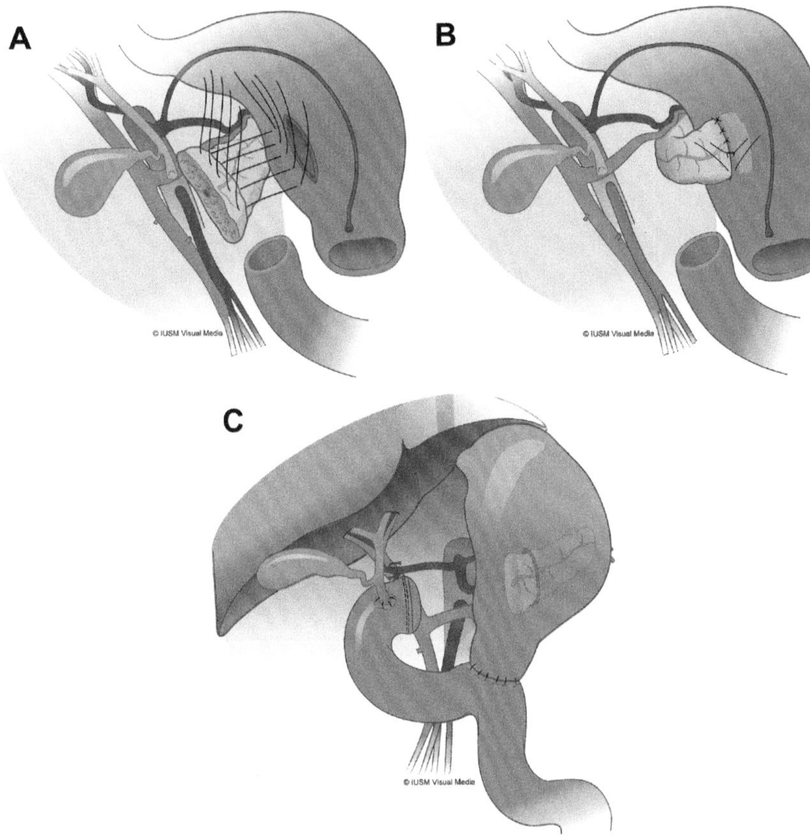

Fig. 1. Technique of pancreaticogastrostomy. (*A*) After mobilization of at least 4 to 6 cm of the pancreas from the splenic artery and vein, a posterior layer of 3-0 silk sutures are placed through the anterior capsule of the pancreas 2 cm from the transaction margin into the seromuscular layer on the left lateral aspect of the size-matched gastrostomy. The gastrostomy is located on the posterior wall of the stomach. Note the clockwise rotation of the stomach around its axis to facilitate this retrogastric reconstruction. (*B*) While the stomach is still rotated, after completing the posterior layer of the anastomosis, the pancreatic remnant is invaginated into the stomach and the anastomosis is completed by an anterior row of 3-0 silk sutures placed 2 cm back from the cut end of the pancreas. Note the mobility required of the remnant pancreas off the splenic artery and vein to facilitate this anastomosis. (*C*) Counterclockwise rotation of the stomach returns it to its normal anatomic configuration and the subsequent pylorojejunostomy is completed. Note the position of the posteriorly placed invaginated pancreaticogastrostomy as seen through the stomach in this drawing.

groups who continue to advocate its benefits [57–61]. Taken as a whole, studies of the best methodologic quality indicate that anastomosis of the pancreatic remnant to either the jejunum or stomach is an equivalent technique with regard to the incidence of major morbidity and postoperative pancreatic leak rates.

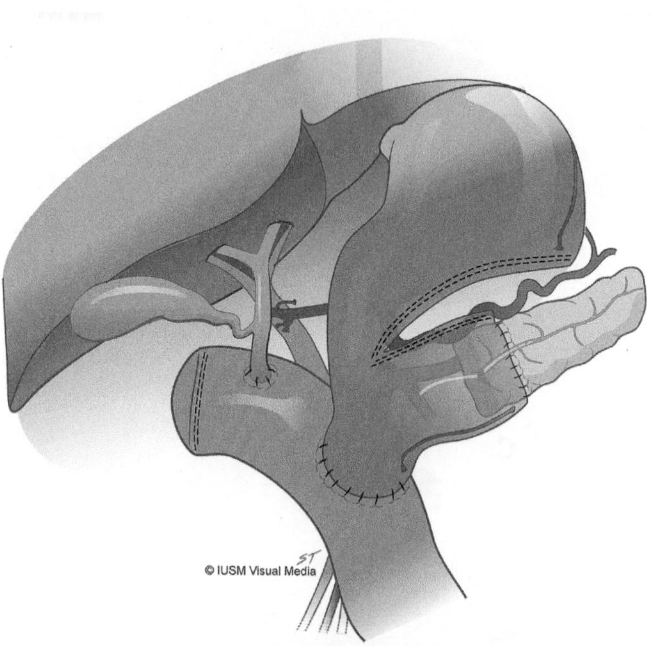

Fig. 2. Gastric partition pancreaticogastrostomy. In this variant, the anastomosis of the pancreas to the stomach is constructed outside the flow of gastric contents into the duodenum by use of a gastric partition staple line. In this technique as described, the anastomosis is constructed using a short (6 cm) internalized pancreatic duct stent (see Fig. 5).

Technique of pancreaticojejunostomy

Although the specific technical modifications of pancreaticojejunostomy described in the literature are detailed and varied, these numerous contributions can be broken down into 3 common variants: (1) end-to-side duct-to-mucosa (Fig. 3A); (2) end-to-side invagination (see Fig. 3B); and (3) end-to-end invagination (see Fig. 3C). In an end-to-side duct-to-mucosa anastomosis, the pancreatic duct is sewn directly to the jejunal mucosa in either an interrupted or running manner using a fine monofilament absorbable suture. Invagination techniques incorporate both the pancreatic duct with varying portions of the pancreatic parenchyma sewn to the full thickness of jejunum in either an end-to-end or end-to-side configuration of the cut end of the pancreas to the jejunum. Although these techniques vary in specifics, they do share common principles including a secure, tension-free anastomosis; adequate blood supply; and pancreatic juice draining directly into the gastrointestinal tract near the biliary anastomosis [26]. The search for the optimal pancreaticojejunostomy has also led to several independent and original suggestions. Most notable are the binding pancreaticojejunostomy described by Peng using mucosal ablation and end-to-end invagination [77–79], a trans-pancreatic U-stitch technique that aims to reduce shear forces during knot

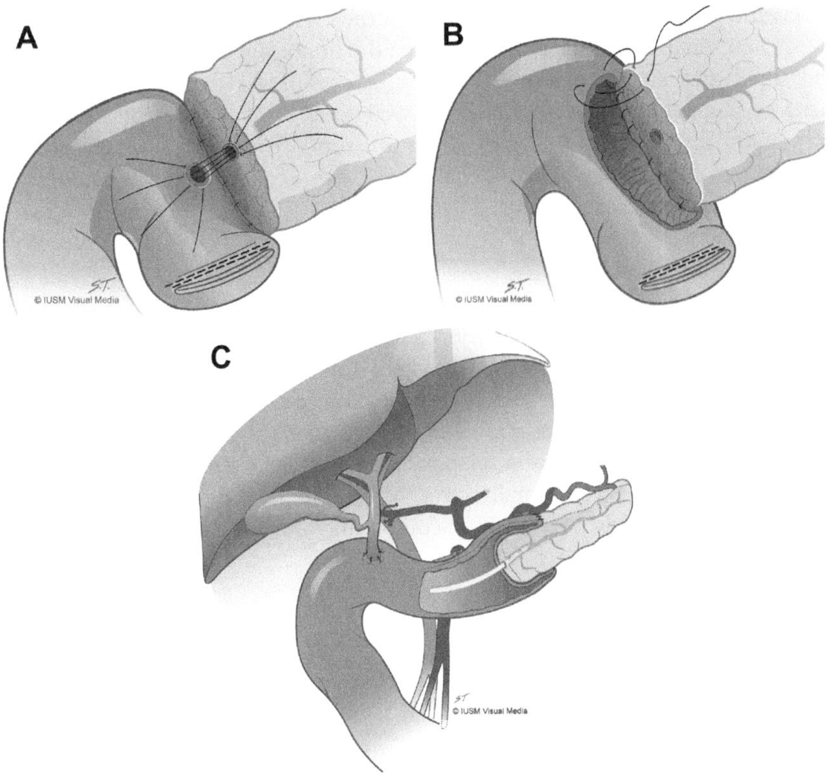

Fig. 3. Common types of pancreaticojejunostomy. (*A*) End-to-side duct to mucosal pancreaticojejunostomy. (*B*) End-to-side invaginated pancreaticojejunostomy. (*C*) End-to-end invaginated pancreaticojejunostomy (with internal transanastomotic stent).

tying [80,81], and modified invagination techniques [82,83]. Despite several nonrandomized and randomized trials [77,84–87], no single investigation has been able to definitively confirm the advantage of one technique over another in reducing the risk of subsequent pancreatic leaks. This clinical equipoise also extends to numerous cohort studies [83,88–94], and appears to be independent of the suggestion that invagination techniques may be superior in patients with soft pancreatic remnants and small pancreatic ducts [38]. With regard to this later point, in a randomized trial of 144 subjects with predominantly soft glands (90%), no benefit was observed in the pancreatic leak rate for either technique [87]. Retrospective studies imply that employing a continuous duct-to-mucosa anastomosis reduces subsequent leaks when compared with an interrupted technique [94,95]. Although a few studies reported superiority of the duct-to-mucosa technique over various invagination approaches [31,42,84], a recent, large, prospective dual-institution trial of 197 subjects reported exactly the opposite conclusion identifying significantly fewer pancreatic fistulas (12% vs 24%, $P < .05$) in the end-to-side invagination cohort [22]. These investigators again highlighted the importance of soft gland texture and small duct size as perhaps the main determining factors in the development of pancreatic leaks. Despite this well-done RCT, judgments based on the totality of the current surgical literature support that duct-to-mucosa and invagination techniques remain equivalent with regard to the incidence of postoperative pancreatic leaks.

Separate jejunal limb

Irrespective of the particular type of pancreaticojejunostomy, some surgeons advocate the use of a dedicated jejunal limb for this anastomosis (Fig. 4). In theory, this technique limits the activation of pancreatic juice enzymes by isolating them from the biliary effluent, which travels though a separate parallel limb in this method of reconstruction. Unfortunately, although some investigators have reported lower rates of pancreatic fistula in small personal series [96–105], neither a recent small retrospective series [106] nor 2 prospective nonrandomized trials [107,108] comparing an isolated Roux loop

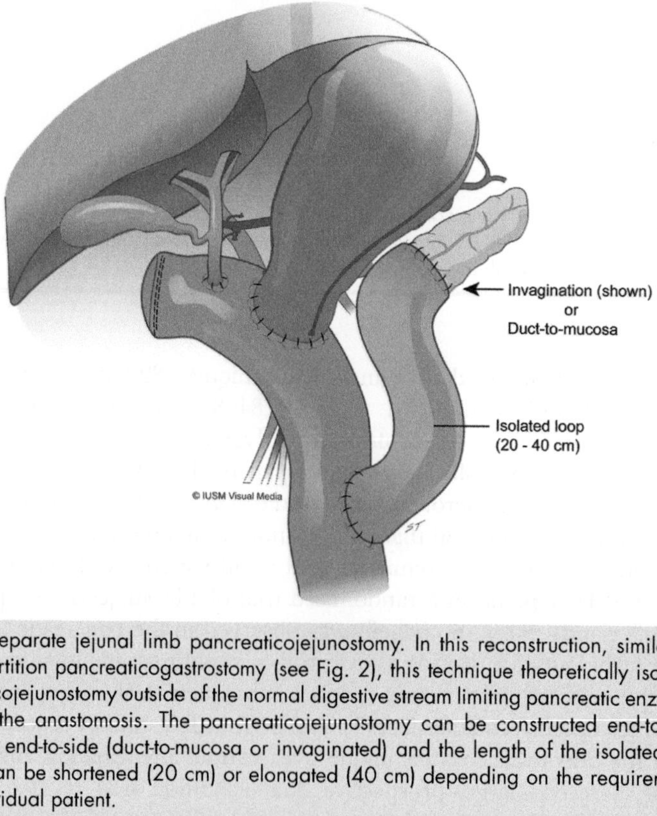

Fig. 4. Separate jejunal limb pancreaticojejunostomy. In this reconstruction, similar to the gastric partition pancreaticogastrostomy (see Fig. 2), this technique theoretically isolates the pancreaticojejunostomy outside of the normal digestive stream limiting pancreatic enzyme activation at the anastomosis. The pancreaticojejunostomy can be constructed end-to-end (as shown) or end-to-side (duct-to-mucosa or invaginated) and the length of the isolated limb of jejunum can be shortened (20 cm) or elongated (40 cm) depending on the requirements for each individual patient.

pancreaticojejunostomy versus a standard pancreaticojejunostomy have identified a benefit in terms of postoperative pancreatic leaks.

Pancreatic duct stenting

The use of transanastomotic stents has several theoretical advantages: (1) diversion of pancreatic juice away from a fresh pancreatico-enteric anastomosis, and (2) protection of the pancreatic duct during suture placement. Potential downside risks include stent migration and pancreatic duct obstruction. As with the previous discussion of technical modifications, although good evidence exists to support the use of transanastomotic stents, a definitive conclusion based on irrefutable level 1 evidence remains lacking.

Internal transanastomotic stenting uses a short (6 cm) silastic stent placed across the pancreaticojejunostomy anastomosis (3 cm into the pancreas and 3 cm into the jejunum) which terminates intraluminally within the jejunal limb or stomach (Fig. 5). External transanastomotic stenting involves delivering a long silastic stent (eg, 5-F pediatric feeding tube) traversing through both the bowel and anterior abdominal wall to allow for complete external drainage and diversion (Fig. 6). Although a recent RCT advocating externalized

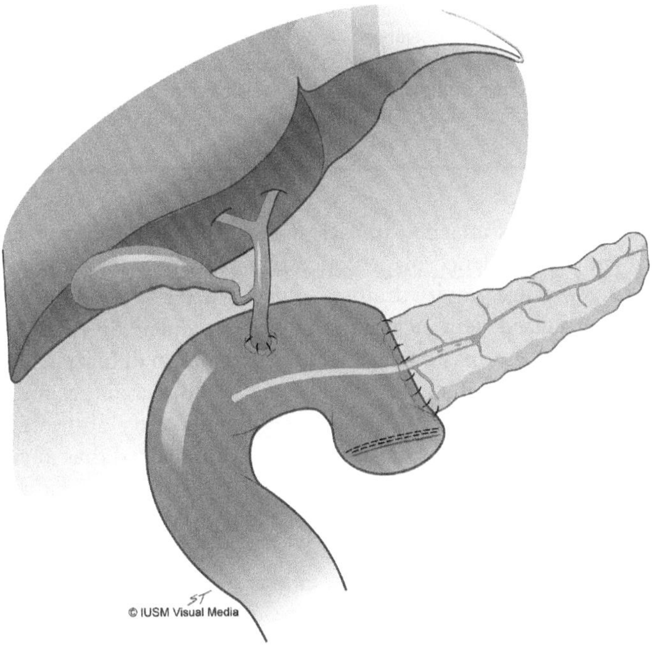

Fig. 5. Short (6 cm), internal transanastomotic pancreatico-enteric stenting. A 6-cm length of silastic pediatric feeding tube (5 or 8 French in size, matched to the internal diameter of the pancreatic duct) is placed approximately 3 cm into the pancreatic duct during anastomotic construction leaving the remaining length (approximately 3 cm) positioned in the biliopancreatic limb.

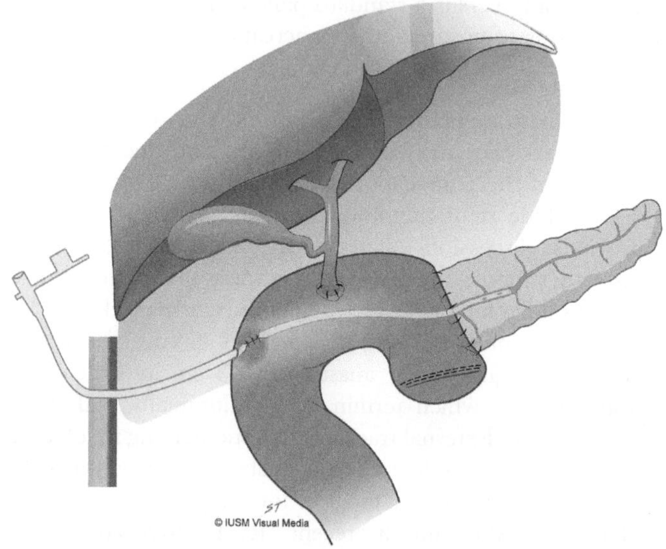

Fig. 6. Long, external transanastomotic pancreatico-enteric stenting. In this technique, a full-length pediatric feeding tube (5 or 8 French in size, matched to the internal diameter of the pancreatic duct) is brought into the jejunum via a Witzel-tunnel technique and placed across the pancreaticojejunostomy during construction. The tube after leaving the biliopancreatic limb via the Witzel tunnel is then brought out through the anterior abdominal wall serving as a controlled pancreatic fistula until healing of the anastomosis, after which it can be removed in the outpatient clinic.

transanastomotic stents attached to a closed suction drainage device reported a reduction in the incidence of postoperative pancreatic fistulas [109], most pancreatic surgeons use gravity drainage only for these stents. Potential advantages of an externalized stent include: (1) a more complete diversion of pancreatic juice away from the anastomosis, and (2) prevention of biliary activation of the pancreatic zymogens. Comparisons of these two techniques are common within the literature, as are studies evaluating the necessity of the stents themselves [24,110–119]. Although cohort studies have indicated that internal stenting may reduce the risk of pancreatic fistula [110,111], subsequent prospective studies in both soft, normal pancreatic glands [112] and in those subjects reconstructed with an isolated jejunal limb [113], or via standard pancreaticojejunostomy [114], found no differences in either the frequency or severity of pancreatic leaks. Although external pancreatic stenting has been associated with a low (0.0% to 4.2%) incidence of pancreatic fistula in several personal series [115–117], it has also been compared with no stenting in multiple study designs. A recent retrospective review failed to identify any advantage to an external transanastomotic stent with regard to pancreatic leak rates [118]. A nonrandomized study of 85 subjects, however, identified a decreased incidence of postoperative pancreatic leaks [119]. In a well-designed RCT of 120 subjects by Poon and colleagues, fewer pancreatic leaks (6.7% vs 2.0%) were found in the subject cohort that used external pancreatic duct stents versus the control group with no stenting. This trial is to be applauded for a tight methodology, including analyzing one specific variable while carefully standardizing the technique of pancreaticojejunostomy (duct-to-mucosa) used [24].

Surprisingly, given the previously mentioned information on the overall utility of pancreatic duct stenting in general, both nonrandomized [120] and randomized [121] prospective clinical trials comparing internal pancreatic stents to external transanastomotic stenting have found no significant benefit to one technique over the other with respect to rate of subsequent pancreatic leaks. A recent publication has reported an increase in the incidence of delayed gastric emptying with the use of pancreatic duct stenting when compared with avoiding stents all together [122]. Taken as a collective, the literature surrounding the use of pancreatic stents remains curious because of its lack of internal inconsistency. Although studies evaluating external transanastomotic pancreatic stents generally support their use, those evaluating internal pancreatic stents have consistently shown no benefit. Oddly, when direct comparisons are made between internal and external stenting, rather than identifying a benefit with external stenting as one would expect based on the individual data, no significant advantage is identified between groups. As a result of these inconsistencies, it remains uncertain if placement of a stent (either internal or external) significantly reduces the rate of postoperative pancreatic fistulas/leaks during pancreaticojejunostomy.

Prophylactic anastomotic drainage

External drainage of pancreatic-enteric anastomosis via either open or closed-suction drainage techniques have a long impassioned history. Although the current trend in general surgery is to minimize their use in a wide variety of complex operations (hepatic, colon, rectal, appendectomy) [123,124], external drainage has remained a fixture in pancreatic surgery. Closed suction drains are classically placed around the pancreatic anastomosis to control a pancreatic leak should one occur, with the hope of transforming an anastomotic leak into a controlled pancreatic fistula thereby avoiding the potential morbid consequences. Without adequate control of a leak (drainage by either a surgeon or interventional radiologist), patients may progress to the development of systemic sepsis, multiorgan failure, and potentially death. Further confounding these unyielding notions is the rather distinct possibility that routine intraperitoneal pancreatic drainage may actually generate leaks from the anastomosis following pancreatoduodenectomy. This leak-generating potential is particularly plausible for closed-suction drainage systems where the suction bulb generates a significant negative pressure to the area surrounding the anastomosis [125,126]. Although this pressure decreases with liquid filling of the reservoir, it can be substantially increased with stripping of a drain (−175 mm Hg), data that have led some surgeons to place their intraperitoneal closed-suction drains to gravity. Because of the high risk associated with not adequately controlling a pancreatic fistula, pancreatic surgeons have been slow to incorporate the results of both a retrospective review [127] and a RCT of 139 subjects to either intraperitoneal drainage or no drainage following pancreatectomy [128]. In this study, Conlon and colleagues found no significant differences in either the number or type of complications, the need for subsequent interventional radiologic drainage or reoperation, or the overall mortality rate between the two subject groups. Although this study has been criticized for several methodological flaws, these compelling findings mandate an appropriately powered, multi-institutional study to carefully examine these issues because the current use of routine intraperitoneal drainage following pancreaticojejunostomy is not based on sound scientific evidence.

In addition to placing the drain, the length of time that a peripancreatic drain is left in place is an additional factor associated with the risk of subsequent pancreatic leaks. Similar to the arguments surrounding routine placement of intraperitoneal drains, this variable is embroiled with a long history of art and tradition. Although some pancreatic surgeons remove drains early based on low drain amylase values, others maintain peripancreatic drainage until the patients are tolerating a regular diet to ensure that a pancreatic fistula is not present with full pancreatic stimulation. A recent RCT has addressed this issue by concluding that fistula rates are lower if the drain is removed on postoperative day 3 provided the drain amylase level is below 5000 IU/L [129]. A link between early drain removal after pancreatoduodenectomy and fewer pancreatic leaks may also be relevant given the observation of a lower institutional pancreatic fistula rate with a generally more rapid drain removal protocol at one institution in the RCT of invagination versus duct-to-mucosa anastomotic techniques [22].

SUMMARY

Despite the overwhelming limitations that plague the literature surrounding the optimal method of reestablishing pancreatico-enteric continuity following a Whipple operation, it is clear that all successful techniques conform to sound surgical principles. These principles include a water-tight and tension-free anastomosis, preservation of adequate blood supply for both organs involved in the anastomosis, and minimal trauma to the pancreas gland. Although surgeon experience, gland texture, and pancreatic duct size are clearly the dominate risk factors from a long list of variables associated with pancreatic leaks following pancreatoduodenectomy, these are nonmodifiable covariates. Although the plethora of current literature cannot provide a single definitive technical solution for restoring pancreatico-enteric continuity, a small number of well-designed RCTs [22,24] support the use of transanastomotic external stenting for high-risk pancreatic glands and an end-to-side invaginated pancreaticojejunostomy. The truth remains that an individual surgeon's mastery of a specific anastomotic technique, in conjunction with a large personal experience, is likely to be the best predictor of a low pancreas leak rate following pancreatoduodenectomy.

References

[1] Whipple AO. A reminiscence: pancreatoduodenectomy. Rev Surg 1963;20:221–5.
[2] Kausch W. Das carcinoma der papilla und seine radikale entfernung. Beitr Klin Chir 1912;78:29–33.
[3] Whipple AO. The rationale of radical surgery for cancer of the pancreas and ampullary region. Ann Surg 1941;114(4):612–5.
[4] Crile G Jr. The advantage of bypass operations over radical pancreaticoduodenectomy in the treatment of pancreatic carcinoma. Surg Gynecol Obstet 1970;130(6):1049–53.
[5] Herter FP, Cooperman AM, Ahlborn TN, et al. Surgical experience with pancreatic and periampullary cancer. Ann Surg 1982;195(3):274–81.
[6] Poon RTP, Fan ST. Decreasing the pancreatic leak rate after pancreaticoduodenectomy. Adv Surg 2008;42:33–48.
[7] Yeo CJ, Cameron JL, Sohn TA, et al. Six hundred fifty consecutive pancreaticoduodenectomies in the 1990s: pathology, complications, and outcomes. Ann Surg 1997;226(3): 248–60.
[8] Poon RTP, Fan ST, Chu KM, et al. Standards of pancreaticoduodenectomy in a tertiary referral centre in Hong Kong: retrospective case series. Hong Kong Med J 2002;8: 249–54.
[9] Neoptolemos JP, Russell RC, Bramhall S, et al. Low mortality following resection for pancreatic and periampullary tumors in 1026 patients: UK survey of specialist pancreatic units. UK Pancreatic Cancer Group. Br J Surg 1997;84(10):1370–6.
[10] Jimenez RE, Fernandez-del Castillo C, Rattner DW, et al. Outcome of pancreaticoduodenectomy with pylorus preservation or with antrectomy in the treatment of chronic pancreatitis. Ann Surg 2000;231(3):293–300.
[11] Bottger TC, Junginger T. Factors influencing morbidity and mortality after pancreaticoduodenectomy: critical analysis of 221 patients. World J Surg 1999;23(2):164–71.
[12] Trede M, Schwall G, Saeger HD. Survival after pancreaticoduodenectomy: 118 consecutive resections without an operative mortality. Ann Surg 1990;211(4):447–58.
[13] Fernandez-del Castillo C, Rattner DW, Warshaw AL. Standards for pancreatic resection in the 1990s. Arch Surg 1995;130(3):295–9.
[14] Cameron JL, Pitt HA, Yeo CJ, et al. One hundred and forty-five consecutive pancreaticoduodenectomies without mortality. Ann Surg 1993;217(5):430–5.
[15] Trede M, Schwall G. The complications of pancreatectomy. Ann Surg 1998;207(1): 39–47.
[16] Cullen JJ, Sarr MG, Ilstrup DM. Pancreatic anastomotic leak after pancreaticoduodenectomy: incidence, significance, and management. Am J Surg 1994;168(4):295–8.
[17] van Berge Henegouwen MI, De Wit LT, Van Gulik TM, et al. Incidence, risk factors, and treatment of pancreatic leakage after pancreaticoduodenectomy: drainage versus resection of the pancreatic remnant. J Am Coll Surg 1997;185(1):18–24.
[18] Grobmyer SR, Rivadeneira DE, Goodman CA, et al. Pancreatic anastomotic failure after pancreaticoduodenectomy. Am J Surg 2000;180(2):117–20.
[19] Buchler MW, Friess H, Wagner M, et al. Pancreatic fistula after pancreatic head resection. Br J Surg 2000;87(7):883–9.
[20] Bassi C, Dervenis C, Buttutini G, et al. Postoperative pancreatic fistula: an international study group (ISGPF) definition. Surgery 2005;138:8–13.
[21] Adams DB. The pancreatic anastomosis: the danger of a leak which anastomotic technique is better? J Gastrointest Surg 2009;13:1182–3.
[22] Berger AC, Howard TJ, Kennedy EP, et al. Does type of pancreaticojejunostomy after pancreaticoduodenectomy decrease rate of pancreatic fistula? A randomized, prospective, dual-institution trial. J Am Coll Surg 2009;208(5):738–47.
[23] Duffas JP, Suc B, Miska S, et al. A controlled randomized multicenter trial of pancreaticogastrostomy or pancreaticojejunostomy after pancreatoduodenectomy. Am J Surg 2005;189(6):720–9.

[24] Poon RT, Fan ST, Lo CM, et al. External drainage of pancreatic duct stent with a stent to reduce leakage rate of pancreaticojejunostomy after pancreaticoduodenectomy: a prospective randomized trial. Ann Surg 2007;246(3):425–35.

[25] Callery MP, Pratt WB, Vollmer CM. Prevention and management of pancreatic fistula. J Gastrointest Surg 2009;13:163–73.

[26] Lai EC, Lau SHY, Lau WY. Measures to prevent pancreatic fistula after pancreaticoduodenectomy. Arch Surg 2009;144(11):1074–80.

[27] Mahvi D. Defining, controlling, and treating a pancreatic fistula. J Gastrointest Surg 2009;13:1187–8.

[28] You D, Jung K, Lee H, et al. Comparison of different pancreatic anastomosis techniques using the definitions of the International Study Group of Pancreatic Surgery: a single surgeon's experience. Pancreas 2009;38(8):896–902.

[29] Oida T, Mimastu K, Kawasaki A, et al. Toward zero pancreatic leakage after pancreaticoduodenectomy for soft pancreas in low-volume pancreatic surgery centers. Hepatogastroenterology 2009;56(91):886–90.

[30] Parr ZE, Sutherland FR, Bathe OF, et al. Pancreatic fistulae: are we making progress? J Hepatobiliary Pancreat Surg 2008;15:1–7.

[31] Bartoli FG, Arnone GB, Ravera G, et al. Pancreatic fistula and relative mortality in malignant disease after pancreaticoduodenectomy: review and statistical meta-analysis regarding 15 years of literature. Anticancer Res 1991;11(5):1831–48.

[32] Strasberg SM, McNevin MS. Results of a technique of pancreaticojejunostomy that optimizes blood supply to the pancreas. J Am Coll Surg 1998;187(6):591–6.

[33] Strasberg SM, Drebin JA, Mokadam NA, et al. Prospective trial of a blood supply-based technique of pancreaticojejunostomy: effect on anastomotic failure in the Whipple procedure. J Am Coll Surg 2002;194(6):746–60.

[34] Hashimoto N, Ohyanagi H. Pancreatic juice output and amylase level in the drainage fluid after pancreaticoduodenectomy in relation to leakage. Hepatogastroenterology 2002;49(44):553–5.

[35] Shyr YM, Su CH, Wu CW, et al. Does drainage fluid amylase reflect pancreatic leakage after pancreaticoduodenectomy? World J Surg 2003;27(5):606–10.

[36] Shrikhande SV, Qureshi SS, Rajnessh N, et al. Pancreatic anastomoses after pancreaticoduodenectomy: do we need further studies? World J Surg 2005;29(12):1642–9.

[37] Molinari E, Bassi C, Salvia R, et al. Amylase value in drains after pancreatic resection as predictive factor of postoperative pancreatic fistula: results of a prospective study in 137 patients. Ann Surg 2007;246(2):281–7.

[38] Marcus SG, Cohen H, Ranson JH. Optimal management of the pancreatic remnant after pancreaticoduodenectomy. Ann Surg 1995;221(6):635–48.

[39] Yeo CJ, Cameron JL, Maher MM, et al. A prospective randomized trial of pancreaticogastrostomy versus pancreaticojejunostomy after pancreaticoduodenectomy. Ann Surg 1995;222(4):580–92.

[40] Sato N, Yamaguchi K, Chijiwa K, et al. Risk analysis of pancreatic fistula after pancreatic head resection. Arch Surg 1998;133(10):1094–8.

[41] Popiela T, Kedra B, Sierzega M, et al. Risk factors of pancreatic fistula following pancreaticoduodenectomy for periampullary cancer. Hepatogastroenterology 2004;51(59):1484–8.

[42] Yang YM, Tian XD, Zhuang Y, et al. Risk factors of pancreatic leakage after pancreatoduodenectomy. World J Gastroenterol 2005;11(16):2456–61.

[43] Murakami Y, Uemura K, Hayasidani Y, et al. A soft pancreatic remnant is associated with increased drain fluid pancreatic amylase and serum CRP levels following pancreatoduodenectomy. J Gastrointest Surg 2008;12(1):51–6.

[44] Kleespies A, Albertsmeier M, Obeidat F, et al. The challenge of pancreatic anastomosis. Langenbecks Arch Surg 2008;393:459–71.

[45] Pratt WB, Callery MP, Vollmer CM Jr. Risk prediction for development of pancreatic fistulas using the ISGPF classification scheme. World J Surg 2008;32(3):419–28.
[46] Lin JW, Cameron JL, Lillemoe KD, et al. Risk factors and outcomes in postpancreaticoduodenectomy pancreaticocutaneous fistula. J Gastrointest Surg 2004;8:951–9.
[47] Gouma DJ, van Greenen RC, van Gulik TM, et al. Rates of complications and death after pancreaticoduodenectomy: risk factors and the impact of hospital volume. Ann Surg 2002;232:786–95.
[48] Yeo CJ, Cameron JL, Lillemoe KD, et al. Does prophylactic octreotide decrease the rates of pancreatic fistula and other complications after pancreaticoduodenectomy? Results of a prospective randomized placebo-controlled trial. Ann Surg 2000;232:419–29.
[49] Yeh TS, Jan YY, Jeng LB, et al. Pancreaticojejunal anastomotic leak after pancreaticoduodenectomy-multivariate analysis of perioperative risk factors. J Surg Res 1997;67:119–25.
[50] Al Sharaf K, Ihse I, Dawiskiba S, et al. Characteristics of the gland remnant predict complications after subtotal pancreaticoduodenectomy. Dig Surg 1997;14:101–6.
[51] Wada K, Traverso LW. Pancreatic anastomotic leak after the Whipple procedure is reduced using the surgical microscope. Surgery 2006;39:736–42.
[52] Waugh JM, Clagett OT. Resection of the duodenum and head of the pancreas for carcinoma: an analysis of thirty cases. Surgery 1946;20:224–32.
[53] Fernàndez-Cruz L, Cosa R, Blanco L, et al. Pancreatogastrostomy with gastric partition after pylorus-preserving pancreatoduodenectomy versus conventional pancreaticojejunostomy: a prospective randomized study. Ann Surg 2008;248(6):930–8.
[54] Mason GR. Pancreatogastrostomy as reconstruction for pancreatoduodenectomy: review. World J Surg 1999;23:221–6.
[55] Declore R, Thomas JH, Pierce GE, et al. Pancreatogastrostomy: a safe drainage procedure after pancreatoduodenectomy. Surgery 1990;108(4):641–7.
[56] Bradbeer JW, Johnson CD. Pancreaticogastrostomy after pancreaticoduodenectomy. Ann R Coll Surg Engl 1990;72(4):266–9.
[57] Sauvanet A, Belghiti J, Panis Y, et al. Pancreaticogastrostomy after pancreatoduodenectomy. HPB Surg 1992;6(2):91–5.
[58] Takano S, Ito Y, Oishi H, et al. A retrospective analysis of 88 patients with pancreaticogastrostomy after pancreaticoduodenectomy. Hepatogastroenterology 2000;47(35):1454–7.
[59] Fabre JM, Arnaud JP, Navarro F, et al. Results of pancreaticogastrostomy after pancreaticoduodenectomy in 160 consecutive patients. Br J Surg 1998;85(6):751–4.
[60] Ihse I, Axelson J, Hansson L. Pancreaticogastrostomy after subtotal pancreatectomy for cancer. Dig Surg 1999;16(5):389–92.
[61] Kapur BM, Misra MC, Seenu V, et al. Pancreaticogastrostomy for reconstruction of pancreatic stump after pancreaticoduodenectomy for ampullary carcinoma. Am J Surg 1998;176(6):274–8.
[62] Pikarsky AJ, Muggia-Sullam M, Eid A, et al. Pancreaticogastrostomy after pancreatoduodenectomy. A retrospective study of 28 patients. Arch Surg 1997;132(3):296–9.
[63] Takao S, Shimazu H, Maenohara S, et al. Modified pancreaticogastrostomy following pancreaticoduodenectomy. Am J Surg 1993;165(3):317–21.
[64] Arnaud JP, Tuech JJ, Cervi C, et al. Pancreaticogastrostomy and pancreaticojejunostomy after pancreaticoduodenectomy. Eur J Surg 1999;165(4):357–62.
[65] Takano S, Ito Y, Watanabe Y, et al. Pancreaticojejunostomy versus pancreaticogastrostomy in reconstruction following pancreaticoduodenectomy. Br J Surg 2000;87(4):423–7.
[66] Wente MN, Shrikhande SV, Muller MW, et al. Pancreaticojejunostomy versus pancreaticogastrostomy: systematic review and meta-analysis. Am J Surg 2007;193(2):171–83.
[67] McKay A, Mackenzie S, Sutherland FR, et al. Meta-analysis of pancreaticojejunostomy versus pancreaticogastrostomy reconstruction after pancreaticoduodenectomy. Br J Surg 2006;93(8):929–36.
[68] Wellner U, Makowiec F, Fisher E, et al. Reduced postoperative pancreatic fistula after pancreatogastrostomy versus pancreaticojejunostomy. J Gastrointest Surg 2009;13(4):745–51.

[69] Kim JH, Yoo BM, Kim JH, et al. Which method should we select for pancreatic anastomosis after pancreaticoduodenectomy? World J Surg 2009;33(2):326–32.
[70] Ramesh H, Thomas PG. Pancreaticojejunostomy versus pancreaticogastrostomy in reconstruction following pancreaticoduodenectomy. Aust N Z J Surg 1990;60(12):973–6.
[71] Bassi C, Falconi M, Molinari E, et al. Reconstruction by pancreaticojejunostomy versus pancreaticogastrostomy following pancreatectomy: results of a comparative study. Ann Surg 2005;242(6):767–71.
[72] Lemaire E, O'Toole D, Sauvanet P, et al. Functional and morphological changes in the pancreatic remnant following pancreaticoduodenectomy with pancreaticogastric anastomosis. Br J Surg 2000;87(4):424–8.
[73] Pessaux P, Aube C, Lebigot J, et al. Permeability and functionality of pancreaticogastrostomy after pancreaticoduodenectomy with dynamic magnetic resonance pancreatography after secretin stimulation. J Am Coll Surg 2002;194(4):454–62.
[74] Konishi M, Ryu M, Kinoshita T, et al. Pathophysiology after pylorus-preserving pancreatoduodenectomy: a comparative study of pancreatogastrostomy and pancreatojejunostomy. Hepatogastroenterology 1999;46(26):1181–6.
[75] Rault A, SaCunha A, Klopfenstein D, et al. Pancreaticojejunal anastomosis is preferable to pancreaticogastrostomy after pancreaticoduodenectomy for long-term outcomes of pancreatic exocrine function. J Am Coll Surg 2005;201(2):239–44.
[76] Strasberg SM, Drebin JA, Soper NJ. Evolution and current status of the Whipple procedure: an update for gastroenterologists. Gastroenterology 1997;113:983–94.
[77] Peng SY, Wang JW, Lau WY, et al. Conventional versus binding pancreaticojejunostomy after pancreaticoduodenectomy: a prospective randomized trial. Ann Surg 2007;245(5):692–8.
[78] Peng SY, Mou YP, Liu YB, et al. Binding pancreaticojejunostomy: 150 consecutive cases without leakage. J Gastrointest Surg 2003;7(7):898–900.
[79] Buc E, Flamein R, Dubois A, et al. Peng's binding pancreaticojejunostomy after pancreaticoduodenectomy: a French prospective study. J Gastrointest Surg 2010;14(4):705–10.
[80] Chen XP, Qiu FZ, Zhang ZW, et al. A new simple and safe technique of end-to-end invaginated pancreaticojejunostomy with transpancreatic U-sutures. Early postoperative outcomes in consecutive 88 cases. Langenbecks Arch Surg 2009;394(4):739–44.
[81] Kleepsies A, Rentsch M, Seeliger H, et al. Blumgart anastomosis for pancreaticojejunostomy minimizes severe complications after pancreatic head resection. Br J Surg 2009;96:741–50.
[82] Ozdemir A, Karakoc D, Hamaloglu E, et al. Pancreaticojejunostomy after pancreaticoduodenectomy: results of a new technique. Hepatogastroenterology 2009;56(90):285–9.
[83] Chen HW, Lai EC, Su SY, et al. Modified technique of pancreatico-jejunal anastomosis with invagination following pancreaticoduodenectomy: a cohort study. World J Surg 2008;32(12):2695–700.
[84] Hosotani R, Doi R, Imamura M. Duct-to-mucosa pancreaticojejunostomy reduces the risk of pancreatic leakage after pancreatoduodenectomy. World J Surg 2002;26(1):99–104.
[85] Langrehr JM, Bahara M, Jacob D, et al. Prospective randomized comparison between a new mattress technique and Cattell (duct-to-mucosa) pancreaticojejunostomy for pancreatic resection. World J Surg 2005;29(9):1111–21.
[86] Lee SE, Yang SH, Jang YJ, et al. Pancreatic fistula after pancreaticoduodenectomy: a comparison between the two pancreaticojejunostomy methods for approximating the pancreatic parenchyma to the jejuna seromuscular layer: interrupted versus continuous stitches. World J Gastroenterol 2007;13(40):5351–6.
[87] Bassi C, Falconi M, Molinari E, et al. Duct-to-mucosa versus end-to-side pancreaticojejunostomy reconstruction after pancreaticoduodenectomy: results of a prospective randomized trial. Surgery 2003;134(5):766–71.
[88] Z'graggen K, Uhi W, Friess H, et al. How to do a safe pancreatic anastomosis. J Hepatobiliary Pancreat Surg 2002;9(6):733–7.

[89] Ibrahim S, Tay KH, Launois B, et al. Triple-layer duct-to-mucosa pancreaticojejunostomy after pancreaticoduodenectomy. Dig Surg 2006;23(5–6):296–302.
[90] Hayashibe A, Kameyama M. The clinical results of duct-to-mucosa pancreaticojejunostomy after pancreaticoduodenectomy in 55 consecutive cases. Pancreas 2007;35(3):273–5.
[91] Peng S, Mou Y, Cai X, et al. Binding pancreaticojejunostomy is a new technique to minimize leakage. Am J Surg 2002;183(3):283–5.
[92] Murakami Y, Uemura K, Hayashidani Y, et al. No mortality after 150 consecutive pancreaticoduodenectomies with duct-to-mucosa pancreaticogastrostomy. J Surg Oncol 2008;97(3):205–9.
[93] Grace PA, Pitt HA, Tompkins RK, et al. Decreased morbidity and mortality after pancreaticoduodenectomy. Am J Surg 1986;151(1):141–9.
[94] Funovics JM, Zoch G, Wenzel E, et al. Progress in reconstruction after resection of the head of the pancreas. Surg Gynecol Obstet 1987;164(4):545–8.
[95] Tsuji M, Kimura H, Konishi K, et al. Management of continuous anastomosis of pancreatic duct and jejuna mucosa after pancreaticoduodenectomy: historical study of 300 patients. Surgery 1998;123(6):617–21.
[96] Hwang TL, Jan YY, Chen MF. Secure pancreaticojejunal anastomosis for the pancreaticoduodenectomy. Hepatogastroenterology 1996;43(7):275–7.
[97] Kingsnorth AN. Safety and function of isolated Roux loop pancreaticojejunostomy after Whipple's pancreaticoduodenectomy. Ann R Coll Surg Engl 1994;76:175–9.
[98] Sikora SS, Posner MC. Management of the pancreatic stump following pancreaticoduodenectomy. Br J Surg 1995;82:1590–7.
[99] Albertson DA. Pancreaticoduodenectomy with reconstruction by Roux-en-Y pancreaticojejunostomy: no operative morality in a series of 25 cases. South Med J 1994;87(2):197–201.
[100] Hilal MA, Malik HZ, Hamilton-Burke W, et al. Modified Cattell's pancreaticojejunostomy, buttressing for soft pancreas and an isolated biliopancreatic loop are safety measurements that improve outcomes after pancreaticoduodenectomy: a pilot study. HPB (Oxford) 2009;11(2):154–60.
[101] Fragulidis GP, Arkadopolos N, Vassiliou I, et al. Pancreatic leakage after pancreaticoduodenectomy: the impact of the isolated jejunal loop length and anastomotic technique of the pancreatic stump. Pancreas 2009;38(7):177–82.
[102] Meyer C, Rohr S, DeManzini N, et al. Pancreatico-jejunal anastomosis with invagination on isolated loop after cephalic pancreaticoduodenectomy. Ann Ital Chir 1997;68(5):613–5.
[103] Papadimtriou JD, Fotopolous AC, Smyrnitis B, et al. Subtotal pancreatoduodenectomy: use of a defunctionalized loop for pancreatic stump drainage. Arch Surg 1999;134(2):135–9.
[104] Khan AW, Agarwal AK, Davidson BR. Isolated Roux loop duct-to-mucosa pancreaticojejunostomy avoids pancreatic leaks in pancreaticoduodenectomy. Dig Surg 2002;19(3):199–204.
[105] Sutton CD, Garcea G, White SA, et al. Isolated Roux-loop pancreaticojejunostomy: a series of 61 patients with zero postoperative pancreatic leaks. J Gastrointest Surg 2004;8(6):701–5.
[106] Perqaiz A, Singhal D, Singh A, et al. Is isolated Roux loop pancreaticojejunostomy superior to conventional reconstruction in pancreaticoduodenectomy? HPB (Oxford) 2009;11(4):326–31.
[107] Casadei R, Zanini N, Pezzilli R, et al. Reconstruction after pancreaticoduodenectomy: isolated Roux loop pancreatic anastomosis. Chir Ital 2008;60(5):641–9.
[108] Kaman L, Sanyal S, Behera A, et al. Isolated Roux loop pancreaticojejunostomy vs single loop pancreaticojejunostomy after pancreaticoduodenectomy. Int J Surg 2008;6(4):306–10.

[109] Lee SE, Ahn YJ, Kim SW. Prospective randomized pilot trial comparing closed suction drainage and gravity drainage of the pancreatic duct in pancreaticojejunostomy. J Hepatobiliary Pancreat Surg 2009;16(6):837–43.

[110] Yoshimi F, Ono H, Asato Y, et al. Internal stenting of the hepaticojejunostomy and pancreaticojejunostomy in patients undergoing pancreaticoduodenectomy to promote earlier discharge from hospital. Surg Today 1996;26(8):665–7.

[111] Shibuya T, Uchiyama K, Imai S, et al. Improvement of pancreaticojejunostomy in pancreaticoduodenectomy. Int Surg 1995;80:57–60.

[112] Imaizumi T, Hatori T, Tobita K, et al. Pancreaticojejunostomy using duct-to-mucosa anastomosis without a stenting tube. J Hepatobiliary Pancreat Surg 2006;13(3):194–201.

[113] Smyrniotis V, Arkadopolous N, Kyriazi MA, et al. Does internal stenting of the pancreaticojejunostomy improve outcomes after pancreaticoduodenectomy? A prospective study. Langenbecks Arch Surg 2010;395(3):195–200.

[114] Winter JM, Cameron JL, Campbell KA, et al. Does pancreatic duct stenting decrease the rate of pancreatic fistula following pancreaticoduodenectomy? Results of a prospective randomized trial. J Gastrointest Surg 2006;10(9):1280–90.

[115] Howard JM. Pancreaticojejunostomy: leakage is a preventable complication of the Whipple resection. J Am Coll Surg 1997;184(5):545–7.

[116] Hamanaka Y, Suzuki T. Total pancreatic duct drainage for leakproof pancreatojejunostomy. Surgery 1994;115(1):22–6.

[117] Mok KT, Wang BW, Liu SI. Management of pancreatic remnant with strategies according to the size of pancreatic duct after pancreaticoduodenectomy. Br J Surg 1999;86(8): 1018–9.

[118] Satoi S, Toyokawa H, Yanagimoto H, et al. Is a nonstented duct-to-mucosa anastomosis using modified Kakita method a safe procedure? Pancreas 2010;39(2):165–70.

[119] Roder JD, Stein HJ, Bottcher KA, et al. Stented versus nonstented pancreaticojejunostomy after pancreaticoduodenectomy. A prospective study. Ann Surg 1999;229(3):41–8.

[120] Ohwada S, Tanahashi Y, Ogawa T, et al. In situ vs. ex situ pancreatic duct stents of duct-to-mucosa pancreaticojejunostomy after pancreaticoduodenectomy with Billroth type I reconstruction. Arch Surg 2002;137(11):1289–93.

[121] Tani M, Kawai M, Hirono S, et al. A prospective randomized controlled trial of internal versus external drainage with pancreaticojejunostomy for pancreaticoduodenectomy. Am J Surg 2010. [Epub ahead of print].

[122] Suzuki S, Kaji S, Koike N, et al. Pancreaticojejunostomy of duct to mucosa anastomosis can be performed more safely without than with a stenting tube. Am J Surg 1009; 198(1):51–54.

[123] Petrowsky H, Demartines N, Roussan V, et al. Evidence-based value of prophylactic drainage in gastrointestinal surgery: a systematic review and meta-analyses. Ann Surg 2004;240(6):1074–85.

[124] Fong Y, Brennan MF, Brown K, et al. Drainage is unnecessary after elective liver resection. Am J Surg 1996;171(1):158–62.

[125] Grobmeyer SR, Graham D, Brennan MF, et al. High-pressure gradients generated by closed-suction surgical drainage systems. Surg Infect (Larchmt) 2002;3(3):245–9.

[126] Whitson BA, Richardson E, Iaizzo PA, et al. Not every bulb is a rose: a functional comparison of bulb suction devices. J Surg Res 2009;156(2):270–3.

[127] Heslin MJ, Harrison LE, Brooks AS, et al. Is intra-abdominal drainage necessary after pancreaticoduodenectomy? J Gastrointest Surg 1998;2(4):373–8.

[128] Conlon KC, Labow D, Leung D, et al. Prospective randomized clinical trial of the value of intraperitoneal drainage after pancreatic resection. Ann Surg 2001;234(4):487–94.

[129] Molinari E, Bassi C, Salvia R, et al. Amylase value in drains for evidenced based fast track in pancreatic surgery: results of a randomized clinical trial [Abstract]. Presented at the 8th Annual Congress of the European HPB Association. Athens, Greece, June 18–20, 2009.

Advances in Surgery 44 (2010) 149–164

ADVANCES IN SURGERY

Adjuvant Chemoradiation Therapy for Pancreas Cancer: Who Really Benefits?

Nipun B. Merchant, MD*, Alexander A. Parikh, MD, Eric H. Liu, MD

Division of Surgical Oncology & Endocrine Surgery, Department of Surgery, Vanderbilt University Medical Center, 597 Preston Research Building, 2220 Pierce Avenue, Nashville, TN 37232-6860, USA

Pancreas cancer remains a major health care problem. In 2009, there were an estimated 42,470 new cases and 35,240 deaths from pancreas cancer, making it the 11th most common cause of cancer but the 4th most common cause of cancer-related death in the United States [1]. Over the past four decades, there has been minimal impact on survival outcomes for this disease, with case fatality rates remaining at approximately 95%.

Most patients with pancreas cancer present with advanced disease at the time of diagnosis, and only 15% to 20% of patients are candidates for potentially curative resection [2–4]. Despite attempted curative resection, the majority of patients eventually recur locally and systemically and ultimately die of the disease, presumably because of the presence of micrometastatic disease present at the time of diagnosis [5–7]. Such a high rate of recurrence implies that surgical resection alone is not adequate and that adjuvant therapies are needed. As a result, much effort has been put into actively pursuing multimodality treatment strategies, including the use of chemotherapy and radiation therapy. The few prospective randomized trials that have been completed and some large retrospective reviews attempting to improve treatment practices regarding adjuvant therapy have failed to establish a definitive standard of care due to study limitations. The purpose of this article is to review the current data in adjuvant and neoadjuvant strategies for pancreas cancer and to better define which patients may benefit from these therapies.

HISTORICAL ADJUVANT TRIALS

Gastrointestinal Tumor Study Group

The standard of care for adjuvant therapy for pancreas cancer in the United States was largely based on the small randomized Gastrointestinal Tumor Study Group (GITSG) trial, published in 1985 [8]. Patients were randomized after resection to observation alone versus bolus 5-fluorouracil (5-FU) chemotherapy

*Corresponding author. *E-mail address:* nipun.merchant@vanderbilt.edu.

0065-3411/10/$ – see front matter
doi:10.1016/j.yasu.2010.05.019

plus split-course radiotherapy (total 40 Gy), followed by weekly 5-FU for 2 years or until disease recurrence was noted. This trial closed early, enrolling only 43 patients over 8 years, with only 30 patients subsequently treated according to the study arm. An interim analysis performed at the time showed a significant improvement in overall median survival in the adjuvant therapy group compared with resection alone (20 months and 11 months, respectively; $P = .035$) with a 2-year survival of 42% versus 15% and 5-year survival of 19% versus 0%, respectively.

As the first such trial reported, trials helped to establish adjuvant chemoradiation therapy (CRT) for patients with resected pancreas cancer as the standard of care in the United States. This trial was, however, fraught with limitations because of its small sample size, slow accrual, and the use of an out-dated split-course radiation regimen and, therefore, is now considered only in historical context.

The European Organisation for Research and Treatment of Cancer

In reaction to the findings of the GITSG trial, the multicenter European Organisation for Research and Treatment of Cancer (EORTC) trial randomized 218 patients with periampullary cancers from 29 European centers to observation alone versus 5-FU plus split-course radiation therapy during radiation. Median survival was not significantly different between the two arms (24.5 vs 19 months, $P = .208$). Although this study was improved by its increased accrual of patients, its results are hard to apply because multiple tumor types were included in the trial. Of the total cohort of patients, 114 patients had pancreas head adenocarcinomas, whereas the others had various periampullary malignancies. Survival outcomes of these different tumor types are clearly disparate and although the two groups were stratified before randomization, this study was not powered or structured to distinguish survival outcomes between the different tumor types. Even for the patients with pancreatic adenocarcinoma, there was a nonsignificant in survival for the adjuvant therapy group (17.1 months vs 12.6 months; $P = .099$); 2-year and 5-year survival for the treatment arm and the observation arm were 37% versus 20% and 23% versus 10%, respectively.

MODERN ADJUVANT THERAPY TRIALS

European Study Group of Pancreas Cancer-1

The early trials sought to answer the question of the benefit of adjuvant in patients with pancreas cancer. The European Study Group of Pancreatic Cancer (ESPAC)-1 trial attempted to answer the question of the role of adjuvant chemotherapy, radiation therapy, or CRT [10–12]. This trial analyzed 289 patients from 53 hospitals in a complicated 2 × 2 factorial study design randomizing resected pancreas cancer patients to (1) observation, (2) adjuvant chemotherapy alone (5-FU, 425 mg/m^2 and leucovorin, 20 mg/m^2 daily for 5 days every 28 days for 6 cycles, for a total of 28 weeks), (3) adjuvant CRT (40 Gy given with 5-FU as a sensitizing agent, using the same schedule as the GITSG trial), or (4) adjuvant CRT followed by chemotherapy. Patients were stratified by margin status at initial randomization. The primary endpoint was to look for an improvement in the 2-year survival of 20% to 40% in patients with negative margins for each of the two randomizations. The investigators estimated that 220 margin-negative patients would give a power of 90% with an α of 0.05 for each randomization procedure. This analysis means that the study was not powered to perform comparisons between each of the arms that result from the 2×2 randomization schema. Because this trial did allow enrollment of margin-positive patients, the accrual plan was to enroll 280 patients in the analysis to reach the goal of 220 margin-negative patients in each arm. In addition to the 2×2 factorial design, an additional 256 patients were allowed "on-study" by the treating physician and allocated to participate in only one of the two randomizations – CRT versus observation or chemotherapy versus observation. These patients were not intended to be part of the planned analysis and thus were appropriately excluded from the final results, which is fortunate, because this cohort included periampullary cancers and non-ductal carcinomas and would have introduced significant heterogeneity into the analysis.

Although a complicated analysis was reported, the major study conclusions of this trial showed that the 5-year overall survival for patients who received chemotherapy versus those who did not was significantly improved (21% vs 8%, $P = .009$) and those who received radiation therapy actually did worse than patients who did not receive radiation therapy (10% vs 20%, $P = .05$). Based on these results, the investigators concluded that adjuvant chemotherapy was beneficial for patients with resected pancreas adenocarcinoma whereas adjuvant CRT was actually detrimental. When the 2×2 factorial arms and the single-randomization arms were analyzed for prognostic factors, the benefit of chemotherapy appeared most pronounced in patients with well-differentiated tumors, lymph node (LN)-positive disease, and margin-negative resection.

The ESPAC-1 trial helped establish a clear role for chemotherapy in the adjuvant setting as well as introduced controversy regarding the role of radiation therapy. The investigators of the trial suggested that the CRT protocol used in this trial may have been detrimental because it delayed the start of full-dose chemotherapy and used a 2-week rest period in the middle of therapy, which is considered suboptimal, because it potentially allowed for growth of tumor cells during that period of time. There were also compliance issues with the CRT administration, with patients receiving variable doses of radiotherapy despite a recommended dose of 40 Gy. Perhaps as important, there was no central review of radiation ports for quality assurance purposes. Therefore, this trial may not adequately evaluate the role of modern radiotherapy regimens in the adjuvant setting.

Additional data from this trial as well as some composite data from subsequent trials, the ESPAC-1 plus trial and the ESPAC-3(v1) trial, were reported in 2009, and recapitulate the results reported in 2004 [13]. The ESPAC-1 plus trial was a cohort of 192 patients who were entered into a randomized comparison between 5-FU and observation alone with clinician's choice of background CRT if indicated. This cohort was conducted as part of the ESPAC-1 trial, adhering to the same eligibility criteria and treatment schedules, and was intended to be additional evidence and therefore was not powered for any analysis apart from the larger ESPAC-1 cohort. The ESPAC-3(v1) trial was initially a three-arm study of adjuvant 5-FU versus gemcitabine versus observation alone. After the publication of the results of the larger ESPAC-1 trial, the observation arm was dropped from ESPAC-3(v2), and some preliminary results were published after accrual of 122 patients to this substudy. The combined analysis of pooled data from each of these component studies again showed the benefit of adjuvant chemotherapy, with overall survival in patients randomized to receive 5-FU exceeding that of patients treated with surgery alone, with a pooled hazard ratio for death of 0.70 in the chemotherapy arm ($P = .003$). The composite 2-year survival rate was reported as 49% for the 5-FU arm, compared with 37% for the observation arm [13].

Charité Onkologie–001

Since the publication of the ESPAC-1 trial, two additional randomized phase III trials reported data providing further insight into the optimal adjuvant therapy for patients with resected pancreas cancer. The first was the Charité Onkologie (CONKO)-001 trial conducted in Germany and Austria, which randomized 368 patients from 88 centers comparing adjuvant chemotherapy with gemcitabine (1000 mg/m^2 weekly, 3 out of 4 weeks for 6 cycles) versus observation alone [14]. Patients were randomized on a 1:1 basis and stratified for resection status (R0 vs R1), T status (T1-2 vs T3-4), and nodal status (N^+ vs N^-). The primary endpoint of the trial was disease-free survival, with a secondary endpoint of overall survival. After a median follow-up time of 53 months, estimated disease-free survival was 13.4 months in the gemcitabine arm compared with 6.9 months in the control arm ($P = .001$), regardless of margin status, tumor size, or nodal involvement. At the time of initial publication, there was no statistically significant benefit seen in overall survival between the two groups. However, at the annual meeting of the American Society of Clinical Oncology (ASCO) in 2008, the updated results showed that patients receiving adjuvant gemcitabine had a median survival rate of 22.8 months versus 20.2 months for patients undergoing surgery alone ($P = .005$) [15]. Estimated 5-year survival for the gemcitabine arm was 21% compared with 9% in the observation arm. This benefit was also likely somewhat diluted by patients receiving gemcitabine at the time of relapse, potentially making the true effect even larger than reported.

Radiation Therapy Oncology Group 9704

RTOG 9704 was a large intergroup study conducted by the Radiation Therapy Oncology Group (RTOG), the Eastern Cooperative Oncology Group (ECOG), and the Southwest Oncology Group (SWOG), inclusive of Canadian affiliates. This trial included 451 patients with adenocarcinoma of the pancreas, with T3 or T4 disease in 75% of patients and node-positive disease in approximately 66% of patients; one-third of patients had positive margins. Randomization was performed after surgery and was stratified by tumor diameter (<3 cm or ≥3 cm) and surgical margins (33% of patients had positive surgical margins). Patients were randomly assigned to either 5-FU (continuous infusion 250 mg/m^2 for 3 weeks, 1 cycle pre-radiation therapy, and 2 cycles post-radiation therapy) or gemcitabine (1000 mg/m^2 weekly for 3 weeks, 1 cycle pre-radiation therapy, and 3 cycles post-radiation therapy) followed by identical CRT regimens (50.4 Gy with continuous infusion of 250 mg/m^2 of 5-FU daily through the course of radiation therapy). Prospective quality assurance procedures were used, including central review of preoperative CT scans and radiation therapy fields before initiation of CRT.

In the final analysis, 451 evaluable patients were included and no difference in overall or disease-free survival between the treatment groups was seen [16]. A subgroup analysis of patients with tumors in the head of the pancreas (eliminating patients with resected body and tail lesions) was performed and showed a significant improvement in median survival for patients receiving gemcitabine compared with those receiving 5-FU (18.8 vs 16.7 months, $P = .047$) and an also an improved 3-year survival (31% vs 22%, respectively). After adjusting for prespecified stratification variables of nodal status, tumor diameter, and surgical margin status, the gemcitabine treatment effect yielded a hazard ratio of 0.80 ($P = .05$). At time of relapse, 82% of patients in the 5-FU group received gemcitabine, so it is speculated that salvage gemcitabine therapy may have weakened the effect observed for overall survival [16]. Based on these results, this adequately powered trial concluded that the addition of gemcitabine to adjuvant 5-FU plus CRT is superior to the addition of 5-FU alone but did not address the issue of whether or not CRT added any benefit to chemotherapy alone.

ESPAC-3(v2)

Taken together, the results of the trials (detailed previously) suggest that patients with resected pancreas cancer are likely to benefit from adjuvant chemotherapy with 5-FU or gemcitabine, irrespective of margin status or nodal status. Further support for this statement comes from ESPAC-3(v2), reported at the ASCO annual meeting in 2009. In this study, more than 1000 patients were randomized to 5-FU 425 mg/m^2 daily × 5 given every 4 weeks with leucovorin 20 mg/m^2 on the same schedule or gemcitabine given on the same schedule as on the CONKO-001 study. There was no difference in disease-free survival or overall survival between the two treatment arms, with 23 months median survival in the 5-FU arm compared with 23.6 months median survival in the gemcitabine arm [17].

EORTC (40013)

Although RTOG 9704 was a well-designed and conducted study, it did not answer the question about the benefit, or perhaps potential detriment, of adding radiation therapy. A new, EORTC randomized phase II trial (40013) comparing gemcitabine alone to gemcitabine plus radiation using modern

CRT techniques (1000 mg/m^2 for 2 cycles followed by weekly gemcitabine 300 mg/m^2 with 50.4 Gy given in 28 fractions of 1.8 Gy) was reported at the 2009 ASCO annual meeting. Ninety patients were randomized to chemotherapy or to CRT. The overall survival for both arms was 24 months; however, there was a significant improvement in local control with the use of CRT [18]. Because local control is of limited benefit when systemic disease is the main driver of survival, it may be difficult to demonstrate benefit for radiation therapy until the systemic treatment of pancreas cancer improves.

PHASE II STUDIES

Virginia Mason Protocol

In 2000, Picozzi and colleagues [19] published their results using a novel, interferon-based adjuvant CRT protocol. Their experimental therapy included radiation therapy (4.5 Gy to 5.4 Gy, 25 fractions over 5 weeks), a 3-drug chemotherapy regimen of continuous infusion 5-FU (200 mg/m^2 daily, days 1 to 35), weekly intravenous bolus cisplatin (30 mg/m^2 daily; days 1, 8, 15, 22, and 29), and subcutaneous interferon-α (3×10^6 units, days 1 to 35). This CRT was followed by continuous infusion 5-FU (200 mg/m^2 daily, weeks 9 to 14 and 17 to 22).

They reported results of 43 patients with a median follow-up of 22 months and showed actuarial overall survival rates for the 1-, 2-, and 5-year periods were 95% (CI, 91% to 98%), 64% (CI, 56% to 72%), and 55% (CI, 46% to 65%), respectively [20]. These impressive results are the highest survival outcomes for patients with pancreas cancer of any adjuvant therapy trial to date. This regimen is criticized, however, for its significant toxicity, with 70% of patients developing grade 3 or 4 toxicities, and 42% of patients requiring hospitalization, virtually all due to gastrointestinal toxicity.

Washington University Interferon-Based Regimen

In response to the results of the Virginia Mason protocol, investigators at Washington University Hospital instituted a phase II, single-arm trial of a modified interferon-based CRT regimen for patients with resectable pancreatic adenocarcinoma [21]. In an attempt to reduce toxicity, this treatment strategy included 3-D conformal radiation (5.4 Gy, 25 fractions over 6 weeks), to limit the volume of bowel in the radiation field, and a simultaneous 3-drug chemotherapy consisting of reduced doses of continuous infusion 5-FU (175 mg/m^2), weekly intravenous bolus cisplatin (25 mg/m^2), and interferon-α (3×10^6 units subcutaneously 3 times per week). To improve the efficacy of the post-CRT phase of treatment, gemcitabine (1000 mg/m^2, 3 of 4 weeks) was used instead of 5-FU.

At a median follow-up of 38 months, the median overall survival was 25 months (CI, 21.5–48.5 months). Actuarial overall survival rates for the 1-, 2- and 3-year periods was 75% (CI, 61%–85%), 56% (CI, 41%–69%), and 41% (CI, 26%–55%), respectively. Although the survival outcomes remain impressive, the toxicity of this regimen was persistent, as 30% of patients failed to complete adjuvant therapy and no patients completed planned therapy without dose modification.

Despite the toxicity, the survival results of both of these interferon-based regimens are promising and cannot be overlooked. The American College of Surgeons Oncology Group (ACOSOG) has recently completed a phase II trial using the Virginia Mason protocol in 89 patients to better clarify the efficacy and toxicity of this aggressive regimen and the results are awaited.

RETROSPECTIVE DATA

Two large retrospective single institutional studies also contribute to our understanding of the role of adjuvant CRT in pancreas cancer and are worth mention. A large review of 616 patients from Johns Hopkins Hospital from 1993 to 2005 compared outcomes of 271 patients who received adjuvant 5-FU based CRT and 345 patients who underwent surgery alone [22]. Patients receiving CRT had significantly improved median survival (21.2 months with CRT vs 14.4 months with surgery alone, $P < .001$). Moreover, even after adjusting for multiple variables, including tumor size, grade, margin, and nodal status, CRT still demonstrated a significant protective effect. A subset analysis suggested that LN-positive patients showed a benefit whereas node-negative patients did not. As a retrospective analysis, there did seem to be selection bias of patients receiving CRT – those receiving CRT tended to be younger, have less comorbid disease, and have fewer post-operative complications.

An analysis from the Mayo Clinic of 472 consecutive patients with negative resection margins from 1975 to 2005 also showed a significant survival benefit with the use of adjuvant CRT [23]. In this study, 274 patients received adjuvant CRT, most receiving concomitant 5-FU, whereas 180 were observed after surgical resection. Radiation doses varied widely, from 13.8 to 60 Gy. Those receiving CRT had improved survival (25.2 vs 19.2 months, $P = .001$) with improved 2-year and 5-year overall survival. Like other single institutional studies, selection bias was a large concern, and in this study, no data were presented regarding the demographic differences between the two groups.

Although these two studies evaluate a large number of patients, they are limited by single-institution biases and by analysis of patients treated over many years, during which time diagnostic capabilities, operative morbidity and mortality, and techniques of delivery of radiation and chemotherapy have improved substantially [24,25].

Surveillance, Epidemiology, and End Results Data

A recent analysis of the Surveillance, Epidemiology, and End Results (SEER) database evaluated 2636 patients with resected pancreas cancer from 1988 to 2003 [26]. Of these, 1123 patients received adjuvant radiation therapy and 1513 did not. With a mean follow-up time of 19 months, median overall survival for patients receiving radiation therapy was 18 months compared with 11 months for the group that did not receive radiation therapy ($P < .01$). Furthermore, the use of radiation therapy was an independent predictor of survival after adjusting for age, race, gender, and tumor grade and stage. The limitations of this study include the lack of data on chemotherapy, margin status, and performance status.

Central pancreas consortium

Given the many intrinsic flaws of the available data, only limited conclusions can be drawn from the disparate results on the use of adjuvant CRT. Some trials suggest that a subset of patients with pancreas cancer benefit from CRT. None of these trials was powered to analyze subsets of patients, however. To overcome some of these limitations, a recent multicenter study from the Central Pancreas Consortium evaluated the outcomes of 747 patients with pancreatic adenocarcinomas who underwent resection at seven high-volume pancreas centers between 1996 and 2006 [27]. Of the 747 patients identified, 374 had surgery alone and 299 had adjuvant CRT. When evaluating the total cohort, patients receiving CRT after surgery had significantly improved survival (20 vs 14.5 months, $P = .001$). On subset and multivariate analysis, patients with LN-positive disease had a significantly improved survival with adjuvant CRT (19.4 vs 10.4 months, $P < .01$), whereas patients who were LN negative did not show any benefit from CRT (22.9 vs 24.2 months, $P = .774$). Patients with both R0 and R1 resection margins benefited from adjuvant CRT. When resection margin and LN status were analyzed together, only the LN-positive patients had a significantly improved survival with CRT, regardless of margin status (R0 or R1). Similarly, LN-negative patients showed no benefit with adjuvant CRT even in patients with R1 resection margins.

The strength of this study comes from the multi-institutional contribution, the large number of subjects, and the inclusion of recent patients undergoing modern surgery and CRT. Single-institutional practice biases are eliminated and its large numbers make subset analyses more meaningful. The study is inherently limited by its retrospective structure and differences in chemotherapeutic regimens, however. Demographic differences between surgery alone and CRT groups included age, margin status, and length of stay after surgery, suggesting that treatment recommendation biases may exist.

Despite these limitations, these data provide valuable information suggesting that adjuvant CRT is beneficial only in the subset of patients who are LN positive. This survival benefit of CRT may be diluted in studies because patients are not stratified by LN or margin status and future trials may need to consider stratification of these patients.

Interpretation of studies

Assembling all the available clinical data into a unified recommendation for adjuvant therapy in patients with resected pancreas cancer has proved a challenge (Table 1) [28]. Clearly, GITSG, EORTC, ESPAC-1, RTOG, and CONKO-001 have established the world opinion of adjuvant therapy, but as a group they failed to define a standard treatment regimen.

Limitations of these trials include small number of patients in the treatment arms (GITSG), poor compliance with the treatment regimens (GITSG,

Table 1
Selected major prospective and retrospective studies of adjuvant therapy for pancreatic adenocarcinoma

	N			All patients		Treatment									
						All pts		R0		R1		LN-		LN+	
Study, year	Obs	Adj	Adjuvant regimen	R1 (%)	LN+ (%)	Obs	Adj	Obs	Adj	Obs	Adj	Obs	Adj	Obs	Adj
GITSG, 1985	22	21	5FU (500mg/m^2 bolus) + 40 Gy Split course XRT	NA	NA	11	20*	-	-	-	-	-	-	-	-
EORTC, 1999	108	110	5FU (25 mg/kg CI)+40 Gy Split course XRT	21	46[$]	12	15.6[$]	-	-	-	-	-	-	-	-
ESPAC-1, 2001	178[†]	175	5FU (500mg/m^2 bolus) + 40 Gy Split course XRT	18	46	16.1[†]	15.5	16.9[†]	15.9	12.1[†]	10.9	-	-	-	-
	235[‡]	238	5-FU (425 mg/m^2) + Leucovorin (20 mg/m^2)	18		14.0	19.7*	15.3	20.7*	10.3	11.0	-	-	-	-
Picozzi et al, 2003	NA	43	5-FU + cisplatin + interferon-α	NA	NA	NA	NA	NA	NA	NA	NA	NA	NA	NA	NA
CONKO-001, 2007	175	179	Gemcitabine (1000 mg/m^2)	17	72	20.2	22.8*	20.8	21.7	14.1	22.1	27.6	34*	18.2	18.5
SEER, 2007	1513	1123	XRT	NA	45	11	18*	NA	NA	NA	NA	-	-	8	17*
Hopkins, 2008	345	271	5FU + 50 Gy XRT	45	80	14.4	21.2*	17	24.3*	11.4	18.3*	15.9	23.2	14.3	20.6
Mayo, 2008	180	274	5FU + 50.4Gy XRT	NA	48	19.2	25.2*	19.2	25.2*	NA	NA	26.4	43.2*	14.4	20.4*
Linehan et al, 2008	NA	53	5FU + cisplatin + interferon-α + 50.4 XRT		77	NA	25	NA	NA	NA	NA	NA	NA	NA	NA
CPC, 2009	374	299	Mainly 5FU +XRT	26	60	14.5	20.0*	15.9	23.4*	8.9	15.0*	24.2	22.9	10.4	19.4*

Abbreviations: Adj, adjuvant therapy; CPC, central pancreas consortium; Obs, surgery alone; XRT, radiation therapy.
*$p<0.05$.
[$]Pancreatic adenocarcinoma only.
[†]No CRT group.
[‡]No chemotherapy group.

EORTC, and ESPAC-1), inclusion of patients with pancreatic adenocarcinoma and other periampullary malignancies (EORTC and ESPAC-1), and flawed randomization schemes (ESPAC-1). In addition, these studies had variable pathologic criteria for study entry–GITSG excluded node-positive patients, the EORTC trial excluded T3 and T4 tumors, and CONKO-001 excluded patients with CA19-9 or carcinoembryonic antigen levels greater than 2.5 normal. Furthermore, despite studying a similar patient population, these studies have at least 22 variations in study design, execution, and analysis [28].

So, with these inherent limitations, how do we best interpret the results? All the trials can be organized around three major issues of adjuvant therapy in resected pancreas cancer:

1. The value of adjuvant chemotherapy (ESPAC-1, CONKO-001, ESPAC-3),
2. The value of adjuvant CRT (GITSG, EORTC, ESPAC-1), and
3. The issue of the choice of chemotherapy when radiation therapy is administered (RTOG).

Role of adjuvant chemotherapy in resected pancreas cancer

The rationale for systemic chemotherapy with or without radiotherapy in the management of resected pancreas cancer is based on the high risk of systemic and locoregional recurrence after surgery alone, demonstrating the systemic nature of this disease from the outset. Both trials evaluating the role of adjuvant chemotherapy therapy, ESPAC-1 and CONKO-001, found significant survival benefit in resected patients. Based on those results, the question is not if systemic chemotherapy should be given but how best to give it. ESPAC-1 showed benefit from 5-FU–based chemotherapy whereas CONKO-001 showed benefit of gemcitabine. The RTOG 9704 trial suggested an advantage of gemcitabine over 5-FU (in the setting of CRT). The ESPAC-3 trial did not find a difference between adjuvant 5-FU and gemcitabine. From these results, current recommendations would include the use of 6 months of adjuvant chemotherapy with 5-FU or gemcitabine as the standard adjuvant therapy for patients with resected pancreas cancer.

Role of radiation therapy in resected pancreas cancer

The rationale to use radiation therapy in the adjuvant setting in patients with resected pancreas cancer is the high local recurrence rates (up to 50%) after surgery alone and even with adjuvant chemotherapy as evidenced by the 34% local recurrence in patients who received gemcitabine therapy in the CONKO-001 trial.

The results of trials examining the role of adjuvant CRT, however, have significantly disparate results and the role of radiation as a component of adjuvant therapy continues to spark considerable debate. The GITSG trial showed a benefit, the EORTC trial showed no benefit, and ESPAC-1 actually showed worse outcomes in patients that received CRT. RTOG 9704 confirmed the benefit of gemcitabine over 5-FU when administering CRT. This trial also showed the importance of adhering to well-defined radiotherapy guidelines, which may actually be a more significant prognostic factor than the choice of chemotherapeutic agent.

Based on these data, no single adjuvant regimen of CRT can claim superiority over another (although gemcitabine chemotherapy should be considered). Where radiation therapy seems most beneficial is in subsets of patients, such as those with LN-positive disease (Central Pancreas Consortium) or patients with an R1 resection who are considered at increased risk for locoregional recurrence.

Neoadjuvant therapy

The benefit of neoadjuvant therapy has been well established in other cancer types, notably esophageal and rectal cancer. Pancreas cancer is emerging as a potential entity that may benefit from pre-resection treatment. The rationale for the neoadjuvant approach are numerous and include early delivery of systemic therapy in what is clearly a systemic disease; delivery of systemic chemotherapy to a well-vascularized tumor bed; potentially downsizing tumors and increasing margin negative resection rates; providing time to identify patients with aggressive tumor biology that may not benefit from surgical resection; and testing the susceptibility of therapies to improve effectiveness of adjuvant therapy. In addition, anastomotic leak rates after neoadjuvant radiation therapy have been shown significantly reduced in patients undergoing pancreaticoduodenectomy [29,30].

A major limitation of treating patients postoperatively includes delay or cancellation of adjuvant therapy if complications occur after pancreas resection, making the neoadjuvant approach more attractive [9,25,31].

Although several trials have been performed examining the use of neoadjuvant therapy, no prospective randomized trial exists (Table 2). Several phase I/II trials, mostly championed by the University of Texas MD Anderson Cancer Center Pancreatic Tumor Study Group, have studied preoperative CRT regimens in patients with potentially resectable pancreas cancer using standardized definitions of resectability, surgical technique, and margin assessment [6,32]. These trials have demonstrated low rates of R1 resection margins, low rates of postoperative local recurrence, survival rates comparable to those reported in the large adjuvant therapy trials, and feasibility in resectable patients.

The neoadjuvant approach has found its place in patients with locally advanced and borderline resectable disease. The ACOSOG has initiated a multicenter, single-arm phase II trial of pre- and postoperative gemcitabine and erlotinib for patients with localized, resectable pancreas cancer (ACOSOG Z5041). This trial will help determine whether or not preoperative treatment is feasible and worthy of further exploration on a larger scale in the cooperative group context.

Challenges for future trials

There are many challenges to optimal clinical trial design to test the question of adjuvant therapy for pancreas cancer [33]. Outcomes in pancreas cancer are

Table 2
Studies of neoadjuvant therapy for pancreatic adenocarcinoma

Study, year	N	Neoadjuvant regimen	Resection rate	Positive margin	Median survival: All patients	Median survival: Resected patients
Yeung et al, 1993[a]	26	MMC, 5-FU + 50.4 Gy	38%	0%	11	NR
Staley et al, 1996	39	5-FU + 50.4 Gy/30 Gy + IORT	100%[c]	18%	19[c]	19
Hoffman et al, 1998[a]	53	5-FU, MMC + 50.4 Gy	45%	33%	11	16
Pisters et al, 1998	35	5-FU + 30 Gy + IORT	57%	10%	NA	25
Pisters et al, 2002	37	Paclitaxel + 30 Gy +IORT	54%	32%	12	19
White, 2004	96	5-FU, 50.4 Gy, ± MMC, ± cis	55%	25%	NA	39
Moutardier et al, 2004	61	Cis, 5-FU + 45–60 Gy	66%	7.5%	13	27
Mornex et al, 2005	41	Cis, 5-FU +50 Gy	63%	NA	12	13
Talamonti et al, 2006	20	Gem + 36 Gy	85%	6%	NA	26
Palmer et al, 2007	24	Gem	38%	25%[b]	9	28
	26	Gem, cis	70%	25%[b]	16	
Evans et al, 2008	86	Gem + 30 Gy	74%	11% (6%[b])	23	34
Varadhachary et al, 2008	90	Cis, Gem +30 Gy	58%	4% (2%[b])	17	31

Abbreviations: Cis, cisplatin; Gem, gemcitabine; IORT, intraoperative radiotherapy; MMC, mitomycin C; NA, not available; NR, not reached.

[a] Also included patients with locally advanced disease.

[b] Posterior (retroperitoneal) margin positive rate.

[c] Only patients who underwent resection were included.

influenced by numerous variables that have not been accounted for in clinical trial design, including margin status, tumor differentiation, and extent of LN involvement. Furthermore, patient selection and inadequate preoperative staging have been the Achilles' heel in studying pancreas cancer. Standardization of surgical technique and pathologic assessment of the resected specimen also remains crucial to the interpretation of studies evaluating adjuvant therapies for resectable pancreas cancer.

This point was recently emphasized in a study to critically evaluate surgical and pathologic quality control and documentation in a national trial of adjuvant therapy [34]. Operative and pathology reports of patients enrolled on ACOSOG Z5031–a multi-institutional protocol of adjuvant CRT (Virginia Mason protocol) after pancreaticoduodenectomy–were rigorously evaluated by four surgical oncologists. Surgical and pathologic variables with the potential to influence staging or outcome were analyzed. An overwhelming absence of consistency of clinical variables associated with the perioperative staging, surgical treatment, and pathologic analyses of patients with pancreas cancer treated with postoperative therapy was identified. Although the independent influence of variability of each of these factors and their documentation on outcome is unknown, the overall effect may lead to heterogeneity among patients treated with adjuvant therapies, the misinterpretation of the results of studies examining the effects of these therapies, and unsatisfactory outcomes. These data reinforce the critical need for optimization and standardization of surgical technique, pathologic analysis of pancreaticoduodenectomy specimens, and associated clinical documentation, suggesting critical areas for improvement in the design of multidisciplinary protocols for patients with resectable pancreas cancer.

Future studies will still need to assess the benefits of adjuvant therapies as well as neoadjuvant approaches. Optimal trial design requires state-of-the-art preoperative imaging to appropriately define resectability based on objective criteria, standard high quality surgery, and pathologic evaluation [6,32]. The design of these trials should take into account the lessons learned from previous trials so that data generated are meaningful and do not suffer from the same mistakes.

References

[1] American Cancer Society. Cancer Facts and Figures 2008 [internet]. Atlanta, GA: ACS; 2008. Available from: http://www.cancer.org. Accessed May 11, 2010.

[2] Golcher H, Brunner T, Grabenbauer G, et al. Preoperative chemoradiation in adenocarcinoma of the pancreas. A single centre experience advocating a new treatment strategy. Eur J Surg Oncol 2008;34(7):756–64.

[3] Kim HJ, Czischke K, Brennan MF, et al. Does neoadjuvant chemoradiation downstage locally advanced pancreatic cancer? J Gastrointest Surg 2002;6(5):763–9.

[4] Tse RV, Dawson LA, Wei A, et al. Neoadjuvant treatment for pancreatic cancer–a review. Crit Rev Oncol Hematol 2008;65(3):263–74.

[5] Greer SE, Pipas JM, Sutton JE, et al. Effect of neoadjuvant therapy on local recurrence after resection of pancreatic adenocarcinoma. J Am Coll Surg 2008;206(3):451–7.

[6] Katz MH, Wang H, Fleming JB, et al. Long-term survival after multidisciplinary management of resected pancreatic adenocarcinoma. Ann Surg Oncol 2009;16(4):836–47.
[7] Lowy AM. Neoadjuvant therapy for pancreatic cancer. J Gastrointest Surg 2008;12(9): 1600–8.
[8] Kalser MH, Ellenberg SS. Pancreatic cancer. Adjuvant combined radiation and chemotherapy following curative resection. Arch Surg 1985;120(8):899–903.
[9] Klinkenbijl JH, Jeekel J, Sahmoud T, et al. Adjuvant radiotherapy and 5-fluorouracil after curative resection of cancer of the pancreas and periampullary region: phase III trial of the EORTC gastrointestinal tract cancer cooperative group. Ann Surg 1999;230(6): 776–82 [discussion: 782–4].
[10] Neoptolemos JP, Kerr DJ, Beger H, et al. ESPAC-1 trial progress report: the European randomized adjuvant study comparing radiochemotherapy, 6 months chemotherapy and combination therapy versus observation in pancreatic cancer. Digestion 1997;58(6): 570–7.
[11] Neoptolemos JP, Dunn JA, Stocken DD, et al. Adjuvant chemoradiotherapy and chemotherapy in resectable pancreatic cancer: a randomised controlled trial. Lancet 2001;358(9293):1576–85.
[12] Neoptolemos JP, Stocken DD, Friess H, et al. A Randomized Trial of chemoradiotherapy and chemotherapy after resection of pancreatic cancer. N Engl J Med 2004;350(12): 1200–10.
[13] Neoptolemos JP, Stocken DD, Tudur SC, et al. Adjuvant 5-fluorouracil and folinic acid vs observation for pancreatic cancer: composite data from the ESPAC-1 and -3(v1) trials. Br J Cancer 2009;100(2):246–50.
[14] Oettle H, Post S, Neuhaus P, et al. Adjuvant chemotherapy with gemcitabine vs observation in patients undergoing curative-intent resection of pancreatic cancer: a randomized controlled trial. JAMA 2007;297(3):267–77.
[15] Neuhaus P, Riess H, Post S, et al. CONKO-001: Final Results of the randomized, prospective, multicenter phase III trial of adjuvant chemotherapy with gemcitabine versus observation in patients with resected pancreatic cancer (PC) [abstract]. J Clin Oncol 2008;26(Suppl 20):LBA4504.
[16] Regine WF, Winter KA, Abrams RA, et al. Fluorouracil vs gemcitabine chemotherapy before and after fluorouracil-based chemoradiation following resection of pancreatic adenocarcinoma: a randomized controlled trial. JAMA 2008;299(9):1019–26.
[17] Neoptolemos J, Büchler M, Stocken DD, et al. ESPAC-3(v2): a multicenter, international, open-label, randomized, controlled phase III trial of adjuvant 5-fluorouracil/folinic acid (5-FU/FA) versus gemcitabine (GEM) in patients with resected pancreatic ductal adenocarcinoma. Presented at the American Society of Clinical Oncology Annual Meeting, Orlando (FL), June, 2009.
[18] Van Laethem JL, Mornex F, Azria D, et al. Adjuvant gemcitabine alone versus gemcitabine-based chemoradiation after curative resection for pancreatic cancer: updated results of a randomized EORTC/FFCD/GERCOR phase II study (40013–22012/9203). Presented at the American Society of Clinical Oncology Annual Meeting, Orlando (FL), June, 2009.
[19] Nukui Y, Picozzi VJ, Traverso LW. Interferon-based adjuvant chemoradiation therapy improves survival after pancreaticoduodenectomy for pancreatic adenocarcinoma. Am J Surg 2000;179(5):367–71.
[20] Picozzi VJ, Kozarek RA, Traverso LW. Interferon-based adjuvant chemoradiation therapy after pancreaticoduodenectomy for pancreatic adenocarcinoma. Am J Surg 2003;185(5): 476–80.
[21] Linehan DC, Tan MC, Strasberg SM, et al. Adjuvant interferon-based chemoradiation followed by gemcitabine for resected pancreatic adenocarcinoma: a single-institution phase II study. Ann Surg 2008;248(2):145–51.
[22] Herman JM, Swartz MJ, Hsu CC, et al. Analysis of fluorouracil-based adjuvant chemotherapy and radiation after pancreaticoduodenectomy for ductal adenocarcinoma of the

pancreas: results of a large, prospectively collected database at the Johns Hopkins Hospital. J Clin Oncol 2008;26(21):3503–10.
[23] Corsini MM, Miller RC, Haddock MG, et al. Adjuvant radiotherapy and chemotherapy for pancreatic carcinoma: the mayo clinic experience (1975–2005). J Clin Oncol 2008;26(21)3511–6.
[24] Cameron JL, Riall TS, Coleman J, et al. One thousand consecutive pancreaticoduodenectomies. Ann Surg 2006;244(1):10–5.
[25] Yeo CJ, Cameron JL, Sohn TA, et al. Six hundred fifty consecutive pancreaticoduodenectomies in the 1990s: pathology, complications, and outcomes. Ann Surg 1997;226(3): 248–57 [discussion: 257—60].
[26] Greco J, Castaldo E, Feurer I, et al. Survival benefit with adjuvant radiation therapy in surgicall resected pancreatic cancer. Preseted at the American Society of Clinical Oncology Gastrointestinal Cancers Symposium. Orlando (FL), January 2007.
[27] Merchant NB, Rymer J, Koehler EA, et al. Adjuvant chemoradiation therapy for pancreatic adenocarcinoma: who really benefits? J Am Coll Surg 2009;208(5):829–38 [discussion: 838–41].
[28] Picozzi VJ, Pisters PW, Vickers SM, et al. Strength of the evidence: adjuvant therapy for resected pancreatic cancer. J Gastrointest Surg 2008;12(4):657–61.
[29] Cheng TY, Sheth K, White RR, et al. Effect of neoadjuvant chemoradiation on operative mortality and morbidity for pancreaticoduodenectomy. Ann Surg Oncol 2006;13(1): 66–74.
[30] Lowy AM, Lee JE, Pisters PW, et al. Prospective, randomized trial of octreotide to prevent pancreatic fistula after pancreaticoduodenectomy for malignant disease. Ann Surg 1997;226(5):632–41.
[31] Spitz FR, Abbruzzese JL, Lee JE, et al. Preoperative and postoperative chemoradiation strategies in patients treated with pancreaticoduodenectomy for adenocarcinoma of the pancreas. J Clin Oncol 1997;15(3):928–37.
[32] Abrams RA, Lowy AM, O'Reilly EM, et al. Combined modality treatment of resectable and borderline resectable pancreas cancer: expert consensus statement. Ann Surg Oncol 2009;16(7):1751–6.
[33] Picozzi VJ. Today's forecast for the Adjuvant Treatment of Pancreatic Cancer: clear or cloudy? Oncology 2007;21(6).
[34] Katz MH, Merchant NB, Brower S, et al. Standardization and documentation of surgical and pathologic variables in a multi-institutional trial of adjuvant therapy for pancreatic cancer: results from ACOSOG Z5031, presented at Gastrointestinal Cancers Symposium. Orlando (FL), January 2010.
[35] Yeung RS, Weese JL, Hoffman JP, et al. Neoadjuvant chemoradiation in pancreatic and duodenal carcinoma. a phase II study. Cancer 1993;72(7):2124–33.
[36] Staley CA, Lee JE, Cleary KR, et al. Preoperative chemoradiation, pancreaticoduodenectomy, and intraoperative radiation therapy for adenocarcinoma of the pancreatic head. Am J Surg 1996;171(1):118–24 [discussion: 124–5].
[37] Hoffman JP, Lipsitz S, Pisansky T, et al. Phase II trial of preoperative radiation therapy and chemotherapy for patients with localized, resectable adenocarcinoma of the pancreas: an Eastern Cooperative Oncology Group Study. J Clin Oncol 1998;16(1): 317–23.
[38] Pisters PW, Abbruzzese JL, Janjan NA, et al. Rapid-fractionation preoperative chemoradiation, pancreaticoduodenectomy, and intraoperative radiation therapy for resectable pancreatic adenocarcinoma. J Clin Oncol 1998;16(12):3843–50.
[39] Pisters PW, Wolff RA, Janjan NA, et al. Preoperative paclitaxel and concurrent rapid-fractionation radiation for resectable pancreatic adenocarcinoma: toxicities, histologic response rates, and event-free outcome. J Clin Oncol 2002;20(10):2537–44.
[40] White RR, Kattan MW, Haney JC, et al. Evaluation of preoperative therapy for pancreatic cancer using a prognostic nomogram. Ann Surg Oncol 2006;13(11):1485–92.

[41] Moutardier V, Magnin V, Turrini O, et al. Assessment of pathologic response after preoperative chemoradiotherapy and surgery in pancreatic adenocarcinoma. Int J Radiat Oncol Biol Phys 2004;60(2):437–43.
[42] Mornex F, Girard N, Scoazec JY, et al. Feasibility of preoperative combined radiation therapy and chemotherapy with 5-fluorouracil and cisplatin in potentially resectable pancreatic adenocarcinoma: The French SFRO-FFCD 97-04 phase II trial. Int J Radiat Oncol Biol Phys 2006;65(5):1471–8.
[43] Talamonti MS, Small W Jr, Mulcahy MF, et al. A multi-institutional phase II trial of preoperative full-dose gemcitabine and concurrent radiation for patients with potentially resectable pancreatic carcinoma. Ann Surg Oncol 2006;13(2):150–8.
[44] Palmer DH, Stocken DD, Hewitt H, et al. A randomized phase 2 trial of neoadjuvant chemotherapy in resectable pancreatic cancer: gemcitabine alone versus gemcitabine combined with cisplatin. Ann Surg Oncol 2007;14(7):2088–96.
[45] Evans DB, Varadhachary GR, Crane CH, et al. Preoperative gemcitabine-based chemoradiation for patients with resectable adenocarcinoma of the pancreatic head. J Clin Oncol 2008;26(21):3496–502.
[46] Varadhachary GR, Wolff RA, Crane CH, et al. Preoperative gemcitabine and cisplatin followed by gemcitabine-based chemoradiation for resectable adenocarcinoma of the pancreatic head. J Clin Oncol 2008;26(21):3487–95.

Advances in Surgery 44 (2010) 165–184

ADVANCES IN SURGERY

Real-Time Glucose Monitoring in the Hospital: Future or Now?

Jeffrey I. Joseph, DO[a,b,*], Brian Hipszer, PhD[a]

[a]Department of Anesthesiology, Artificial Pancreas Center, Jefferson Medical College, Thomas Jefferson University, 565 Jefferson Alumni Hall, 1020 Locust Street, Philadelphia, PA 19107, USA
[b]Anesthesiology Program for Translational Research, Jefferson Medical College, Thomas Jefferson University, Suite 6215 Gibbon, 111 South 11th Street, Philadelphia, PA 19107, USA

Hyperglycemia and hypoglycemia commonly occur in hospitalized patients despite significant nursing time and resources devoted to glucose control [1–8]. Twenty-one percent of the 32,000 per month point-of-care (POC) glucose measurements at the authors' university hospital are above 200 mg/dL and 4% are below 70 mg/dL (query of RALS database for the entire month of November 2009). Each measurement above and below the clinically acceptable range requires nursing and physician time to assess the patient, make an adjustment in therapy, and document the event in the medical record.

The concentration of blood glucose (BG) fluctuates significantly over time because of changes in nutrient intake, endogenous glucose production, endogenous insulin release, insulin sensitivity, cellular metabolism, and the patient's ability to develop a stress response [3,7,9–11]. Perioperative hyperglycemia, hypoglycemia, and glycemic variability may lead to increased morbidity, mortality, length of stay, and cost in high-risk patient populations [1,2,6,12,13]. Safe and effective glycemic management requires vigilance, clinical judgment, and frequent adjustments in therapy [9].

Continuous glucose monitoring (CGM) systems are being developed for operating rooms, critical care units, and general floors of the hospital that measure and display the concentration of blood, plasma, or interstitial fluid (ISF) glucose every 1 to 15 minutes [9,14–25]. Real-time glucose trend data will be displayed at the bedside using a 1-, 3-, or 6-hour window. In the near future, high-risk patients could be continuously monitored from hospital admission through discharge to facilitate the timely detection and prevention of hyperglycemia and hypoglycemia [9,26,27].

The CGM sensor and display will travel with the patient from the emergency department or operating room to the critical care unit, radiology

*Corresponding author. Department of Anesthesiology, Jefferson Medical College, Thomas Jefferson University, 565 Jefferson Alumni Hall, 1020 Locust Street, Philadelphia, PA 19107. *E-mail address:* jeffrey.joseph@jefferson.edu.

0065-3411/10/$ – see front matter
doi:10.1016/j.yasu.2010.05.016

department, and general floor. Caregivers will observe the CGM display during each patient encounter to assess the current glucose concentration; direction of glucose change (increasing, decreasing, or stable); and rate of glucose change (slow, fast, or stable) [9,15,28–31]. The time and dose of insulin administration will be more appropriately matched with nutrient delivery and the current metabolic state of the patient [26].

Caregivers will easily recognize a high-risk situation by observing a rapidly increasing or decreasing glucose trend on the bedside CGM display [32]. Programmable threshold and rate of change alarms will warn the critical care or general floor nurse of impending hypoglycemia, well before the onset of symptoms. The incidence of mild to moderate hypoglycemia will be minimized. Severe and prolonged hypoglycemia will be eliminated [26,27].

HYPERGLYCEMIA IN THE HOSPITAL

Hyperglycemia develops when carbohydrate absorption from the intestine, hepatic glucose production (gluconeogenesis and glycogenolysis), renal glucose production, and parenteral glucose infusion exceed the cellular uptake of glucose and the elimination of glucose by the kidneys [3,7,11,33–37]. The pancreas, liver, intestine, autonomic nervous system, and brain form an integrated system that maintains the concentration of arterial BG within a narrow range (70–130 mg/dL) despite dynamic changes in food intake and cell metabolism. Beta cells within the islets of Langerhans rapidly alter the rates of insulin synthesis and release in direct response to a changing BG concentration. An increase in the arterial BG concentration causes an increase in the portal vein insulin concentration and a decrease in the portal vein glucagon concentration, leading to increased hepatic glucose uptake and decreased hepatic glucose production [3].

Glucose molecules rapidly move from the plasma to the ISF by simple diffusion, and then enter the cytosol of most cells (neurons, Schwann cells, red blood cells) by facilitated diffusion. In contrast, the transport of ISF glucose into the cytosol of skeletal muscle and adipose tissue cells requires activation of glucose transporters, which is achieved through the interaction of insulin with receptors on the surface of the cells. The pharmacodynamic affects of insulin on the rate of glucose transport into skeletal muscle and adipose tissue cells (insulin sensitivity) can increase or decrease rapidly because of changes in insulin receptor number, receptor function, cell function, capillary blood flow, pH, and temperature [26,38,39].

Approximately 7.5% of the United States population has diabetes. Twenty-two million Americans have type 2 diabetes, 1 million have type 1 diabetes, and 135,000 have gestational diabetes. One quarter to one third of patients with type 2 diabetes is undiagnosed and untreated. An additional 30% of the adult United States population has prediabetes, defined as impaired fasting glucose or impaired glucose tolerance. Many patients with prediabetes and undiagnosed diabetes develop hyperglycemia and glycemic variability during their hospital stay [3,40,41].

In addition, many patients without diabetes or prediabetes (ie, preadmission fasting BG < 100 mg/dL or hemoglobin A_{1c} < 6.5%) develop hyperglycemia in the hospital, during the stressful portion of a medical illness or surgical procedure, a condition known as "hospital-related hyperglycemia" or "stress hyperglycemia" [3,10,11,33,40–42]. The hallmark of this condition is decreased insulin sensitivity in hepatic, skeletal muscle, and adipose tissues. The degree of insulin resistance has been correlated with increased levels of catecholamines, tissue factors, cytokines, corticosteroids, bacteria toxins, and hypothermia [43].

Hepatic glucose production is increased and skeletal muscle and adipose tissue glucose uptake decreased in proportion to the level of metabolic stress. This response is maximal immediately after surgery and wanes over the following 1 to 3 days. Hyperglycemia is amplified by the administration of intravenous (IV) glucose solutions and the administration of catecholamine and steroid medications [43,44]. A prolonged or bimodal stress response may signify the onset of infection or a surgical complication.

The optimal BG range in a specific medical or surgical patient population remains controversial. The range from 100 to 180 mg/dL has traditionally been recommended to minimize the risk for hypoglycemia and the adverse effects of hyperglycemia. BG levels 160 to 180 mg/dL often exceed the kidney's ability to reabsorb glucose, leading to glycosuria, dehydration, and electrolyte abnormality [9]. A high rate of dilute urine production can give the clinician a false sign of adequate hydration status, when the patient is actually dehydrated.

Observational studies in the intensive care unit (ICU) demonstrate a strong relationship between the degree of hyperglycemia and increased morbidity, mortality, length of stay, and cost. Many of these studies document a decreased risk for nosocomial infection, renal failure, and ICU mortality when insulin is titrated to maintain the average BG level less than 200, less than 150, or less than 110 mg/dL [1–3,6,7,45,46]. Outcome data supporting intensive insulin therapy (IIT) and tight BG control are most consistent in diabetic and nondiabetic patients undergoing cardiac surgery [8]. The reports by Furnary and colleagues [46,47] clearly demonstrate a decreased rate of infection, arrhythmia, and mortality when glycemia is maintained at less than 150 mg/dL for 3 days during and after cardiac surgery.

Several prospective randomized trials in the ICU demonstrate decreased morbidity and mortality when hyperglycemia is controlled in the near-normal range (70–110 mg/dL) with hourly adjustments in insulin therapy [8,48,49]. More recent clinical trials have not demonstrated an outcome benefit in ICU patients managed with ITT titrated to maintain BG in the low-normal range compared with the mild hyperglycemia range [50–52].

Current clinical methods of BG monitoring and ITT have not been able consistently to achieve the desired BG range without an unacceptably high rate of severe hypoglycemia [50]. A typical ICU patient's BG level is outside of the target BG range more than 50% of the time. The high prevalence of hyperglycemia and hypoglycemia has been consistent from hospital to hospital despite detailed management protocols, frequent manual BG measurements, and adjustments in insulin therapy [2,4–8,12,32,49,50,53,54].

Results from the available clinical trials performed in the ICU should be interpreted with caution because of the variability in type of blood sampled (ie, capillary, arterial, peripheral venous, or central venous); blood sample handling; and type of analyzer used for glucose monitoring (ie, central laboratory, ICU blood gas analyzer, or POC glucose meter and strip technology) [55]. The NICE-SUGAR trial, for example, did not determine the influence of blood sample type and analyzer type on the glucose measurement. This influence is especially important because the mean glucose difference between the IIT group and conventional treatment group was 23 mg/dL and more than half of the BG measurements overlapped [50].

HYPOGLYCEMIA IN THE HOSPITAL

Hypoglycemia develops when the rate of glucose leaving the plasma (glucose uptake by the cells and excretion by the kidneys) exceeds the rate of glucose entering the plasma (hepatic glycogenolysis, hepatic and renal gluconeogenesis, gastrointestinal absorption, and IV glucose infusion) [4]. Neurons within the brain, spinal cord, and periphery require a constant supply of glucose to maintain homeostasis. The ISF glucose concentration surrounding a neuron may become inadequate if the plasma glucose concentration is low, capillary blood flow is low, or cell metabolism is high [2].

Most hospitalized patients develop a strong physiologic response to a rapid or gradual fall in BG concentration (onset begins when BG fall below 90 mg/dL). The response becomes very intense when the BG level decreases below 50 mg/dL. The signs and symptoms of hypoglycemia may be mild or pronounced, depending on the BG level, rate of change, and patient physiology [4–6].

The hypothalamus responds to neuroglycopenia by stimulating the secretion of growth hormone and by increasing sympathetic nervous system activity, leading to increased secretion of epinephrine, norepinephrine, and cortisol from the adrenal glands and glucagon from the pancreas. Endogenous glucose production and cardiac output greatly increase, leading to rapid delivery of glucose to the ISF surrounding the hypothalamus [4–6].

Patients with long-standing diabetes often do not develop the typical physiologic response to hypoglycemia, a condition known as "hypoglycemia unawareness" [4]. General anesthetics, sedatives, and cardiovascular medications also attenuate the body's response to hypoglycemia. Severe and prolonged neuroglycopenia (<20–30 mg/dL) causes progressive deterioration of cell function with eventual apoptosis. Neuron death can occur in 30 minutes when a low glucose concentration is combined with low tissue blood flow. Surgical patients with a history of hypoglycemia unawareness are at increased risk and require more frequent monitoring and vigilance [9].

The actual frequency, severity, and duration of hypoglycemic episodes in the hospital is unknown because of the low frequency of BG monitoring in patients with diabetes and the lack of BG monitoring in patients without a diagnosis of diabetes. Hypoglycemic episodes with mild signs and symptoms (commonly defined as a POC glucose measurement < 70 mg/dL) are underreported and poorly documented in the hospital's medical record. The signs and symptoms of hypoglycemia are often mistaken for other conditions or masked by anesthesia, sedation, cardiovascular medications, and illness [2,4–7].

Patients who experience one or more hypoglycemic episodes in the hospital are at increased risk for morbidity, mortality, length of stay, and cost [2,6,50,56–60]. Variables that may adversely affect clinical outcome are (1) lowest BG concentration, (2) maximum rate of BG change, (3) duration of hypoglycemia, (4) recurrent hypoglycemia, (5) glycemic variability, and (6) low tissue blood flow [53,61–63]. Increased catecholamines and sympathetic tone may induce cardiac arrhythmia or worsen myocardial-cerebral-renal ischemia. Hypoglycemia may also be a marker of suboptimal clinical care, decreased physiologic reserve, severe malnutrition, diffuse cancer, or severe hepatic-renal disease [7].

A retrospective review of 4368 patients with diabetes treated on the general floors of a university hospital revealed the incidence of hypoglycemia (BG < 50 mg/dL) was 7.7%. Every day with a hypoglycemic episode increased length of stay by 2.5 days. The odds of inpatient mortality and mortality within 1 year of hospital discharge increased 85% and 66%, respectively, for each additional day with a hypoglycemic episode. In-hospital mortality increased threefold for every 10 mg/dL decrease in the lowest BG recorded during the hospital admission [64].

Varghese and colleagues [65] performed a prospective observational study of patients admitted to a university hospital and managed with insulin or oral diabetes medication. Of the 2174 hospitalized patients studied over the 3-month period, 28% were managed with oral diabetes medication and 72% only with insulin. Seventy-seven percent were managed on the general floors and 33% in the critical care units. Two-hundred and six patients had 484 hypoglycemic episodes (BG < 70 mg/dL). Four percent of the hypoglycemia events (19 of 484) were associated with an adverse event: 10 patients had a loss of consciousness or seizure temporally related to hypoglycemia. Forty-three percent of the patients developed recurrent hypoglycemia during their hospital stays [65].

Critical care patients managed with IIT targeted to the near-normal BG range are at increased risk for hypoglycemia. Hypoglycemia is most common when the mean BG level is low and glycemic variability is high. Critical care units that maintain a mean BG greater than 140 mg/dL have a low incidence of hypoglycemia [2–8,48–50,66]. The American Diabetes Association and the Association of Academic Clinical Endocrinologists recently changed their guidelines because of the 6.8% incidence of severe hypoglycemia in the IIT group of the NICE-SUGAR study. The new guidelines recommend a higher target BG range (140–180 mg/dL) and greater vigilance to minimize the risk for hypoglycemia [41,50,56,67].

FREQUENCY OF BG MONITORING

Multiple glucose measurements per hour are required to characterize the glycemic pattern accurately in a hospitalized patient. In reality, the BG concentration is measured before meals and before bedtime in most hospitalized patients with diabetes. Glucose is not typically measured during the overnight period from 2200 to 0700. Few patients are treated aggressively with IIT and hourly glucose monitoring [9,26]. Approximately 5 minutes of a caregiver's time is required to obtain a patient blood sample and measure the concentration of glucose using a POC meter. Clinical application of an IIT protocol with hourly measurements requires more than 2 hours of a caregiver's time to monitor the BG concentration of an individual patient [68]. The risk for severe and prolonged hypoglycemia is greatly increased, however, when the frequency of monitoring is low, especially on the general floors [5,6].

The average and maximum rate of BG change in hospitalized patients managed in the ICU and general floors have not been well characterized. The concentration of BG changes slowly (<1 mg/dL/min) more than 90% of the time in ambulatory patients with diabetes. The maximum rate of change is rarely greater than 3 mg/dL/min [9,18]. In the hospital, however, the concentration of glucose can fall faster than 3 mg/dL/min following a large IV dose of insulin, an abrupt decrease in nutrient delivery, or an acute increase in insulin sensitivity [20,54,69,70]. BG monitoring once per hour in the critical care environment of the hospital may be insufficient to eliminate the risk for hypoglycemia [5,8].

CURRENT METHODS OF GLUCOSE MONITORING

Most hospitalized patients at risk for hyperglycemia or hypoglycemia have their BG tested using capillary blood obtained by lancing the fingertip. The use of capillary blood may produce an erroneous glucose measurement because of tissue edema, low peripheral perfusion, small sample size, and contamination from cleaning solution or carbohydrate on the skin surface [71–77]. In general, fingerstick capillary blood samples should be avoided when an accurate BG measurement is required for safe patient management.

Hospitals have not standardized or optimized methods of blood sample collection, handling, or analysis to ensure an accurate and reliable glucose measurement. Preanalytical and analytical errors are additive [71–74,78–80]. Adherence to one validated method of sample acquisition, handling, and analysis is required to ensure measurement accuracy and uniformity.

Frequent sample acquisition from a radial artery, peripheral venous catheter, or central venous catheter (CVC) is limited because of blood loss, acquisition difficulties, the risk of infection, and time constraints. Blood loss from hourly radial artery catheter sampling exceeds 80 mL/day when 3 mL of dead-space blood is discarded with each sample. Blood loss from hourly CVC sampling exceeds 200 mL/day when 10 mL of dead-space blood is wasted [9,26,27]. Closed sampling systems (VAMP System, Edwards LifeSciences, Irvine, CA,

USA, and SafeSet Blood Sampling System, Hospira, Lake Forest, IL, USA) facilitate frequent blood sample acquisition without loss of dead-space blood.

Sample acquisition from a vascular catheter becomes difficult when fibrous protein, platelets, and formed clot obstructs the catheter tip or occludes the vein. Frequent sampling increases the incidence of obstruction, whereas irrigation with a heparin or saline solution mitigates clot formation. Most hospitals limit sampling from a CVC to decrease the risk for infection [9,26].

Blood simultaneously sampled from the fingertip, radial artery, peripheral vein, superior vena cava, right atrium, and pulmonary artery has a different glucose concentration [81–84]. The difference can be caused by the variable rate of glucose uptake by different tissue beds, the appearance of glucose from the gut following a meal, the release of glucose from the liver and kidneys, the mixing of blood with glucose-containing or glucose-free IV fluids, and changes in the plasma volume. In general, the concentration of glucose in blood sampled from the radial artery is 6 mg/dL greater than peripheral venous blood and 10 to 60 mg/dL greater than blood sampled from the superior vena cava. The concentration of glucose in fingerstick capillary blood samples tends to be higher than simultaneously measured radial artery, peripheral venous, and superior vena cava samples [83,84]. Blood sampled from the inferior vena cava and right atrium often has the highest concentration because of hepatic glucose output.

A clean and fresh sample of arterial or venous whole blood increases the accuracy and precision of glucose measurement. Blood sampled from a vascular catheter and stopcock, however, may be contaminated with glucose-free or glucose-containing solution traveling through the IV tubing or a collateral vein. Diluted blood samples are common in the clinical setting despite withdrawing a volume 2.5 times greater than the volume of the tubing and catheter (ie, dead-space volume) before obtaining the sample. Blood sampled from the proximal port of a CVC catheter is commonly contaminated with solutions infused into the middle and distal infusion ports, especially during positive pressure mechanical ventilation [26,84]. Identification of a contaminated sample can be difficult when monitoring infrequently. Measuring potassium, hemoglobin, or hematocrit in the blood sample can often provide evidence of dilution or contamination.

Sitting for 1 hour at room temperature, the glucose concentration of whole blood sample in a standard blood collection tube decreases 10%. A collection tube that contains sodium fluoride to inhibit glycolysis is recommended considering the long and variable time between sample collection at the bedside and testing in hospital laboratory. A hemolyzed blood sample may artificially lower the plasma glucose concentration because of dilution with intracellular fluid. The glucose concentration of a centrifuged specimen is 15% higher than a noncentrifuged specimen because of movement of proteins out of the plasma [26,76,80].

Hospital protocols should standardize the type of glucose analyzer and method of sample acquisition. Glucose measurements from a POC meter,

ICU analyzer, and central laboratory analyzer may be significantly different, depending on the method of sample application, type of enzyme, chemistry of assay, type of transducer, and method of calibration. The accuracy, precision, and sensitivity of each analyzer may differ when measuring samples of whole blood or plasma in the hypoglycemic, euglycemic, and hyperglycemic ranges [85]. The accuracy and precision of glucose measurement using POC glucose meter and strip technologies are much lower than blood gas analyzers and central laboratory analyzers, especially in the hypoglycemia range [76]. In addition, some analyzers are affected by changes in hematocrit, oxygen, pH, temperature, acetaminophen, uric acid, ascorbic acid, and carbohydrates that resemble glucose (eg, maltose) [77,82,83,86,87].

There is great clinical need for a real-time glucose monitoring system that can automatically measure the concentration of glucose with accuracy, precision, and ease of clinical use. Automation and standardization of the glucose measurement process has the potential to decrease nursing time and improve BG control, clinical outcome, safety, and cost.

CGM SYSTEMS FOR THE HOSPITAL

In-hospital CGM systems are being developed to measure the concentration of glucose in the blood, plasma, or ISF several times per hour. Each type of CGM system has unique advantages and limitations when used to monitor patients in the critical care and general floor environments [9,14–26,88,89]. Early studies in the hospital evaluated subcutaneous tissue ISF glucose sensors commercialized for the ambulatory patient with diabetes. More recent studies have focused on sensors that measure glucose in the blood [90–92].

Vascular catheter CGM systems

Vascular catheter CGM systems may become the standard-of-care for the monitoring of glucose levels in critical care environments of the hospital. The systems automatically transfer a sample of whole blood from a vascular catheter to an external flow-through glucose sensor. Several systems produce a large volume of blood loss, whereas other systems flush the sample back into the bloodstream to avoid blood loss. Blood is the typical body fluid used for glucose measurement in the hospital. CGM systems that measure glucose in blood may overcome may of the limitations of subcutaneous tissue ISF monitoring systems. However, frequent sample acquisition from a vascular catheter can be problematic because of activation of platelets and clotting factors, leading to protein deposition and thrombus formation within the sensor, tubing, catheter, and vessel lumen [15,26].

The GlucoScout (International Biomedical, Austin, TX, USA) has Food and Drug Administration (FDA) approved labeling to measure the concentration of glucose every 5 minutes for 72 hours using blood automatically sampled from a radial artery, peripheral vein, or CVC. Each blood sample is transported to an external sterile flow-through glucose-oxidase electrochemical sensor and returned back into the bloodstream followed by a 6-mL infusion of glucose-salt solution [93,94].

The sensor is calibrated before clinical use using a glucose-free salt solution (0 mg/dL) and a glucose-containing salt solution (83 mg/dL). The glucose solution is used to recalibrate the sensor before each sample acquisition [25,93,94]. The accuracy and precision of the GlucoScout measurement are comparable with plasma glucose measurements made with a central laboratory glucose analyzer [15]. The real-time CGM measurements can be used to adjust insulin therapy in the operating room, critical care, and general floor environments.

Many hospitals add heparin to the flush solution (1 unit/mL) to minimize the risk for catheter and vessel thrombosis. Heparin is often omitted from the flush solution to avoid heparin-induced thrombocytopenia or thrombosis, leading to an increased incidence of peripheral venous catheter and vein thrombosis. The volume of infused flush solution averages 23 mL/h when sampling every 20 minutes, 41 mL/h when sampling every 10 minutes, and 77 mL/h when sampling every 5 minutes. Frequent sampling and flushing into a radial artery may cause premature catheter failure and hand edema, whereas samples obtained from the proximal lumen of a CVC may be contaminated with fluids infused through a more distal lumen.

The GlucoClear Intravenous Blood Glucose (IVBG) Monitor was jointly developed by Edwards LifeSciences (Irvine, CA, USA) and DexCom (San Diego, CA, USA). The IVBG system transports a small volume of blood into the lumen of an IV catheter, measures the concentration of BG using a sterile enzyme-based electrochemical sensor, and returns the sample back into the bloodstream [26]. A small volume of glucose-salt-heparin solution is used to flush the sample back into the vessel lumen and perform a one-point sensor calibration. The measurement process and calibration are automated and standardized to ensure accuracy and precision. The very small sample volume is optimal for sample acquisition from a peripheral vein. GlucoClear accuracy is comparable with plasma glucose measurements made with a central laboratory glucose analyzer. The glucose trend data are displayed at the bedside on a large screen. Threshold alarms can be programmed to facilitate the early detection of hyperglycemia and hypoglycemia. The GlucoClear IVBG is available for clinical use in the European Union and should receive FDA approval for commercialization in the United States in 2010.

The Optiscanner (Optiscan Biomedical, Hayward, CA, USA) transports blood from a vascular catheter to an external monitor, centrifuges the sample to extract plasma, and measures the concentration of glucose using mid-infrared spectroscopy. Almost the entire blood sample is returned back into the bloodstream followed by a small amount of flush solution (blood loss is <10 mL/day). A large and diverse library of plasma spectra where used to produce a universal calibration algorithm. The mid-infrared measurement of plasma has low scattering and a high signal-to-noise ratio. Clinical trial data demonstrated satisfactory accuracy, sensitivity, and specificity for CGM in the critical care setting [95].

Unlike the previous CGM systems, the Biostator (Miles Laboratories, Elkhart, IN, USA), STG-22 (Nikkiso, Tokyo, Japan), and Glucostator (GmbH, Osburg, Germany) transport blood at a slow and constant rate from a dual-lumen vascular catheter to a flow-through glucose-oxidase electrochemical sensor and then to a waste container. Blood loss often exceeds 100 mL/day. The CGM systems measure, display, and record the concentration of BG every 1 to 5 minutes. In addition to being a glucose sensor, the devices function as a closed-loop artificial pancreas system. Computer algorithms direct the IV infusion of insulin and glucose to automatically maintain the BG level in the desired target range. Safe and effective performance has been demonstrated in the operating room, ICU, and general floors of the hospital. No serious adverse events have been published in the peer literature related to frequent monitoring or closed-loop insulin delivery. Unfortunately the systems are large, complex, difficult to maintain, and currently do not have FDA approval for clinical use in the United States [91,92,96–100].

Intravascular CGM systems

The GlucCath (GluMetrics, Irvine, CA, USA) glucose monitoring system consists of a small-diameter optical fiber tipped with a glucose-sensitive hydrogel surrounded by a hemocompatible porous membrane. The distal portion of the optical fiber is inserted into the lumen of a peripheral vein using standard techniques and dwells within the bloodstream for 2 to 3 days. The optical fiber is connected to a bedside monitor that contains a light source, detector, battery, electronics, and display. The concentration of plasma glucose is measured continuously then averaged to provide the clinician with an updated glucose level every 1 to 2 minutes [26,89].

Glucose molecules pass through the porous membrane to interact with a fluorescent dye, a fluorescence quencher, and a boronic acid–based glucose receptor combined within a hydrogel matrix. The boric-acid receptor provides high specificity for the D-glucose molecule. In the absence of glucose, the quencher-receptor is tightly associated with the dye inhibiting fluorescence. In the presence of glucose, the interaction between the quencher and the dye is weakened, resulting in a rapid increase in fluorescence that is proportional to the concentration of glucose.

The fluorescence chemistry was optimized to produce the highest accuracy and sensitivity in the euglycemic and hypoglycemic ranges. There is a large and rapid change in the fluorescent signal following a small change in the BG level. The fluorescent signal changes 6% as the BG changes from 250 to 400 mg/dL, providing a resolution of ± 10 mg/dL. The signal changes 37% as the BG changes from 50 to 200 mg/dL, providing a resolution of ± 2 mg/dL. Long-term stability permits infrequent calibration using a venous blood sample and a reference BG measurement.

The GlucCath has performed well when inserted into the peripheral veins of volunteer subjects and hospitalized patients. Ninety-eight percent of the GlucCath measurements in the volunteer study less than 75 mg/dL were within

± 15 mg/dL of the reference values and 95% of the measurements greater than 75 mg/dL were within ± 20% of the reference values. These results exceed the International Organization for Standardization criteria for clinical accuracy (standard 15197). Ninety-five percent of the paired glucose measurements were within zone A of the Clarke Error Grid and the mean absolute relative difference (MARD) was 7.97% (GluMetrics, personal communication, November 2009). The GlucCath is currently undergoing clinical trials in United States hospitals and should receive FDA approval for commercialization in 2010.

The DIRAMO System for Continuous Blood Glucose Monitoring (Flowsion Medical, Nordborg, Denmark) consists of a small-diameter dialysis catheter that is inserted into the lumen of a peripheral vein for up to 72 hours [26]. Glucose molecules diffuse through the pores of a blood-dwelling dialysis catheter into the glucose-free dialysate solution. The glucose-enriched perfusate then reacts with glucose-oxidase enzyme and luminescent compounds located within an external microfluidic reaction chip. The glucose concentration is measured continuously and detected optically by a chemiluminescent sensor. The concentration of glucose is proportional to the luminescence intensity. Slow and precise transport of dialysate solution through the dialysis catheter ensures complete equilibration with the plasma glucose. The glucose measurements are averaged and displayed every minute on a bedside monitor.

Subcutaneous tissue ISF CGM systems

The Glucoday (A. Menarini Diagnostics, Firenze, Italy) uses a small-diameter dialysis catheter inserted in the subcutaneous tissue of the abdomen. The monitor measures, displays, and records the concentration of ISF glucose every 3 minutes for 48 hours. Glucose molecules diffuse through the small-pore membrane from the ISF into the dialysate solution. The solution is transported to an external flow-through glucose-oxidase electrochemical sensor and then to a waste container. The glucose sensor is calibrated using external high-low controls and a reference BG measurement once per day [14,18].

The Glucoday is commercially available for monitoring glucose in the operating room, ICU, and general floors of the hospital in the European Union. The CGM glucose measurements have not correlated closely with time-matched BG measurements made with a reference BG analyzer. The low correlation is most pronounced for several hours after catheter insertion and during periods of rapid glucose change. In addition, dialysis catheters are prone to fracture and premature failure after insertion into the subcutaneous tissue of surgical patients [18]. Other dialysis catheter CGM systems use infrared spectroscopy or a physical change to measure the concentration of glucose [101–104].

Needle-type subcutaneous tissue ISF CGM systems may be optimal for patients managed on the general floors of the hospital where ambulation and ease of clinical use are most important. The CGM sensor's thin electrode is easily inserted into the subcutaneous tissue with minimal discomfort. The electrode is connected to a miniature sensor that contains electronics, a transmitter, and rechargeable battery. Data are wirelessly transmitted from the patient-worn sensor to a bedside controller and display.

The Guardian RT (Medtronic Diabetes, Northridge, CA, USA), DexCom Seven (DexCom, San Diego, CA, USA), and Navigator (Abbott Diabetes Care, Alameda, CA, USA) have FDA-approved labeling for measuring the concentration of glucose in the ISF of ambulatory patients with diabetes. These devices report an estimate of the plasma glucose concentration every 5 minutes for 3 to 7 days with a reported MARD between 10% and 30% [14,19,20,23,26–28,30,88,105,106]. The abdomen, flank, thigh, buttocks, upper arm, and chest are common insertion sites. Physicians are using the real-time CGM glucose trend data to monitor heart surgery and major general surgery patients without FDA-approved labeling for these patient populations. The anterior thigh and upper-outer buttocks are common glucose sensor insertion sites in patients undergoing surgery of the abdomen and thorax [16,17].

Current CGM systems require one or more hours of run-in time after insertion because of an unstable sensor-tissue interface. Sensitivity often decreases and fluctuates for several hours after electrode insertion because of tissue injury and inflammation [107]. CGM accuracy depends greatly on the method of calibration. Reference BG measurements should be obtained for calibration only when the blood-tissue glucose level is stable (eg, a rate of change <0.5 mg/dL/min). Frequent recalibration may be required in some patients because of ongoing changes in the sensor-tissue interface, membrane, enzyme, or electrochemistry [108,109].

A change in ISF glucose may lag a BG change by 10 to 30 minutes (average, 12 minutes) [23,109]. Reference BG measurements can be time-shifted when used for calibration of an ISF glucose sensor [110–112]. Some CGM sensors correlate closely with time-matched reference BG measurements (eg, MARD <10%; R^2 >0.94). The reason why some ISF sensors correlate poorly with reference BG measurements is not well understood [17,26,107,109]. The inaccuracies associated with this technology led the FDA to limit labeling to adjunctive clinical use. The real-time information from these devices cannot be used to adjust insulin therapy. An adjustment in therapy requires a confirmatory BG measurement using a patient blood sample and reference glucose analyzer [28,30,108,113].

The use of CGM in the hospital has the potential to prevent hypoglycemia while minimizing exposure to hyperglycemia [32,70,106]. A caregiver could assess a patient's risk for hypoglycemia during each encounter by glancing at the bedside display. A steep downward slope of the glucose trend data is easily recognized as a high-risk clinical situation requiring increased vigilance [32]. Timely information allows the caregiver to intervene with oral or IV carbohydrate to prevent severe or prolonged hypoglycemia [9,26].

All CGM systems alarm when the glucose level exceeds preset high or low thresholds. Several systems have alarm algorithms that predict the onset of hypoglycemia 20 to 30 minutes into the future [28,106,114]. Sensitivity and specificity for hypoglycemia detection are improved when the algorithm considers the rate of change and threshold [115]. False alarms, missed hypoglycemia events, and data loss can be decreased by averaging multiple CGM sensors. Two or more sensor output signals that move in parallel can be processed in real-time to improve accuracy and robustness, whereas signals that deviate significantly from the mean can be used to detect sensor malfunction [116]. There is a trade-off between the number of sensors, complexity, practicality, and cost.

The CGM systems described require invasive methods for glucose monitoring. Noninvasive systems currently under development attach to the skin surface and use near-infrared spectroscopy, electrical impedance, and physical changes to estimate the concentration of glucose in the dermis and subcutaneous tissue. These systems have been limited by low sensitivity, specificity, signal-to-noise ratio, and difficulty maintaining a stable sensor-tissue interface [117].

GLUCOSE SENSOR AUGMENTED INSULIN DELIVERY

Current glycemic management practices require manual blood sample acquisition and testing to assess glycemic control and adjust therapy. CGM systems are poised to replace POC glucose testing, providing the standardization required to reduce the variability in blood sampling and handling while reducing the workload involved in frequent glucose monitoring.

These systems will measure and display BG in real-time and alarm for impending hypoglycemia and hyperglycemia while caregivers titrate the delivery of insulin and glucose based on this information. Manpower issues may limit routine manual insulin adjustments to once per hour with additional adjustments in the rate of insulin delivery when the CGM alarms.

Typically, IIT using the IV infusion of insulin and frequent (eg, hourly) glucose monitoring is reserved for patients in critical care settings. Using current and historical glucose measurements, the insulin infusion rate is adjusted to bring the patient's glucose level into a desired range safely and expeditiously. Current algorithms used to adjust insulin therapy are only applicable to patients who are not eating (but may be receiving enteral or parenteral nutrition). Numerous algorithms have been described and compared in the literature [70,118–126].

At the present time, Hospira (Lake Forest, IL, USA) is pursuing the integration of EndoTool glucose management software into its Symbiq smart infusion pump and Cardinal Health (Dublin, OH, USA) is collaborating with GlucoTec (Greenville, SC, USA) to combine the Alaris line of IV pumps with the Glucommander Plus glucose management system. Combining intelligent infusion systems with CGM systems will facilitate the transfer of data between the devices. These integrated systems will recommend an insulin dose adjustment based on the CGM glucose trend but still require human intervention to adjust therapy [38,113,115,127].

Future systems will also integrate infusion pumps that deliver IV glucose, IV parenteral nutrition, and enteral tube feedings to optimize nutrition in addition to maintaining glycemic control [9,26,27,34–37,128]. Algorithms will use pharmacokinetic-dynamic models of regular insulin [39], glucose, total parenteral nutrition, partial parenteral nutrition, tube feeding nutrients, and meals to enhance insulin dose recommendations and alarms. These systems will also facilitate research to determine the affects of controlling glucose, insulin, or nutrition on clinical outcome following major surgery.

Finally, fully automated systems will automatically adjust the dose of IV insulin and IV glucose every few minutes to clamp the BG level in the desired range. Closed-loop control will enhance safety and effectiveness when the clinical situation is changing rapidly [9,24,97–99,128–132]. Lessons learned in the hospital will help to advance research toward an artificial pancreas for the ambulatory patient with insulin-dependent diabetes [133,134].

References

[1] Krinsley JS. Association between hyperglycemia and increased hospital mortality in a heterogeneous population of critically ill patients. Mayo Clin Proc 2003;78(12): 1471–8.

[2] Krinsley JS, Grover A. Severe hypoglycemia in critically ill patients: risk factors and outcomes. Crit Care Med 2007;35(10):2262–7.

[3] Clement S, Braithwaite SS, Magee MF, et al. Management of diabetes and hyperglycemia in hospitals. Diabetes Care 2004;27(2):553–91.

[4] Cryer PE. Hypoglycaemia: the limiting factor in the glycaemic management of the critically ill? Diabetologia 2006;49(8):1722–5.

[5] Braithwaite SS, Buie MM, Thompson CL, et al. Hospital hypoglycemia: not only treatment but also prevention. Endocr Pract 2004;10(Suppl 2):89–99.

[6] Fischer KF, Lees JA, Newman JH. Hypoglycemia in hospitalized patients: causes and outcomes. N Engl J Med 1986;315(20):1245–50.

[7] Wexler DJ, Meigs JB, Cagliero E, et al. Prevalence of hyper- and hypoglycemia among inpatients with diabetes: a national survey of 44 U.S. hospitals. Diabetes Care 2007;30(2):367–9.

[8] Van den Berghe G, Wouters P, Weekers F, et al. Intensive insulin therapy in the critically ill patients. N Engl J Med 2001;345(19):1359–67.

[9] Joseph JI. Management of the diabetic surgical patient. In: Goldstein BJ, Müller-Wieland D, editors. Type 2 diabetes: principles and practice. 2nd edition. New York: Informa Healthcare; 2007. p. 475–90.

[10] Capes SE, Hunt D, Malmberg K, et al. Stress hyperglycaemia and increased risk of death after myocardial infarction in patients with and without diabetes: a systematic overview. Lancet 2000;355(9206):773–8.

[11] Mizock BA. Alterations in carbohydrate metabolism during stress: a review of the literature. Am J Med 1995;98(1):75–84.

[12] Inzucchi SE. Clinical practice. Management of hyperglycemia in the hospital setting. N Engl J Med 2006;355(18):1903–11.

[13] Lipshutz AK, Gropper MA. Perioperative glycemic control: an evidence-based review. Anesthesiology 2009;110(2):408–21.

[14] Vriesendorp TM, DeVries JH, Holleman F, et al. The use of two continuous glucose sensors during and after surgery. Diabetes Technol Ther 2005;7(2):315–22.

[15] Ganesh A, Hipszer B, Loomba N, et al. Evaluation of the VIA blood chemistry monitor for glucose in healthy and diabetic volunteers. J Diabetes Sci Technol 2008;2(2):182–93.

[16] Hipszer B, Furlong KJ, Lessin JB, et al. Continuous glucose monitoring in the perioperative period. Anesthesiology 2006;105:A583.

[17] Hipszer B, Chervoneva I, Gratch DM, et al. The performance of subcutaneous glucose sensors in surgical patients. J Diabetes Sci Technol 2008;2(2):A71.

[18] De Block C, Manuel-Y-Keenoy B, Van Gaal L, et al. Intensive insulin therapy in the intensive care unit: assessment by continuous glucose monitoring. Diabetes Care 2006;29(8): 1750–6.
[19] Murakami A, Gutierrez MA, Lage SHG, et al. A continuous glucose monitoring system in critical cardiac patients in the intensive care unit. Comput Cardiol 2006;233–6.
[20] Corstjens AM, Ligtenberg JJ, van der Horst IC, et al. Accuracy and feasibility of point-of-care and continuous blood glucose analysis in critically ill ICU patients. Crit Care 2006;10(5):R135.
[21] Bochicchio GV, Bochicchio KM, Lettich K, et al. Cutting edge technology in tight glycemic control (TGC). Crit Care Med 2007;35:A142.
[22] Monsod TP, Flanagan DE, Rife F, et al. Do sensor glucose levels accurately predict plasma glucose concentrations during hypoglycemia and hyperinsulinemia? Diabetes Care 2002;25(5):889–93.
[23] Aussedat B, Dupire-Angel M, Gifford R, et al. Interstitial glucose concentration and glycemia: implications for continuous subcutaneous glucose monitoring. Am J Physiol Endocrinol Metab 2000;278(4):E716–728.
[24] Chee F, Fernando T, van Heerden PV. Closed-loop glucose control in critically ill patients using continuous glucose monitoring system (CGMS) in real time. IEEE Trans Inf Technol Biomed 2003;7(1):43–53.
[25] Widness JA, Kulhavy JC, Johnson KJ, et al. Clinical performance of an in-line point-of-care monitor in neonates. Pediatrics 2000;106(3):497–504.
[26] Joseph JI, Hipszer B, Mraovic B, et al. Clinical need for continuous glucose monitoring in the hospital. J Diabetes Sci Technol 2009;3(6):1309–18.
[27] Joseph JI, Goldstein BJ. Future management approaches: new devices on the horizon for glucose monitoring and medication delivery. In: Goldstein BJ, Muller-Wieland D, editors. Type 2 diabetes: principles and practice. 2nd edition. New York: Informa Healthcare; 2007. p. 561–74.
[28] Reach G. Continuous glucose monitoring and diabetes health outcomes: a critical appraisal. Diabetes Technol Ther 2008;10(2):69–80.
[29] Rodbard D. Interpretation of continuous glucose monitoring data: glycemic variability and quality of glycemic control. Diabetes Technol Ther 2009;11(Suppl 1):S55–67.
[30] Kovatchev BP, Gonder-Frederick LA, Cox DJ, et al. Evaluating the accuracy of continuous glucose-monitoring sensors: continuous glucose-error grid analysis illustrated by TheraSense freestyle navigator data. Diabetes Care 2004;27(8):1922–8.
[31] Umpierrez GE, Smiley D, Zisman A, et al. Randomized study of basal-bolus insulin therapy in the inpatient management of patients with type 2 diabetes (RABBIT 2 trial). Diabetes Care 2007;30(9):2181–6.
[32] Ryan MT, Savarese VW, Hipszer B, et al. Continuous glucose monitor shows potential for early hypoglycemia detection in hospitalized patients. Diabetes Technol Ther 2009;11(11):745–7.
[33] Esposito K, Nappo F, Marfella R, et al. Inflammatory cytokine concentrations are acutely increased by hyperglycemia in humans: role of oxidative stress. Circulation 2002;106(16):2067–72.
[34] Plank LD, Hill GL. Energy balance in critical illness. Proc Nutr Soc 2003;62(2):545–52.
[35] De B, Chapman M, Fraser R, et al. Enteral nutrition in the critically ill: a prospective survey in an Australian intensive care unit. Anaesth Intensive Care 2001;29(6):619–22.
[36] Heyland DK, MacDonald S, Keefe L, et al. Total parenteral nutrition in the critically ill patient: a meta-analysis. JAMA 1998;280(23):2013–9.
[37] McMahon MM, Miles JM. Glycemic control and nutrition in the intensive care unit. Curr Opin Clin Nutr Metab Care 2006;9(2):120–3.
[38] Steed RD, Davidson PC, Bode BW, et al. Computer-controlled intravenous insulin infusion using intermittent bedside glucose monitoring: one year's experience. Diabetes 1986;35(Suppl 1):32A.

[39] Hipszer B, Joseph J, Kam M. Pharmacokinetics of intravenous insulin delivery in humans with type 1 diabetes. Diabetes Technol Ther 2005;7(1):83–93.
[40] ACE/ADA Task Force on Inpatient Diabetes. American college of endocrinology and American diabetes association consensus statement on inpatient diabetes and glycemic control. Endocr Pract 2006;12(4):458–68.
[41] Garber AJ, Moghissi ES, Bransome ED Jr, et al. American college of endocrinology position statement on inpatient diabetes and metabolic control. Endocr Pract 2004;10(1): 77–82.
[42] Turina M, Fry DE, Polk HC Jr. Acute hyperglycemia and the innate immune system: clinical, cellular, and molecular aspects. Crit Care Med 2005;33(7):1624–33.
[43] Yu WK, Li WQ, Li N, et al. Influence of acute hyperglycemia in human sepsis on inflammatory cytokine and counterregulatory hormone concentrations. World J Gastroenterol 2003;9(8):1824–7.
[44] Lukins MB, Manninen PH. Hyperglycemia in patients administered dexamethasone for craniotomy. Anesth Analg 2005;100(4):1129–33.
[45] Finney SJ, Zekveld C, Elia A, et al. Glucose control and mortality in critically ill patients. JAMA 2003;290(15):2041–7.
[46] Furnary AP, Gao G, Grunkemeier GL, et al. Continuous insulin infusion reduces mortality in patients with diabetes undergoing coronary artery bypass grafting. J Thorac Cardiovasc Surg 2003;125(5):1007–21.
[47] Furnary AP, Zerr KJ, Grunkemeier GL, et al. Continuous intravenous insulin infusion reduces the incidence of deep sternal wound infection in diabetic patients after cardiac surgical procedures. Ann Thorac Surg 1999;67(2):352–60 [discussion: 360–2].
[48] Van den Berghe G, Wouters PJ, Bouillon R, et al. Outcome benefit of intensive insulin therapy in the critically ill: insulin dose versus glycemic control. Crit Care Med 2003;31(2):359–66.
[49] Van den Berghe G, Wilmer A, Hermans G, et al. Intensive insulin therapy in the medical ICU. N Engl J Med 2006;354(5):449–61.
[50] NICE-SUGAR Study Investigators, Finfer S, Chittock DR, et al. Intensive versus conventional glucose control in critically ill patients. N Engl J Med 2009;360(13):1283–97.
[51] Gandhi GY, Nuttall GA, Abel MD, et al. Intensive intraoperative insulin therapy versus conventional glucose management during cardiac surgery: a randomized trial. Ann Intern Med 2007;146(4):233–43.
[52] Preiser JC. Restoring normoglycaemia: not so harmless. Crit Care 2008;12(1):116.
[53] Wintergerst KA, Buckingham B, Gandrud L, et al. Association of hypoglycemia, hyperglycemia, and glucose variability with morbidity and death in the pediatric intensive care unit. Pediatrics 2006;118(1):173–9.
[54] Bode BW, Braithwaite SS, Steed RD, et al. Intravenous insulin infusion therapy: indications, methods, and transition to subcutaneous insulin therapy. Endocr Pract 2004;10(Suppl 2): 71–80.
[55] Mraovic B. Analysis: continuous glucose monitoring during intensive insulin therapy. J Diabetes Sci Technol 2009;3(4):960–3.
[56] Moghissi ES, Korytkowski MT, DiNardo M, et al. American association of clinical endocrinologists and American diabetes association consensus statement on inpatient glycemic control. Endocr Pract 2009;15(4):353–69.
[57] Stagnaro-Green A, Barton MK, Linekin PL, et al. Mortality in hospitalized patients with hypoglycemia and severe hyperglycemia. Mt Sinai J Med 1995;62(6):422–6.
[58] Vriesendorp TM, DeVries JH, van Santen S, et al. Evaluation of short-term consequences of hypoglycemia in an intensive care unit. Crit Care Med 2006;34(11):2714–8.
[59] Newton CA, Young S. Financial implications of glycemic control: results of an inpatient diabetes management program. Endocr Pract 2006;12(Suppl 3):43–8.
[60] Wiener RS, Wiener DC, Larson RJ. Benefits and risks of tight glucose control in critically ill adults: a meta-analysis. JAMA 2008;300(8):933–44.

[61] Egi M, Bellomo R, Stachowski E, et al. Variability of blood glucose concentration and short-term mortality in critically ill patients. Anesthesiology 2006;105(2):244–52.
[62] Monnier L, Mas E, Ginet C, et al. Activation of oxidative stress by acute glucose fluctuations compared with sustained chronic hyperglycemia in patients with type 2 diabetes. JAMA 2006;295(14):1681–7.
[63] Auer RN. Hypoglycemic brain damage. Metab Brain Dis 2004;19(3-4):169–75.
[64] Turchin A, Matheny ME, Shubina M, et al. Hypoglycemia and clinical outcomes in patients with diabetes hospitalized in the general ward. Diabetes Care 2009;32(7):1153–7.
[65] Varghese P, Gleason V, Sorokin R, et al. Hypoglycemia in hospitalized patients treated with antihyperglycemic agents. J Hosp Med 2007;2(4):234–40.
[66] Inzucchi SE, Siegel MD. Glucose control in the ICU–how tight is too tight? N Engl J Med 2009;360(13):1346–9.
[67] Griesdale DE, de Souza RJ, van Dam RM, et al. Intensive insulin therapy and mortality among critically ill patients: a meta-analysis including NICE-SUGAR study data. CMAJ 2009;180(8):821–7.
[68] Aragon D. Evaluation of nursing work effort and perceptions about blood glucose testing in tight glycemic control. Am J Crit Care 2006;15(4):370–7.
[69] Logtenberg SJ, Kleefstra N, Snellen FT, et al. Pre- and postoperative accuracy and safety of a real-time continuous glucose monitoring system in cardiac surgical patients: a randomized pilot study. Diabetes Technol Ther 2009;11(1):31–7.
[70] Goldberg PA, Siegel MD, Sherwin RS, et al. Implementation of a safe and effective insulin infusion protocol in a medical intensive care unit. Diabetes Care 2004;27(2):461–7.
[71] Desachy A, Vuagnat AC, Ghazali AD, et al. Accuracy of bedside glucometry in critically ill patients: influence of clinical characteristics and perfusion index. Mayo Clin Proc 2008;83(4):400–5.
[72] Kanji S, Buffie J, Hutton B, et al. Reliability of point-of-care testing for glucose measurement in critically ill adults. Crit Care Med 2005;33(12):2778–85.
[73] Fahy BG, Coursin DB. Critical glucose control: the devil is in the details. Mayo Clin Proc 2008;83(4):394–7.
[74] Soo Hoo GW. Tight blood glucose control in the ICU: how best to measure glucose control? Chest 2008;133(1):316–7 [author reply 317].
[75] Sylvain HF, Pokorny ME, English SM, et al. Accuracy of fingerstick glucose values in shock patients. Am J Crit Care 1995;4(1):44–8.
[76] Dungan K, Chapman J, Braithwaite SS, et al. Glucose measurement: confounding issues in setting targets for inpatient management. Diabetes Care 2007;30(2):403–9.
[77] Slater-MacLean L, Cembrowski G, Chin D, et al. Accuracy of glycemic measurements in the critically ill. Diabetes Technol Ther 2008;10(3):169–77.
[78] NCCLS. Point-of-care blood glucose testing in acute and chronic care facilities; approved guideline—second edition. NCCLS document C30-A2 (ISBN 1-56238-471-6). Wayne (PA); 2002.
[79] Finkielman JD, Oyen LJ, Afessa B. Agreement between bedside blood and plasma glucose measurement in the ICU setting. Chest 2005;127(5):1749–51.
[80] Nichols JH. What is accuracy and how close must the agreement be? Diabetes Technol Ther 2005;7(3):558–62.
[81] Nayak PP, Morris K, Lang H, et al. Lack of agreement between arterial and central venous blood glucose measurement in critically ill children. Intensive Care Med 2009;35(4):762–3.
[82] Karon BS, Gandhi GY, Nuttall GA, et al. Accuracy of Roche accu-chek inform whole blood capillary, arterial, and venous glucose values in patients receiving intensive intravenous insulin therapy after cardiac surgery. Am J Clin Pathol 2007;127(6):919–26.
[83] Karon BS, Griesmann L, Scott R, et al. Evaluation of the impact of hematocrit and other interference on the accuracy of hospital-based glucose meters. Diabetes Technol Ther 2008;10(2):111–20.

[84] Flood J, Joseph J, Kim L, et al. Glucose levels in blood simultaneously sampled from the radial artery, vena cava, and fingertip. Anesthesiology 2007;107:A1123.
[85] Torjman MC, Jahn L, Joseph JI, et al. Accuracy of the hemocue portable glucose analyzer in a large nonhomogeneous population. Diabetes Technol Ther 2001;3(4):591–600.
[86] Boyd JC, Bruns DE. Quality specifications for glucose meters: assessment by simulation modeling of errors in insulin dose. Clin Chem 2001;47(2):209–14.
[87] Mahoney JJ, Ellison JM. Assessing glucose monitor performance: a standardized approach. Diabetes Technol Ther 2007;9(6):545–52.
[88] Goldberg PA, Siegel MD, Russell RR, et al. Experience with the continuous glucose monitoring system in a medical intensive care unit. Diabetes Technol Ther 2004;6(3):339–47.
[89] Torjman MC, Dalal N, Goldberg ME. Glucose monitoring in acute care: technologies on the horizon. J Diabetes Sci Technol 2008;2(2):178–81.
[90] Schaller R, Feichtner F, Kohler H, et al. A novel automated discontinuous venous blood monitoring system for ex vivo glucose determination in humans. Biosens Bioelectron 2009;24(7):2239–45.
[91] Yamashita K, Okabayashi T, Yokoyama T, et al. The accuracy of a continuous blood glucose monitor during surgery. Anesth Analg 2008;106(1):160–3.
[92] Yamashita K, Okabayashi T, Yokoyama T, et al. Accuracy and reliability of continuous blood glucose monitor in post-surgical patients. Acta Anaesthesiol Scand 2009;53(1):66–71.
[93] Lucisano JY, Edelman SV, Quinto BD, et al. Development of a biosensor-based, patient-attached blood glucose monitoring system. Proc Am Chem Soc 1997;76:256.
[94] VIA Medical Corporation. VIA blood chemistry monitor for glucose VIA V-GLU 1 operator's manual. San Diego (CA); VIA Medical Corporation: 1998.
[95] Krinsley J, Zheng P, Hall D, et al. ICU validation of the optiscanner, a continuous glucose monitoring device: 255. Crit Care Med 2006;34(12):A67.
[96] Okabayashi T, Hnazaki K, Nishimori I, et al. Continuous post-operative blood glucose monitoring and control using a closed-loop system in patients undergoing hepatic resection. Dig Dis Sci 2008;53(5):1405–10.
[97] Kadish AH. A servomechanism for blood sugar control. Biomed Sci Instrum 1963;1:171–6.
[98] Ozyol MB, Herfarth C, Kerner W, et al. Postoperative blood-sugar regulation in pancreatectomized patients using the artificial "beta cell.". Chirurg 1979;50(4):227–32.
[99] Schwartz SS, Horwitz DL, Zehfus B, et al. Use of a glucose controlled insulin infusion system (artificial beta cell) to control diabetes during surgery. Diabetologia 1979;16(3):157–64.
[100] Gin H, Catargi B, Rigalleau V, et al. Experience with the biostator for diagnosis and assisted surgery of 21 insulinomas. Eur J Endocrinol 1998;139(4):371–7.
[101] Rossetti P, Porcellati F, Fanelli CG, et al. Evaluation of the accuracy of a microdialysis-based glucose sensor during insulin-induced hypoglycemia, its recovery, and post-hypoglycemic hyperglycemia in humans. Diabetes Technol Ther 2006;8(3):326–37.
[102] Plank J, Schaller R, Ellmerer M, et al. Continuous glucose monitoring using the SCGM1 system in postcardiothoracic surgery patients. Crit Care 2006;10:P254.
[103] Heise HM, Kondepati VR, Damm U, et al. Microdialysis based monitoring of subcutaneous interstitial and venous blood glucose in type 1 diabetic subjects by mid-infrared spectrometry for intensive insulin therapy. Optical Diagnostics Sensing VIII 2008;6863:686308.1–686308.11.
[104] Heise HM, Damm U, Bodenlenz M, et al. Bedside monitoring of subcutaneous interstitial glucose in healthy individuals using microdialysis and infrared spectrometry. J Biomed Opt 2007;12(2):024004.
[105] McGarraugh G. The chemistry of commercial continuous glucose monitors. Diabetes Technol Ther 2009;11(Suppl 1):S17–24.
[106] Allen HF, Rake A, Roy M, et al. Prospective detection of hyperglycemia in critically ill children using continuous glucose monitoring. Pediatr Crit Care Med 2008;9(2):153–8.

[107] Joseph J, Torjman MC. Implantable glucose sensors. In: Wnek GE, Bowlin GL, editors. Encyclopedia of biomaterials. New York: Marcel-Dekker Publisher; 2004. p. 683–92.
[108] CLSI. Performance metrics for continuous interstitial glucose monitoring; approved guideline. CLSI document POCT05-A (ISBN 1-56238-685-9). Wayne (PA); 2008.
[109] Rebrin K, Steil GM. Can interstitial glucose assessment replace blood glucose measurements? Diabetes Technol Ther 2000;2(3):461–72.
[110] Hipszer B, Joseph JI. Lag associated with interstitial glucose sensors used in a diabetic surgical patient. Anesthesiology 2006;105:A584.
[111] Simon B, Treat V, Marco C, et al. A comparison of glycaemic variability in CSII vs. MDI treated type 1 diabetic patients using CGMS. Int J Clin Pract 2008;62(12):1858–63.
[112] Lodwig V, Heinemann L, Glucose Monitoring Study Group. Continuous glucose monitoring with glucose sensors: calibration and assessment criteria. Diabetes Technol Ther 2003;5(4):572–86.
[113] Garg SK. The future of continuous glucose monitoring. Diabetes Technol Ther 2009;11(Suppl 1):S1–3.
[114] McGarraugh G, Bergenstal R. Detection of hypoglycemia with continuous interstitial and traditional blood glucose monitoring using the FreeStyle navigator continuous glucose monitoring system. Diabetes Technol Ther 2009;11(3):145–50.
[115] Brauker J. Continuous glucose sensing: future technology developments. Diabetes Technol Ther 2009;11(Suppl 1):S25–36.
[116] Ward WK, Casey HM, Quinn MJ, et al. A fully implantable subcutaneous glucose sensor array: enhanced accuracy from multiple sensing units and a median-based algorithm. Diabetes Technol Ther 2003;5(6):943–52.
[117] Chuang H, Trieu M, Hurley J, et al. Pilot studies of transdermal continuous glucose measurement in outpatient diabetic patients and in patients during and after cardiac surgery. J Diabetes Sci Technol 2008;2(4):595–602.
[118] Furnary AP, Wu Y, Bookin SO. Effect of hyperglycemia and continuous intravenous insulin infusions on outcomes of cardiac surgical procedures: the Portland Diabetic Project. Endocr Pract 2004;10(Suppl 2):21–33.
[119] Trence DL, Kelly JL, Hirsch IB. The rationale and management of hyperglycemia for inpatients with cardiovascular disease: time for change. J Clin Endocrinol Metab 2003;88(6):2430–7.
[120] Chase JG, Shaw G, Le Compte A, et al. Implementation and evaluation of the SPRINT protocol for tight glycaemic control in critically ill patients: a clinical practice change. Crit Care 2008;12(2):R49.
[121] Davidson PC, Steed RD, Bode BW. Glucommander: a computer-directed intravenous insulin system shown to be safe, simple, and effective in 120,618 h of operation. Diabetes Care 2005;28(10):2418–23.
[122] Saager L, Collins GL, Burnside B, et al. A randomized study in diabetic patients undergoing cardiac surgery comparing computer-guided glucose management with a standard sliding scale protocol. J Cardiothorac Vasc Anesth 2008;22(3):377–82.
[123] Blaha J, Kopecky P, Matias M, et al. Comparison of three protocols for tight glycemic control in cardiac surgery patients. Diabetes Care 2009;32(5):757–61.
[124] Braithwaite SS, Clement S. Algorithms for intravenous insulin delivery. Curr Diabetes Rev 2008;4(3):258–68.
[125] Bequette BW. Analysis of algorithms for intensive care unit blood glucose control. J Diabetes Sci Technol 2007;1(6):813–24.
[126] Steil GM, Deiss D, Shih J, et al. Intensive care unit insulin delivery algorithms: why so many? How to choose? J Diabetes Sci Technol 2009;3(1):125–40.
[127] Cochran S, Miller E, Dunn K, et al. Endotool software for tight glucose control for critically ill patients [abstract supplement]. Crit Care Med 2006;34(12):A68.
[128] Hovorka R. Continuous glucose monitoring and closed-loop systems. Diabet Med 2006;23(1):1–12.

[129] Albisser AM, Leibel BS, Ewart TG, et al. An artificial endocrine pancreas. Diabetes 1974;23(5):389–96.
[130] Chase JG, Shaw GM, Lin J, et al. Targeted glycemic reduction in critical care using closed-loop control. Diabetes Technol Ther 2005;7(2):274–82.
[131] Chee F, Fernando T, van Heerden PV. Closed-loop control of blood glucose levels in critically ill patients. Anaesth Intensive Care 2002;30(3):295–307.
[132] Watson BG, Elliott MJ, Pay DA, et al. Diabetes mellitus and open heart surgery. A simple, practical closed-loop insulin infusion system for blood glucose control. Anaesthesia 1986;41(3):250–7.
[133] Weinzimer SA, Steil GM, Swan KL, et al. Fully automated closed-loop insulin delivery versus semiautomated hybrid control in pediatric patients with type 1 diabetes using an artificial pancreas. Diabetes Care 2008;31(5):934–9.
[134] Renard E, Costalat G, Chevassus H, et al. Closed loop insulin delivery using implanted insulin pumps and sensors in type 1 diabetic patients. Diabetes Res Clin Pract 2006;74(Suppl 2):S173–7.

Advances in Surgery 44 (2010) 185–198
ADVANCES IN SURGERY

Minimally Invasive Thyroid and Parathyroid Operations: Surgical Techniques and Pearls

Brian Hung-Hin Lang, MS, FRACS
Division of Endocrine Surgery, Department of Surgery, University of Hong Kong Medical Centre, Queen Mary Hospital, 102 Pokfulam Road, Pokfulam, Hong Kong SAR, China

Over the last decade, new modern technologies increasingly have been proposed and applied in thyroid and parathyroid operations. Some of these new technologies include intraoperative neuromonitoring of the recurrent laryngeal nerve (RLN), quick intraoperative parathyroid hormone assay, and application of new energy devices such as ultrasonic shears and endoscopic visualization and magnification. The overall objectives of these technologies are to not only increase the safety and quality of thyroid surgery but also improve patient outcomes [1]. With the help of these new technologies and with the wider acceptance and greater demand by the public and surgeons for endoscopic and minimally invasive procedures, increasing varieties of minimally invasive thyroidectomy (MIT) and parathyroidectomy (MIP) techniques have been described. Since the first reported case of endoscopic parathyroidectomy in 1996 by Michel Gagner [2], over 20 different approaches in MIT and MIP had been reported [3].

To those not so familiar with these MIT and MIP approaches, they can be categorized into two main groups, namely the direct/cervical and the indirect/extracervical approaches, according to the site of incision made relative to the neck area [4]. The former are considered truly minimally invasive, as small skin incisions are made directly over the neck. These approaches allow direct access to the thyroid and parathyroid glands. On the other hand, the latter often are considered endoscopic rather than truly minimally invasive, because incisions are made far from the neck and so they require more tissue extensive dissection to gain access to the neck [5]. The indirect/extracervical approaches are generally technically more challenging because of the limited working space and frequent instrument collisions. There is also a comparatively longer learning curve and initial operating time. However, the indirect/extracervical approaches do offer better cosmetic results, because scars can be hidden by clothing. These approaches have been popular in Asian countries, where scarlessness in the neck is preferred.

E-mail address: blang@hkucc.hku.hk.

0065-3411/10/$ – see front matter
doi:10.1016/j.yasu.2010.05.012

For the purpose of this article, MIT and MIP will be considered separately. The two actually deal with different disease entities, and each MIT approach also can be applied to MIP. The MIP section will focus on the surgical principles rather than detailed description of each surgical approach. For each approach, a brief technical description will be given and will be followed by discussing its major advantages, disadvantages, and reported outcomes.

MIT

Direct/cervical approaches

Minimally invasive video-assisted thyroidectomy

Minimally invasive video-assisted thyroidectomy (MIVAT) was developed by Miccoli and colleagues [6] in Pisa, Italy in 1998. MIVAT is a minimally invasive procedure that is comprised of an endoscopic part and an open part. The patient is put under either general anesthesia with orotracheal intubation or locoregional anesthesia with bilateral deep cervical plexus block. The patient is put in a supine position with his or her neck in neutral position. The operating team consists of three surgeons. The operator stands on the opposite side of the excised lobe with the first assistant holding the camera and the second assistant retracting the wound. A 2 cm central neck incision is made 2 cm above the sternal notch. The midline then is exposed by means of two army–navy retractors and incised longitudinally for 3 to 4 cm. The entire procedure is performed gasless with the operating field maintained by means of two retractors held by the second assistant. The thyroid lobe is bluntly dissected away from strap muscles and pushed inferomedially by one of the retractors. With the help of a 5 mm 30 endoscope, the upper pedicle is visualized, and individual vessels are divided with ultrasonic shears. Once the upper pedicle has been divided securely and the external branch of the superior laryngeal nerve has been identified, the entire upper pole is pulled up and gradually delivered to the main wound. The rest of the lobe then is dissected in the subcapsular plane like an open procedure. For bilateral resection, the procedure is repeated in the opposite side. No drain is required, and glue is used to seal the skin.

Table 1 summarizes the major advantages and disadvantages using this approach. The MIVAT technique has been adopted by various groups. It is applicable in most benign thyroid conditions and low-risk papillary thyroid carcinoma (PTC). Because it is possible to combine a central compartment neck dissection, this approach is ideal for prophylactic thyroidectomy in asymptomatic patients with the rearranged during transfection germ-line mutation. In MIVAT, the only important limiting factor appears to be the size of the thyroid removed, because only a small neck incision is made. Glands exceeding 25 to 30 mL measured by ultrasound or nodules larger than 3.5 cm often are excluded [7].

Lateral endoscopic approach

This approach first was described by Henry in Marseille, France, in 1999 [8]. Unlike the conventional thyroidectomy, the thyroid lobe is being approached laterally (ie, via the plane between the carotid sheath and the strap muscles) [9].

Table 1
Summary of major advantages and disadvantages with various approaches in minimally invasive thyroidectomy

MIT approaches	Authors (year)	Special equipment	Major advantages	Major disadvantages
Direct/Cervical				
MIVAT	Miccoli et al (1999) [6]	Endoscope, ultrasonic shears	Good long-term data are available; bilateral resection is possible	At least 2 experienced assistants required
Lateral endoscopic	Henry and Sebag (2006) [8]	Endoscope, CO_2 insufflation	Direct view of the vital structures (eg, RLN and parathyroid glands)	Applicable to unilateral thyroid resection only
Mini-incision	Gosnell et al (2004) [10]	None required	Techniques adopted similar to open procedure, minimally invasive	Applicable to unilateral thyroid resection only
Indirect/Extracervical				
Infraclavicular	Shimizu et al (1998) [13]	Flexible endoscope, ultrasonic shears	Large-sized tumors can be resected	Main wound is prone to hypertrophy; contralateral thyroid resection is difficult
Axillary	Ikeda et al (2000) [16]	Endoscope, ultrasonic shears	Scars can be completely hidden by clothing, relatively short distance when lesion-side arm is fully abducted	Collision of instruments; contralateral thyroid resection is difficult
Chest	Ohgami et al (2000) [24]	Endoscope, ultrasonic shears	Multiangle approach is possible	Parasternal wound is prone to hypertrophy
ABBA	Shimazu et al (2003) [25]	Endoscope, ultrasonic shears, CO_2 insufflation	Multiangle approach is possible	Excessive flap dissection leading to discomfort and pain
BABA	Choe et al (2007) [27]	Endoscope, ultrasonic shears, CO_2 insufflation	Good surgical ergonomics, as instruments are perpendicular to each other; bilateral resection is made easier	Excessive flap dissection leading to discomfort, paresthesia, and pain
PAA	Lee et al (2009) [28]	Endoscope, ultrasonic shears, CO_2 insufflation, special designed retractors	Good surgical ergonomics while avoiding periareolar dissections	Excessive flap dissection leading to discomfort and pain, possible facial nerve injury
Robot-assisted				
Axillary	Kang et al (2009) [29]	da Vinci robot	3-dimensional endoscopic view, more flexible instruments	High costs
BABA	Lee et al (2009) [31]	da Vinci robot	3-dimensional endoscopic view, more flexible instruments	High costs

Abbreviations: ABBA, axillo-bilateral-breast approach; BABA, bilateral axillo-breast approach; MIT, minimally invasive thyroidectomy; MIVAT, minimally invasive video-assisted thyroidectomy; PAA, postauricular and axillary approach; RLN, recurrent laryngeal nerve.

Therefore, this approach only can be applied to unilateral resection or hemithyroidectomy. The procedure begins with a 10 mm incision along the medial border of the sternocleidomastoid muscle (SCM), and the dissection then is deepened and extended along the lateral space of the thyroid lobe. Two 3 mm ports then are inserted above and below the 10 mm incision along the SCM. The operating space is maintained with low pressure (8 mm Hg) CO_2 insufflation. One major advantage of using the lateral approach is that the key structures and landmarks such as the esophagus, trachea, inferior thyroid artery, parathyroid glands, and the RLN can be identified readily and protected during dissection. Through the magnified endoscopic view, small vascular branches can be skeletonized and cauterized, maintaining a bloodless field. Once the lobe is entirely freed, the specimen is extracted through the 10 mm incision.

Table 1 summarizes the major advantages and disadvantages using this approach. If the frozen section or definitive pathology reveals malignancy, however, the patient will need to have a conventional cervicotomy. Furthermore, because of its relatively stringent inclusion criteria, only up to 5% of patients requiring surgery are eligible for this approach. Nevertheless, a series of over 100 cases was recently reported by Slotema and colleagues [4], and there were five open conversions and five patients requiring open completion total thyroidectomy because of diagnosis of cancer.

Mini-incision

This approach first was described by Gosnell and colleagues [10] at Royal North shore Hospital, Sydney, Australia. It was developed from their techniques in MIP. The procedure is essentially an open technique, and the success of the procedure relies on the good use of head light, loupe magnification, and small retractors. The procedure begins with a small (2.5 cm) lateral incision placed directly over the nodule. A subplatysmal space is developed to allow the skin incision to be moved around the neck and over the relevant area of dissection. Like the lateral endoscopic approach, it uses the plane between SCM and strap muscles. The middle thyroid vein is divided, and the dissection is deepened down to the prevertebral plane. Once the strap muscles are dissected from the thyroid lobe by retracting them medially, the lateral surface of the thyroid gland is visualized. The isthmus is divided, and that allows full mobilization of the resected lobe. The skin incision then is retracted in a cephalad direction, and the upper pole is divided. The lower pole is mobilized by careful capsular dissection with preservation of the inferior parathyroid gland on its vascular pedicle. At this stage, the thyroid nodule is delivered through the incision, allowing the critical lateral dissection to be undertaken close to the skin surface. Capsular dissection is continued until the RLN is encountered. The nerve is preserved by continuing the mobilization of the gland superiorly, and the superior parathyroid is gently dissected away from the thyroid capsule on its vascular pedicle. The ligament of Berry is divided, and the thyroid lobe is removed through the small incision. The skin incision is closed subcuticularly.

Table 1 summarizes the major advantages and disadvantages of this approach. Because this is essentially an open procedure, it is associated with a relatively short learning curve. Similar to the lateral endoscopic approach, however, if frozen section or definitive pathology reveals malignancy, the patient will need a conventional cervicotomy. Over 200 cases have been reported using this method with minimal morbidity [11,12].

Extracervical approaches

Infraclavicular approach

This approach initially was described by Shimizu and colleagues [13,14] in Tokyo in 1998, and the aim was to make the surgery scarless in the neck. It is also known as video-assisted neck surgery (VANS), and to date, close to 1000 cases have been performed by Shimizu and colleagues [15]. The procedure involves making a 30 mm skin incision below the inferior border of the clavicle on the side of the thyroid lesion, followed by raising a skin flap from the incision to thyroid area under either direct or endoscopic vision. The working space is then either maintained with a skin lifting device or low-pressure CO_2 insufflation. One or two 5 mm ports are inserted lateral to the main incision. The rest of the dissection is done similarly to an open procedure. In most instances, dissection of the gland is performed with ultrasonic shears, and the specimen is retrieved in a bag via the 30mm incision, leaving no scar in the neck.

Table 1 summarizes the major advantages and disadvantages using this approach. This technique has been criticized for not being able to fully hide the scars by clothing (which defeats the purpose of performing extracervically) and the fact that the main wound is usually more prone to hypertrophy. Nevertheless, large thyroid tumors of up to 7 cm in size have been resected successfully [15].

Axillary approach

Since the first report by Ikeda and colleagues in 2000, this has become one of the most popular extracervical approaches, and it is widely practiced by different investigators, including the author's group [16–22]. The operation is performed either with gas or without gas insufflation. For the gasless approach, a skin lifting device often is used. Similar to other extracervical approaches, a skin flap is raised to the thyroid area via the axillary incision. In the author's approach, patients are placed in a supine position under general anesthesia. The neck is slightly extended and the lesion-side arm is raised above the head and fixed for the shortest distance from axilla to anterior neck (Fig. 1). A 4 to 6 cm-sized vertical skin incision is made in the axilla for the insertion of a 30° endoscope and endoscopic instruments. One 10 mm trocar is incorporated into the main wound, and a second 5 mm trocar is placed 4 to 5 cm medial to the lower end of the axillary wound. Dissection is approached through the space between two arms of SCM. An external retractor is inserted through the skin incision in the axilla (Fig. 2). Under endoscopic visualization, the upper pole of the thyroid is drawn downward, and the superior thyroid

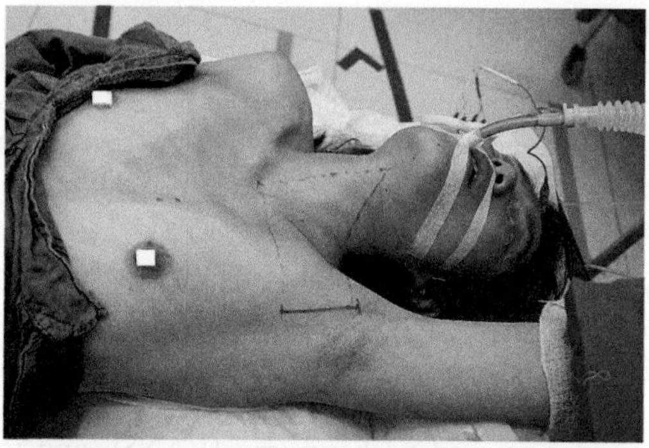

Fig. 1. The patient's neck has been extended, and the lesion-side arm has been raised above the head and fixed for the shortest distance from axilla to anterior neck.

vessels are identified and individually divided close to thyroid lobe using the ultrasonic shears (Fig. 3). The lower pole is dissected from the adipose tissue and cervical thymic tissue, and the inferior thyroid vein is divided close to the thyroid gland. The lobe then is retracted medially, and the perithyroidal fascia is divided and sharply dissected using an endoscopic dissector. The inferior thyroid artery is divided close to the thyroid gland using ultrasonic shears, and the whole cervical course of the RLN is traced (Fig. 4). After excision, the specimen usually is retrieved through the axillary wound, and the operating field is irrigated (Fig. 5). If bilateral resection is required, the contralateral lobe can be resected by adopting the medial approach. This avoids inserting more ports. In the author's experience, the operating time is 90 min for unilateral resection and 120 to 150 min for bilateral resection.

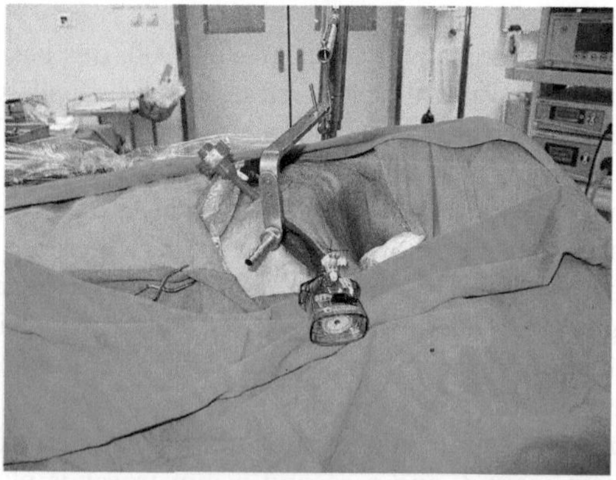

Fig. 2. A special lifting device has been inserted into the left axillary wound for the gasless approach. A 10 mm port has been incorporated into the main wound, and another 5 mm port has been inserted 6 cm medial and 2 cm below the main axillary wound. This arrangement allows good angulations between instruments.

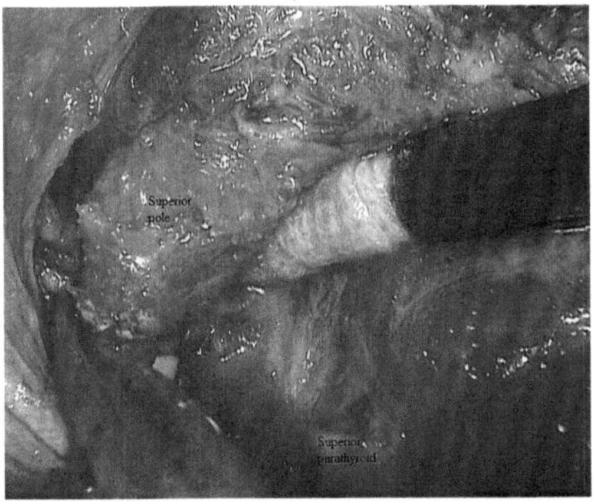

Fig. 3. Endoscopic lateral view of the thyroid gland using the gasless transaxillary approach. The upper pole of the right thyroid lobe is divided by the ultrasonic shears with the thyroid lobe being retracted inferomedially.

Table 1 summarizes the major advantages and disadvantages of using this approach. Total thyroidectomy with or without central neck dissection is possible with this approach, and therefore many low-risk PTC currently are managed using this approach. Over 600 benign and malignant cases have been reported using this method with comparable complication rates as open thyroidectomy [23].

Chest approach

This approach first was described by Ohgami and colleagues in 2000 [24]. Two incisions are placed bilaterally in the infraclavicular region or upper

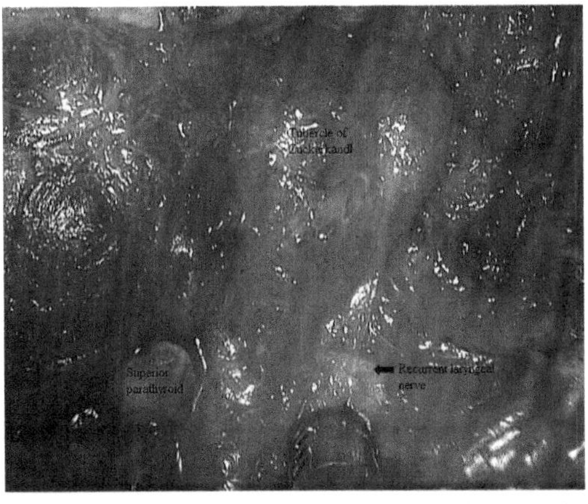

Fig. 4. Endoscopic lateral view of the thyroid gland using the gasless transaxillary approach. It depicts the recurrent laryngeal nerve (*black arrow*) lying below the tubercle of Zuckerkandl after the thyroid lobe has been retracted medially.

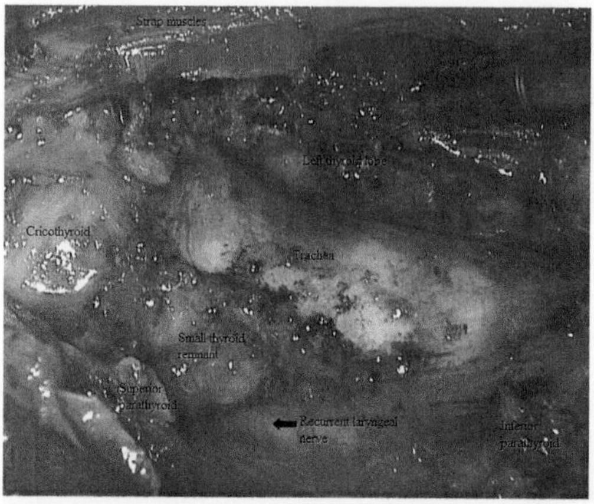

Fig. 5. The anatomic landmarks after endoscopic removal of the right thyroid lobe using the gasless transaxillary approach.

circumareolar areas. The subcutaneous space in the breast area and the subplatysmal space in the neck are bluntly dissected through the incisions, and the camera port is inserted on the ipsilateral side of the thyroid lobe to be removed. CO_2 is insufflated at a pressure up to 6 mm Hg to create the operative space. An additional third port is inserted infraclavicularly. The anterior border of the sternocleidomastoid is dissected out. The strap muscles then are divided longitudinally. Dissection of the thyroid is commenced inferiorly and then proceeds to the posterior and lateral aspects of the gland. Division of the thyroid vessels and parenchyma is performed endoscopically using an ultrasonically activated scalpel. As the gland is elevated, the cervical course of the RLN can be visualized and protected. For unilateral resection, the isthmus is divided with ultrasonic shears. Hemostasis is achieved; a suction drain is left in place, and the skin is closed subcuticularly. Table 1 summarizes the major advantage and disadvantage of this approach. Similar to the infraclavicular approach, these wounds tend to hypertrophy, and some postoperative bruising appears inevitable. Furthermore, some female patients prefer no dissection around the breast area.

Axillo-bilateral-breast approach

This first was described by Shimazu and colleagues in 2003 [25]. It has been called the hybrid approach, because it is essentially a combined axillary and breast approach [26]. The main reason for this approach is it improves the angulations between the endoscopic instruments relative to the thyroid gland. Under general anesthesia, the patient's neck is slightly extended. The arm on the tumor side is first abducted, and the legs are parted such that the camera person can stand between the legs. A 2.5 cm incision is made along the upper margin of the areola on the tumor side. After blunt dissection of the subcutaneous tissue of the breast, a subplatysmal working space is created with a balloon dissector. Following insertion of a 10 mm trocar through the incision, the working space is inflated with CO_2 gas at 4 to 6 mm Hg, and a 10-mm telescope is inserted through the trocar. Two additional 10 mm trocars are inserted through the axillary incision on the tumor side and through the incision at the upper margin of the areola on the opposite side, respectively. The working space is made wide to the level of thyroid cartilage in the upper side and to the medial edge of each SCM in the lateral sides. The strap muscles and SCM are separated, and the strap muscles on the tumor side are transected using the ultrasonic shears. The lower pole is mobilized, and the isthmus is divided. The lobe is retracted upward and dissected from the trachea and surrounding connective tissue in the lateral margin of the lobe. For larger lesions, the camera can be placed in the axillary port for better visualization of the upper pole. The rest is performed in a similar way as other endoscopic procedures. The resected specimen is retrieved with a plastic bag. Divided strap muscles are sutured. Table 1 summarizes the major advantages and disadvantages of using this approach.

Bilateral axillo-breast approach

Like the axillo-bilateral-breast approach (ABBA), the bilateral axillo-breast approach (BABA) is also a combined axillary and breast approach, except one more axillary port on the opposite side is inserted. This first was reported by Choe and colleagues [27] in 2007. Under general anesthesia, the patient is placed in supine position with the neck extended using a pillow. Both arms are mildly abducted to provide for insertion of 5 mm ports. Diluted (1:200,000) epinephrine solution is injected into the subcutaneous space in both breasts and the subplatysmal space in the neck to reduce bleeding during dissection. After making two incisions on both upper circumareolar areas, subcutaneous and subplatysmal dissections are performed bluntly with the use of a Rochester clamp and vascular tunneler. The working space is extended to the level of the thyroid cartilage superiorly and to the medial border of each sternocleidomastoid muscle laterally. After establishing the required working space, the ports (12 mm) are inserted. The working space is maintained with CO_2 insufflation at pressure of 5 to 6 mm Hg. The remaining dissection is completed with the visual guidance of the flexible endoscope. Two 5 mm ports are inserted into each axilla. Strap muscles are split in the middle. After full visualization of the cricothyroid membrane, the isthmic portion of the thyroid gland, and the central lymph node group, the isthmus is dissected. This procedure results in optimal retraction of the thyroid tissue for dissection of its lateral and posterior aspects. Thyroidectomy is performed using Harmonic Scalpel (Johnson & Johnson Medical, Cincinnati, OH, USA) under full visualization of superior and inferior thyroidal arteries, parathyroid glands, and RLNs. The resected specimen then is retrieved via the 12 mm port. Table 1 summarizes the major advantages and disadvantages of this approach. With this approach, total thyroidectomy and central neck dissection is technically feasible, and so low-risk PTC can be managed using this approach. This approach, however, often has been criticized for being very invasive, and a few patients do complain of prolonged paresthesias over the chest area and some hardening of skin along the subcutaneous or subplatysmal tracks.

Postauricular and axillary approach

To avoid excessive dissection around the areolar areas (which some female patients may not accept), the postauricular and axillary approach (PAA) was developed by Lee and colleagues [28] in 2009. This is a challenging but nevertheless innovative procedure. The neck is extended, and both arms are abducted for the insertion of the axillary ports. The operator stands on the side of the lesion; the camera is placed on the opposite side, and two assistants are situated at the head of the patient. A 21-gauge spinal needle is used to subcutaneously infiltrate the subplatysmal space of the neck and the subcutaneous space of the axillary and anterior chest area with diluted epinephrine solution (0.1 mL of epinephrine [1:1000] in 200 mL of normal saline). A 12 mm axillary incision is made, and the subplatysmal space is dissected bluntly by using a vascular tunneler. The working space is extended superiorly, laterally, and inferiorly to the level of the thyroid cartilage, the medial border of each SCM, and the anterior chest, respectively. After establishing the required working space, a 12 mm trocar is inserted, and the operative space under the flap is insufflated with low-pressure CO_2 (5–6 mm Hg). Another incision is made on the contralateral axillary region, and a 5 mm trocar is inserted. By using 5 mm ultrasonic shears, the rest of the dissection is completed with the visual guidance of a 5 mm flexible videoscope. Bilateral postauricular incisions are made, and two 5 mm trocars are inserted. By using a monopolar dissector, a midline incision is made between the strap muscles from the level of the thyroid cartilage to the suprasternal notch. During the dissection, the bilateral strap muscles are retracted laterally with right-angled graspers via the postauricular ports, and the isthmus is divided. The thyroid lobe is retracted medially. The superior vessels of the thyroid gland are coagulated, and the inferolateral side of the thyroid gland is approached; the RLN and parathyroid glands are protected. The resected specimen is pulled out through the 12 mm axillary port by using a plastic bag. A frozen section of the resected specimen is tested for confirmation of suspected pathology. Experience with this approach remains relatively limited. Table 1 summarizes the major advantage and disadvantage of this approach. This is a novel approach to the thyroid gland, but like ABBA and BABA, PAA has been criticized for its invasiveness. To date, only a few dozen cases had been reported. The marginal or cervical branches of both facial nerves are prone to traction injury; therefore this approach has not been popular so far.

ROBOT-ASSISTED THYROIDECTOMY

The addition of the robot such as the da Vinci surgical system could possibly be a major step in making extracervical approaches more ergonomic for surgeons. The added benefits of using the robot include the three-dimensional view of the operating field, the more flexible endoscopic instruments with seven degrees of freedom and 90° articulation, the improvement in tactile sense, and filtering hand tremors [29]. Kang and colleagues [30] recently reported their experience of 200 robot-assisted cases using the gasless transaxillary approach for low-risk PTC with concomitant central neck dissection and reported good short-term results in terms of less pain and increased patient satisfaction. A separate group also reported similar results using the BABA technique [31]. To date, the robot only has been applied in the extracervical and not in the cervical approaches. The use of the robot has been criticized for being too expensive, but perhaps with higher volumes, the costs might be lowered. With more centers worldwide acquiring robots, it is expected that the number of robot-assisted thyroidectomies will increase over time. Certainly, the author's group has started using the robot in some select cases (Fig. 6).

MIP

MIP has now become the standard approach for surgical management of primary hyperparathyroidism. It is the approach of choice for patients diagnosed with primary hyperparathyroidism caused by a solitary parathyroid adenoma, and it is fast becoming an alternative approach in parathyroid reoperations. Like MIT, it comes in various forms and under various names; these include total endoscopic approach, video-assisted approach, radio-guided approach and mini-incision approach. In principle, however, they are similar, as they involve surgical excision of one single abnormal parathyroid gland (ie, adenoma) without disturbing the other three parathyroid glands. Therefore, a better collective name for them should be the focused approach. Although the extracervical approaches have been described for both unilateral

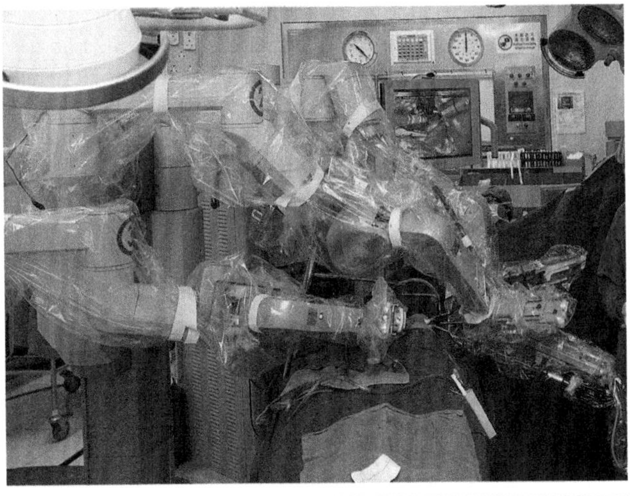

Fig. 6. The four robotic arms being inserted through the axillary incision and the chest cannula.

and bilateral neck explorations, they have not been adopted widely [32]. Among the endocrine surgeons, the most popular approach remains the open mini-incision approach with no video assistance.

The mini-incision approach in MIP is technically similar to the one in MIT. Essentially a 2 cm incision is made at the medial border of SCM. The site of incision is marked after performing a bedside ultrasound in the operating theater. The incision site is placed close to the localized parathyroid adenoma such that minimal tissue dissection is required. Like the mini-incision approach in MIT, a subplatysmal space is developed, and the plane between SCM and strap is opened up. Once the common carotid artery is identified, it is important to dissect all the way down to the prevertebral fascia medial to the artery such that the thyroid lobe and parathyroid glands can be retracted medially. At this point, the parathyroid adenoma usually is identified and carefully excised in whole.

MIP is an operation associated with low morbidity and high success rates (>95%), but the operating surgeon should be meticulous, familiar with the anatomy, and experienced. Unlike the traditional open method where all four parathyroid glands are identified, MIP requires accurate preoperative localization of the abnormal parathyroid gland before it can be attempted. This is because in MIP, the operating surgeon would not have the benefit of examining the other three parathyroid glands; therefore, there is a possibility of missing underlying multiglandular disease such as double adenomas or four-gland hyperplasia. In the author's center, over 70% of patients with newly diagnosed primary hyperparathyroidism will be eligible for MIP because of a positive preoperative localization by Tc99 m sestamibi or ultrasound [33]. To further improve the surgical success of MIP and to minimize the possibility of persistent or recurrent HPT after MIP, some have advocated the routine use of various surgical adjuncts such as radioguided probes or a quick intraoperative parathyroid hormone assay at the time of operation, but to date, their routine use remains questionable because of the marginal benefit and the high cost-to-benefit ratio. Nevertheless, MIP with or without the use of adjuncts, when performed in experienced hands has an equivalent success rate of greater than 95%, as the conventional four-gland exploration, and has all the benefits one expects from minimally invasive surgery.

SUMMARY

With advances in technology and greater demand for minimally invasive procedures, novel minimally invasive approaches to thyroid and parathyroid glands increasingly have been described and practiced worldwide. For the MIT approaches, the direct/cervical approaches truly can be considered minimally invasive, as they require less surgical dissection than the conventional thyroidectomy. The indirect/extracervical approaches, however, only can be considered endoscopic, however, because they generally do require greater surgical dissection. Still, among the indirect/extracervical approaches, the axillary approach appears the preferred choice, as it requires the least amount of dissection while offering the advantage of being scarless in the neck. The addition of the robot such as the de Vinci surgical system could make some of the extracervical approaches technically less challenging and improve patient outcomes. Unlike MIT, MIP has become the standard approach for surgical management of primary hyperparathyroidism caused by localized solitary parathyroid adenoma.

References

[1] Dralle H. Impact of modern technologies on quality of thyroid surgery. Langenbecks Arch Surg 2006;391:1–3.
[2] Gagner M. Endoscopic subtotal parathyroidectomy in patients with primary hyperparathyroidism. Br J Surg 1996;83:875.
[3] Dionigi G, Rovera F, Boni L. Commentary on transoral access for endoscopic thyroid resection. Surg Endosc 2009;23(2):454–5.
[4] Slotema ET, Sebag F, Henry JF. What is the evidence for endoscopic thyroidectomy in the management of benign thyroid disease? World J Surg 2008;32:1325–32.
[5] Henry JF. Minimally invasive thyroid and parathyroid surgery is not a question of the length of the incision. Langenbecks Arch Surg 2008;393:621–6.
[6] Miccoli P, Berti P, Conte M, et al. Minimally invasive surgery for thyroid small nodules: preliminary report. J Endocrinol Invest 1999;22:849–51.
[7] Miccoli P, Berti P, Ambrosini CE. Perspectives and lessons learned after a decade of minimally invasive video-assisted thyroidectomy. ORL J Otorhinolaryngol Relat Spec 2008;70:282–6.
[8] Henry JF, Sebag F. Lateral endoscopic approach for thyroid and parathyroid surgery. Ann Chir 2006;131(1):51–6.
[9] Palazzo FF, Sebag F, Henry JF. Endocrine surgical technique: endoscopic thyroidectomy via the lateral approach. Surg Endosc 2006;20:339–42.
[10] Gosnell JE, Sackett WR, Sidhu S, et al. Minimal access thyroid surgery: technique and report of the first 25 cases. ANZ J Surg 2004;74:330–3.
[11] Palazzo F, Sywak MS, Sidhu SB, et al. Safety and feasibility of thyroid lobectomy via a lateral 2.5-cm incision with a cohort comparison of the first 50 cases: evolution of a surgical approach. Langenbecks Arch Surg 2005;390:230–5.
[12] Lundgren C, Stalberg P, Grodski S, et al. Minimally invasive thyroid surgery (MITS) for diagnostic excision of solitary thyroid nodules. Asian J Surg 2007;30:250–4.
[13] Shimizu K, Akira S, Tanaka S. Video-assisted neck surgery: endoscopic resection of benign thyroid tumors aiming at scarless surgery on the neck. J Surg Oncol 1998;69:178–80.
[14] Shimizu K, Akira S, Jasmi AY, et al. Video-assisted neck surgery: endoscopic resection of thyroid tumors with a very minimal neck wound. J Am Coll Surg 1999;188:697–703.
[15] Shimizu K, Tanaka S. Asian perspective on endoscopic thyroidectomy—a review of 193 cases. Asian J Surg 2003;26:92–100.
[16] Ikeda Y, Takami H, Sasaki Y, et al. Endoscopic neck surgery by the axillary approach. J Am Coll Surg 2000;191:336–40.
[17] Udomsawaengsup S, Navicharern P, Tharavej C, et al. Endoscopic transaxillary thyroid lobectomy: flexible vs. rigid laparoscope. J Med Assoc Thai 2004;87(S2):S10–4.
[18] Chantawibul S, Lokechareonlarp S, Pokawatana C. Total video endoscopic thyroidectomy by an axillary approach. J Laparoendosc Adv Surg Tech A 2003;13:295–9.
[19] Yoon JH, Park CH, Chung WY. Gasless endoscopic thyroidectomy via an axillary approach: experience of 30 cases. Surg Laparosc Endosc Percutan Tech 2006;16:226–31.
[20] Jung EJ, Park ST, Ha WS, et al. Endoscopic thyroidectomy using a gasless axillary approach. J Laparoendosc Adv Surg Tech A 2007;17:21–5.

[21] Witzel K. The axillary access in unilateral thyroid resection. Langenbecks Arch Surg 2007;392:617–21.
[22] Duncan TD, Rashid Q, Speights F, et al. Endoscopic transaxillary approach to the thyroid gland: our early experience. Surg Endosc 2007;21:2166–71.
[23] Kang SW, Jeong JJ, Yun JS, et al. Gasless endoscopic thyroidectomy using trans-axillary approach; surgical outcome of 581 patients. Endocr J 2009;56:361–9.
[24] Ohgami M, Ishii S, Arisawa Y. Scarless endoscopic thyroidectomy: breast approach for better cosmesis. Surg Laparosc Endosc Percutan Tech 2000;10:1–4.
[25] Shimazu K, Shiba E, Tamaki Y, et al. Endoscopic thyroid surgery through the axillo-bilateral-breast approach. Surg Laparosc Endosc Percutan Tech 2003;13:196–201.
[26] Tan CT, Cheah WK, Delbridge L. Scarless (in the neck) endoscopic thyroidectomy (SET): an evidence-based review of published techniques. World J Surg 2008;32:1349–57.
[27] Choe JH, Kim SW, Chung KW, et al. Endoscopic thyroidectomy using a new bilateral axillo-breast approach. World J Surg 2007;31:601–6.
[28] Lee KE, Kim HY, Park WS, et al. Postauricular and axillary approach endoscopic neck surgery: a new technique. World J Surg 2009;33:767–72.
[29] Kang SW, Jeong JJ, Yun JS, et al. Robot-assisted endoscopic surgery for thyroid cancer: experience with the first 100 patients. Surg Endosc 2009;23(11):2399–406.
[30] Kang SW, Jeong JJ, Nam KH, et al. Robot-assisted endoscopic thyroidectromy for thyroid malignancies using a gasless transaxillary approach. J Am Coll Surg 2009;209:e1–7.
[31] Lee KE, Rao J, Youn YK. Endoscopic thyroidectomy with the da Vinci robot system using the bilateral axillary breast approach (BABA) technique: our initial experience. Surg Laparosc Endosc Percutan Tech 2009;19:71–5.
[32] Ikeda Y, Takami H. Endoscopic parathyroidectomy. Biomed Pharmacother 2000;54: 52s–6s.
[33] Lo CY, Lang BH, Chan WF, et al. A prospective evaluation of preoperative localization by technetium-99m sestamibi scintigraphy and ultrasonography in primary hyperparathyroidism. Am J Surg 2007;193(2):155–9.

Advances in Surgery 44 (2010) 199–228

ADVANCES IN SURGERY

ELSEVIER
MOSBY

What's New in Neoadjuvant Therapy for Breast Cancer?

Georgia M. Beasley, MD, John A. Olson Jr, MD, PhD*

Department of Surgery, Duke University Medical Center, Box 3118, Durham, NC 27710, USA

Neoadjuvant therapy for breast cancer, or treatment preceding surgical removal of the tumor and lymph nodes, was first described in patients with locally advanced breast cancer in the late 1970s [1]. The proposed goals of neoadjuvant therapy were to downstage inoperable tumors and improve locoregional control. With the widespread use of breast cancer screening, breast cancers are increasingly being diagnosed at earlier stages. As such, patients presenting with locally advanced breast cancer are less commonly seen than before; data from the American National Cancer Institute's Surveillance, Epidemiology, and End Results (SEER) program show that only 7% of all breast cancer patients have American Joint Committee on Cancer (AJCC) Stage III disease at diagnosis [2,3]. Recently, the indications for neoadjuvant therapy have been expanded to include patients with operable and early-stage disease [4,5]. The use of neoadjuvant therapy has rapidly become the preferred treatment for many subsets of patients with breast cancer and not just those with locally invasive or inflammatory breast cancers in whom the role of neoadjuvant therapy is well established. However, there are currently many unresolved clinical questions regarding the use of neoadjuvant therapy in initially operable breast cancer, including demonstration of equivalent survival to standard therapy (surgery followed by chemotherapy +/− radiation), implications for staging, and appropriate assessment of response. Here the authors review the goals of neoadjuvant therapy, discuss the benefits and disadvantages of neoadjuvant therapy as well as issues related to staging and prognostic markers, and identify areas of focus for future research.

GOALS OF NEOADJUVANT THERAPY IN BREAST CANCER

Primary chemotherapy has been established as the standard of care for patients with locally advanced and inflammatory breast cancers [6]. The use of preoperative systemic chemotherapy has been shown to induce response and help achieve local control with the addition of subsequent surgery and radiation therapy. Anthracycline-based regimens in this population improved survival

*Corresponding author. *E-mail address*: jaomd@duke.edu.

0065-3411/10/$ – see front matter
doi:10.1016/j.yasu.2010.05.013

rates up to 25% at 10 years compared with historical experience and local therapy alone [7,8]. Given the success in the inoperable and locally advanced population, the use of preoperative systemic therapy has subsequently been investigated in patients who present with initially operable breast cancer. The primary goal of this approach (also known as neoadjuvant therapy) in these patients is to potentially surgically downstage disease to enable breast-conserving surgery (BCS) for women who might otherwise require a mastectomy. Another potential goal is to expose micrometastases to early systemic chemotherapy early in the treatment course to improve distant disease-free and overall survival. Of importance, tumor response can be monitored during neoadjuvant therapy with the potential to alter treatment based on individual response. In examining the data to determine how well neoadjuvant therapy for operable breast cancer achieves the aforementioned goals, potential disadvantages to this approach must also be considered. Specifically with the use of neoadjuvant chemotherapy (NAC), there should be no significant difference in local recurrence, distant recurrence, disease progression, or survival compared with standard adjuvant (postoperative) chemotherapy. In addition, neoadjuvant therapy must not interfere or disrupt definitive surgery or radiation therapy. Each of these issues has been addressed and is reviewed here.

Breast conservation

The ability of preoperative systemic therapy to decrease tumor size (also known as downstage) and increase rates of BCS has been examined in several randomized and nonrandomized clinical trials [4,5,9–12]. The clinical efficacy of preoperative chemotherapy to surgically downstage tumors is dependent on tumor response to chemotherapy. Several trials have demonstrated that a majority of patients (roughly 70%–80%) have a clinical response to induction chemotherapy in both the breast and axilla [4]. Complete clinical response in this situation is being defined as complete disappearance of the palpable or imageable tumor in the breast following preoperative systemic therapy, with partial clinical response being defined as tumor shrinkage greater than 50%. Pathologic complete response, defined as no tumor remaining in the breast on histopathology following preoperative systemic therapy occurs in 3% to 46% of patients, depending on the particular agents used [13]. Table 1 summarizes data from several large randomized trials. Given that a large portion of patients do respond to neoadjuvant therapy, studies have examined whether response to chemotherapy can lead to breast conservation therapy. In 2 large randomized trials comparing preoperative versus postoperative [11,12] chemotherapy, a higher percentage of patients were able to be treated with breast conservation therapy in the preoperative chemotherapy arms. Specifically in the National Surgical Adjuvant Breast and Bowel Project B18 (NSABP-18), physicians were required to specify the type of surgery planned before initiation of treatment. Sixty-nine (27.0%) of the 256 women for whom a mastectomy had been planned before randomization ultimately had BCS after NAC [5]. It is interesting that when the 2 groups (preoperative vs postoperative chemotherapy)

Table 1
Preoperative chemotherapy trials

Trial	Year	Type	No. of patients	Chemotherapy regimen	cCR	pCR	BCS
NSABP-18 [4,38]	1997	RCT	1523	AC→S vs S→AC	36%	13%	67% vs 60%
EORTC 10902 [12]	2001	RCT	698	FEC→S vs S→FEC	6.60%	4%	23% vs 18%
NSABP-27 [29]	2003	RCT	2411	AC→S vs AC→D→S vs AC→S→D	40.1%/63.6%	13.7%/26%	
Gerpar-DUO [30]	2005	RCT	913	dd AD→D vs AD	31.2% vs 55.7%	7% vs 14.3%	58.1% vs 63.4%
ECTO Trial [10]	2001	RCT	1355	S→A→CMF vs S→AP→CMF vs AP→CMF→S	49% in AP→CMF→S	17% in AP→CMF→S	65% in AP→CMF→S

Abbreviations: AC, doxorubicin, cyclophosphamide; BCS, breast conservation surgery; cCR, complete clinical response; CMF, cyclophosphamide, methotrexate, fluorouracil; D, docetaxel; FEC, fluorouracil, epirubicin, cyclophosphamide; pCR, pathologic complete response; P, paclitaxel; RCT, randomized controlled trial; S, surgery.

were compared with respect to type of operation performed, the frequency of BCS was greater in the preoperative group (67% vs 60%; $P = .002$). Of patients in the preoperative chemotherapy group in the European Organization for Research and treatment of Cancer Trial (EORCT) 10902 trial, 57 (23%) underwent BCS and not the planned mastectomy, versus 14 patients (18%) who underwent mastectomy and not the planned BCS [12]. Defining the true rate of conversion from mastectomy to BCS is difficult, reflecting differences in both the inclusion criteria and the selection criteria used to identify candidates for BCS in several reported studies [14–20]. The reported proportions of patients who have BCS (as opposed to mastectomy) after NAC range from 13% to 83% [14–21].

The true benefit of neoadjuvant therapy in terms of BCS is difficult to estimate. Many factors weigh on the decision for BCS and the outcome, including patient preference, surgeon philosophy, and surgical skill. Because the preoperative determination of eligibility for BCS is also not an exact process, the true conversion from mastectomy to BCS is imprecise. Further, for patients who are good or marginal candidates for tumor shrinkage may increase the ability to obtain clear margins with less tissue resected at first attempt. These parameters have not been measured in clinical trials, making assessment of this effect impossible.

While one important benefit of chemotherapy may be that selected patients can be treated with breast conservation therapy after responding to chemotherapy, there are concerns about local-regional recurrence and ipsilateral breast tumor recurrence that must be addressed [22,23]. Clinical assessment of tumor response may demonstrate tumor shrinkage as a result of chemotherapy, but there is no absolute proof that the tumor has actually shrunken in size. Thus, treating downstaged tumors with more breast-conserving modalities may result in a higher false-negative rate of tumor-negative surgical margins. Concerns over the rates of locoregional recurrence in using breast conservation therapy after NAC may be well founded. Specifically, in the NSABP-B18 trial, the rates of ipsilateral breast recurrence were 10.7% in 503 women treated with lumpectomy in the preoperative group and 7.6% in the 448 women treated with lumpectomy in the postoperative group at a median follow-up of 9.5 years [11]. Although this difference was not statistically significant, there were significant data in the preoperative chemotherapy group regarding locoregional recurrence. The breast recurrence rate was higher in patients who were originally mastectomy candidates and were converted to BCS (15.7%) compared with those who were candidates for BCS initially (9.9%) ($P = .04$) [11]. In the European Organization for the Research and Treatment of Cancer (EORTC) 10902 trial, patients who were converted from needing mastectomy to having breast-conserving therapy because of downstaging of the tumor did worse in terms of overall survival (hazard ratio [HR] = 2.53; 95% confidence interval [CI] = 1.02–6.25) compared with patients who were initially planned to receive breast-conserving therapy and were treated accordingly [12]. Patient characteristics were examined to try and explain the observed difference in disease outcome. Of the patients who were downstaged (and thus had breast-conserving therapy), 35% were clinically node-negative before the start of chemotherapy versus 46% in the group in which breast-conserving therapy was already feasible before the administration of chemotherapy. After chemotherapy, the pathologic node-negative rates were 63% and 51%, respectively. In this particular study, nodal status did not seem to explain the difference in disease outcome. Although these data in patients converted from needing mastectomy to having breast-conserving therapy may suggest recurrence rates are higher when a smaller surgery is performed, the data could also be interpreted to suggest larger tumors have a more aggressive biologic behavior. In fact, other studies have failed to observe an increase in the rate of local recurrence following neoadjuvant therapy. For example, the Milan group reported a 5-year ipsilateral breast tumor recurrence rate of 7% after BCS and NAC [9]. A meta-analysis of 9 randomized studies examining approximately 4000 subjects that compared neoadjuvant and adjuvant chemotherapy also explored this issue [24]. This meta-analysis did report that the use of preoperative chemotherapy to convert patients to a breast-conserving approach is associated with an increase in the relative risk of locoregional recurrence for patients treated with neoadjuvant therapy. In that analysis, neoadjuvant therapy was statistically significantly associated with an increased risk of locoregional disease recurrences (risk ratio [RR] = 1.22, 95% CI = 1.04–1.43), compared with adjuvant therapy [24]. The difference, however, could largely be explained by trials in which breast conservation was achieved with the use of radiation alone and surgery was never performed after neoadjuvant therapy. Radiation alone was used in these studies when lesions were no longer identified on mammography or clinical examination. Thus, while higher rates of local recurrences may not occur when surgical breast conservation is used, certainly these findings argue for the benefit of surgical resection of the primary tumor site in addition to radiation even when a complete clinical response has been achieved.

Other retrospective studies have examined patterns of local-regional recurrence among patients treated with breast conservation therapy after NAC [22]. A study from The University of Texas M.D. Anderson Cancer Center examined the outcome of 340 patients with stage II or III noninflammatory disease who underwent breast conservation therapy after preoperative chemotherapy. The study examined patterns of locoregional recurrence (LRR) and ipsilateral breast tumor recurrence (IBTR). The observed 5-year actuarial rates of LRR-free and IBTR-free survival (91% and 95%, respectively) were similar for patients undergoing breast conservation surgery without NAC. At median follow-up of 63 months, 9% developed LRR. Of interest, clinical N2 or N3 disease, lymphovascular space invasion, a multifocal or break up pattern of residual disease, and residual disease greater than 2 cm were all associated with locoregional recurrence. However, clinical T stage did not correlate with breast recurrence except in cases when T3/T4 tumors responded to chemotherapy by breaking into smaller parts and leaving a multifocal pattern of disease. Patients who have a multifocal pattern of residual tumor have a local recurrence of up to 20% [22]. The results of this study demonstrate that breast conservation surgery is a safe and effective alternative to mastectomy for appropriately selected patients treated with NAC. Specifically, large tumors that respond to chemotherapy with a multifocal pattern of residual tumor should not be considered for BCS.

Defining the optimal selection criteria for breast conservation therapy after NAC remains to be determined, although studies such as the M.D. Anderson study discussed in the previous paragraph have provided insight. The same group went on to develop a prognostic index to help refine selection criteria and to serve as a general framework for clinical decision making for patients treated by breast-conserving therapy after NAC [25]. The prognostic index was able to help identify a small percentage of patients (4%) at high risk for local recurrence. In March 2007, the National Cancer Institute organized a symposium to evaluate issues relevant to locoregional treatment of patients receiving preoperative chemotherapy including breast conservation surgery [23]. In general, patients who have any of the following factors after NAC should not be considered candidates for breast conservation: gross multicentric disease, diffuse calcifications, residual tumor size in excess of 5 cm, residual skin edema, direct skin involvement, chest wall fixation, or medical contraindications to the use of radiotherapy [22,23]. One particularly concerning situation highlighted by the M.D. Anderson trial is that chemotherapy may not produce a uniform response of cancer but rather a multifocal pattern, leaving clusters of viable tumor cells at a distance from the central tumor site. Multifocality of the primary tumor has been shown in up to 16.3% of patients undergoing neoadjuvant therapy, although other estimates are not as high [26]. Breast conservation therapy should not be offered to patients who have this type of response. In addition to these recommendations, the primary tumor location should be marked early in the course of neoadjuvant therapy to ensure tumor bed localization at the time of surgery, especially after a complete response has been achieved. Restaging of the disease before a surgical procedure has also been advocated [23]. Finally, BCS should only be performed when clearly negative margins can be obtained and when whole-breast radiation can be performed after breast conservation surgery [23].

Treatment of micrometastatic disease

In addition to breast-conserving therapy, neoadjuvant therapy has potential other benefits. Preoperative therapy may have a more favorable effect on survival compared with postoperative chemotherapy. The proposed rationale is that systemic micrometastases may be exposed to early systemic therapy. Neoadjuvant therapy has been found to lead to better control of systemic residual disease in results from animal models [27–29]. These animal models show an increase of circulating growth-stimulating factors after the removal of the primary tumor in murine models [27–29]. In these models, adjuvant systemic therapy administered before the removal of the primary tumor impaired this increase in cell-kinetic mechanisms and improved survival [30,31]. However, there has yet to be definitive evidence that a survival benefit exists for patients undergoing neoadjuvant versus adjuvant systemic chemotherapy [4,10,11,15]. In fact, the rates of distant recurrence, disease progression, and survival have been demonstrated to be comparable in patients undergoing NAC followed by surgery versus the more traditional approach of surgery followed by chemotherapy.

Distant recurrence, disease progression, and survival

In terms of survival, there seems to be no advantage for neoadjuvant therapy before surgery compared with systemic chemotherapy after surgery [4,10,11,21,32,33]. None of these trials, including EORTC trial 10902 and NSABP-B18, has been able to show a positive effect of preoperative chemotherapy in terms of progression-free or overall survival. Two trials, conducted by Mauriac and Scholl [15,34–38], initially reported a significant positive effect of preoperative chemotherapy on progression-free and overall survival, but after a longer period of follow-up the significant benefit of preoperative chemotherapy on survival had disappeared. In a recent update on the NSABP-B18 trial with up to 16-year follow-up, there were no statistically significant differences in disease-free survival and overall survival between the 2 groups [39]. However, there were trends in favor of preoperative chemotherapy for disease-free survival and overall survival in women younger than 50 years (HR = 0.85, $P = .09$ for disease-free survival; HR = 0.81, $P = .06$ for overall survival). In this follow-up article, women younger than 50 years seemed to benefit from preoperative versus postoperative chemotherapy. In contrast, women 50 years and older had better outcomes with postoperative chemotherapy. Proposed reasons for these findings are speculative but relate to estrogen receptor (ER) status. Younger women are more likely to have ER-negative tumors, and there may be a benefit to early initiation of adjuvant chemotherapy in premenopausal women with ER-negative tumors [40,41]. In the adjuvant setting, data suggest that the absolute benefits from chemotherapy are greater with ER-negative tumors compared with ER-positive tumors [42]. ER-negative tumors also may have a higher pathologic response rate to chemotherapy than ER-positive tumors [43,44]. This result may in part explain why younger women seemed to have a greater benefit from preoperative chemotherapy. Whether younger patients ultimately gain a survival benefit from neoadjuvant therapy remains to be determined, but certainly deserves further study.

Additional data on the possible survival advantage of neoadjuvant therapy are available. In a meta-analysis of 9 trials and 3946 patients, no statistically or clinically significant differences were found between neoadjuvant therapy and adjuvant therapy arms in the end points of death (summary RR = 1.00, 95% CI = 0.90–1.12), disease progression (summary RR = 0.99, 95% CI = 0.91–1.07), or distant disease recurrence (summary RR = 0.94, 95% CI = 0.83–1.06) [20]. These data suggest that the effect of systemic therapy on overall survival is dependent more on the chemosensitivity of the primary lesion [45–47] and other biologic factors related to the tumor than on the timing of chemotherapy (before or after surgery). Data clearly show that both clinical and pathologic response to NAC are correlated with survival. In the NSABP B18 trial, the rate of disease-free survival at 9 years was 64% in patients with complete clinical responses after neoadjuvant therapy compared with 46% in nonresponders ($P = .0008$). In addition, the disease-free survival at 9 years in patients who achieved complete pathologic response was 75% compared with 58% for incomplete responders ($P = .0005$). Patients who obtain the greatest survival advantage from NAC are those who experience a complete response of their primary tumor and axillary lymph nodes [4,48]. Given that response to neoadjuvant therapy is a prognostic marker for disease-free and overall survival, another potential benefit of neoadjuvant therapy is the ability to monitor tumor response and alter individual treatment plans to improve tumor response.

Optimizing response to neoadjuvant chemotherapy

Improving pathologic response to NAC has been explored by the addition of newer agents, dose-dense administration, using alternative schedules, and switching the treatment based on lack of initial response. In early trials of neoadjuvant therapy, agent choice and schedule mimicked those of adjuvant therapy, and mainly doxorubicin and cyclophosphamide (AC) regimens were used. Trials showing benefit with the use of taxanes in the adjuvant therapy setting were followed by their application to neoadjuvant use [49,50]. Early studies in the neoadjuvant setting demonstrated the use of docetaxel in sequence with an AC regimen was feasible, with pathologic complete response (pCR) rates ranging from 5% to 14% [51]. The NSABP-B27 trial was designed to determine the effect of adding docetaxel (T) to preoperative AC on tumor response rates, disease-free survival, and overall survival. Preoperative T added to AC significantly increased the proportion of patients having pCR compared with preoperative AC alone (26% vs 13%, respectively; $P < .0001$) [39]. However, Protocol B-27 results demonstrated that the addition of T to AC did not significantly affect disease-free survival or overall survival. Another study examined the schedule of drug administration. Sequential AC plus docetaxel therapy was found to be more effective at inducing pCR than dose-dense (concurrent) doxorubicin and docetaxel [21]. The B-27 trial also examined the role of surgery performed between the administration of AC and docetaxel, and found no difference between any of the arms in terms of disease-free or overall survival [32]. Capecitabine and gemcitabine have also recently been incorporated into neoadjuvant trials, with fewer mature data available [52–54]. While further studies can examine the role of optimal drug scheduling, neoadjuvant therapy can provide additional benefits by acquiring early information on tumor response and biology of the disease.

One of the proposed benefits to neoadjuvant therapy is the ability to monitor tumor response; this would allow treatment to be altered when no tumor response occurs. In the GEPARTRIO trial, patients were treated with 2 cycles of neoadjuvant docetaxel, doxorubicin, and cyclophosphamide. Of the 2090 patients treated, 622 (29.8%) had clinically stable (nonresponding) disease and were randomly assigned to receive 4 more cycles of the same regimen versus 4 cycles of a noncross-resistant regimen of vinorelbine and capecitabine before surgery [55,56]. The pCR rate was not improved by switching the chemotherapy regimen, suggesting that tumors were broadly chemoresistant. In the Aberdeen trial, 34% of 145 patients enrolled failed to demonstrate a clinical response after 4 cycles of anthracycline-based chemotherapy [57]. After the initial 4 cycles, these patients with stable or progressive disease were switched to docetaxel for 4 cycles followed by surgery; the pCR in this group of patients was 1.8%, which compared with 15% in patients who experienced a partial or complete clinical response to anthracycline-based chemotherapy and were randomized to receive additional anthracycline-based chemotherapy. This result is in accordance with the GEPARTRIO trial, which showed that altering the type of chemotherapy may not improve response in broadly chemoresistant disease. It is interesting that the Aberdeen trial also examined the role of extended NAC in patients who were partial or complete clinical responders to the initial 4 cycles of anthracycline-based chemotherapy. Patients who had a complete or partial response after initial chemotherapy were randomized to either 4 more cycles of anthracycline-based chemotherapy or 4 cycles of docetaxel. Pathologic complete response, disease-free survival, and overall survival were significantly improved in those assigned to receive docetaxel therapy compared with those who continued with the anthracycline-based therapy alone. The pCR rate in those assigned to the anthracycline-based/docetaxel arm was 30.8% (vs 15% in those randomized to 4 more cycles of anthracycline-based chemotherapy). This result likely reflects the inherent chemoresistance of some tumors regardless of agent, and suggests a role for the addition of other agents if patients respond to initial treatment, in an effort to achieve a pCR. However, for clinical nonresponders altering the treatment has not been shown to alter response rates or survival. Despite the lack of improvement by altering treatment, patients with disease progression during initial treatment should still be switched to an alternative regimen, offered surgery if the tumor is resectable, or considered for investigational treatments. In addition to the application of these cytotoxic chemotherapy regimens, there is some evidence for response to preoperative endocrine and biologically targeted agents [58–60].

NEOADJUVANT CHEMOTHERAPY VERSUS NEOADJUVANT ENDOCRINE AND TARGETED THERAPY

In adjuvant therapy, molecular tests can assess the estimated risk of recurrence in patients with early-stage breast cancer and identify distinct biologic classes of tumor [60]. Prognostic tests that use gene profiles have been developed, and are currently being used in the United States to provide information about risk of recurrence and death as well as potentially providing information to guide therapy [61]. The best characterized molecular predictive markers are the ER, the progesterone receptor (PR), and the human epidermal growth factor receptor 2 (HER2). Adjuvant therapies targeting these receptors have been found to reduce mortality and improve outcomes [62–67]. In fact, endocrine therapy, in the form of tamoxifen or aromatase inhibitors are among the most active drugs available for women with hormone receptor–positive breast cancer. Meta-analyses performed by the Early Breast Cancer Trialists' Collaborative Group (EBCTG) have shown that tamoxifen given as adjuvant therapy reduces the annual breast cancer death rate by 31%, largely irrespective of the use of chemotherapy and of age (<50, 50–69, ≥70 years), PR status, or other tumor characteristics [68]. Further, aromatase inhibitor therapy has emerged as a more active alternative to tamoxifen [58,59,69–71]. It is clear that endocrine therapy is the first and most effective targeted agent for the 75% of women whose breast cancer expresses ER and/or PR. Both endocrine and targeted therapies have also been explored in a neoadjuvant setting.

Neoadjuvant endocrine therapy is a logical therapy for women with endocrine-sensitive tumors, which is approximately 75% of patients [72,73]. Initial experience with tamoxifen showed that primary endocrine therapy can achieve clinical responses of 50% or greater and convert inoperable patients to operability. Third-generation aromatase inhibitors have largely replaced tamoxifen for this indication due to greater efficacy observed with the use of aromatase inhibitors [58,59,69–71]. Neoadjuvant aromatase inhibitor studies have documented response rates between 37% and 60% and have demonstrated statistically significant improvements in breast conservation rates up to 50% in some patients [58,59,70]; rates comparable if not exceeding that of NAC. A summary of 3 randomized controlled studies is presented in Table 2. One randomized trial explored the efficacy of NAC agents versus neoadjuvant endocrine therapy in achieving clinical response and BCS in patients with ER-positive breast cancer [74]. At 3 months, there was no statistically significant difference in overall response between the 2 groups (62% response in endocrine group and 63% in chemotherapy group). At 36 months (after surgery), there was no significant difference in the incidence of local recurrence (3.3% endocrine vs 3.4% chemotherapy). In a recent phase 2 multicenter study of neoadjuvant aromatase inhibitor therapy with letrozole, 62% of patients experienced a clinical response [75]. Other trials have examined a combination of gonadotropin releasing hormone analogue (GnRH) and letrozole in the neoadjuvant setting. The pCR was 3% and the breast conservation rate 42% [76]. Of note, a longer duration of neoadjuvant endocrine therapy seems to be associated with higher response rates. In patients treated with extended durations of preoperative letrozole, tumor responses continued to occur for up to 12 to 24 months [77]. The variability in response rates from early studies has led to attempts to try and identify particular patient populations that will benefit from response.

Logically speaking, endocrine therapy should be reserved for patients with endocrine-sensitive tumors. In a phase 3 randomized trial, patients with low ER expression had minimal response to either letrozole or tamoxifen [78]. In

Table 2
Preoperative endocrine therapy trials

Trial	Year	Type	No. of patients	Chemotherapy regimen	cCR	pCR	BCS
IMPACT [69]	2001	RCT	330	A vs T vs T+A→S	3% vs 4% vs 3%		46% s 26% vs 22%
PROACT [23]	2006	RCT	451	A→S vs T→S			47.2% vs 38.3%
PO24 [70]	2001	RCT	337	L→S vs T→S	10% vs 4%	1.3% vs 1.8%	45% vs 35%

Abbreviations: A, anastrozole; L, letrozole; S, surgery; T, tamoxifen.

that same trial, patients with intermediate ER expression had higher response rates to letrozole as opposed to tamoxifen, further demonstrating improved efficacy for aromatase inhibitors. A randomized trial comparing the 3 Food and Drug Administration–approved aromatase inhibitors is being conducted by the American College of Surgeons Oncology Group (ACOSOG Z1031) to identify whether differences exist between these agents in the neoadjuvant setting. In addition to ER status, evaluation of Ki-67 might also predict which patients will benefit from neoadjuvant endocrine therapy. The decline in Ki-67 after preoperative endocrine therapy might predict long-term outcome [79]. Recently, a prognostic algorithm has been developed that incorporates information on Ki-67, ER, and stage derived from the postneoadjuvant endocrine therapy tumor specimen to identify patients with such a low relapse rate that they can consider forgoing adjuvant chemotherapy [80]. Preoperative endocrine therapy has traditionally been reserved for women thought not to be able to tolerate chemotherapy. Recent data suggest that tumor biology, rather than age or infirmity of the host, might better drive the decision between neoadjuvant endocrine and chemotherapy. Whether neoadjuvant endocrine therapy can replace NAC in selected patients and result in similar outcomes remains to be determined. In addition, patients with ER-negative tumors may have improved outcomes with chemotherapy compared with patients with ER-positive tumors [44].

While the role for neoadjuvant endocrine therapy is still being defined, data clearly show that endocrine therapy alone is insufficient for control of local tumor growth. Although breast conservation rates are high following neoadjuvant endocrine therapy as opposed to NAC, patients not undergoing surgery were found to have significantly higher locoregional relapse rates (23% vs 8%) in a study comparing tamoxifen alone with tamoxifen plus surgery [81]. Patients not undergoing surgery also had a worse overall and breast cancer mortality, indicating that surgery should be offered to patients who receive primary endocrine therapy, regardless of response.

Amplification of the HER2 gene or overexpression of the cell-surface protein has been associated with a poor prognosis [66]. Approximately 20% of breast cancers overexpress HER2. Trastuzumab (Herceptin) is a monoclonal antibody directed against the extracellular domain of HER2. In patients with HER2-positive early breast cancer, trastuzumab improves response rates of disease-free and overall survival [82–84]. Trastuzumab has been explored in the neoadjuvant setting as well [85–87]. In one trial, 42 patients with HER2-positive disease with operable breast cancer were randomly assigned to either 4 cycles of paclitaxel followed by 4 cycles of fluorouracil, epirubicin, and cyclophosphamide, or to the same chemotherapy with simultaneous weekly trastuzumab for 24 weeks. Of the 42 randomized patients, 26% in the chemotherapy arm achieved pCR compared with 65.2% in the trastuzumab plus chemotherapy arm ($P = .016$) [86,87]. Early reports from a similarly designed randomized neoadjuvant study in HER2-positive breast cancer patients also show a dramatic improvement in pCR with the addition of Herceptin [87].

There are some concerns about the use of anthracyclines with trastuzumab causing cardiac toxicity [88]. The combination of trastuzumab with epirubicin is currently under evaluation in the ACOSOG 1041 trial. These early trials of neoadjuvant trastuzumab certainly are encouraging, and trastuzumab should be included into neoadjuvant regimens for patients with HER2-positive disease.

Multiple other targeted agents are currently in development. Another HER2 monoclonal antibody in development is pertuzumab [89]. Lapatinib is a reversible small-molecule tyrosine-kinase inhibitor directed against HER2 [90]. Other novel approaches to overcoming chemoresistance include targeted agents directed at inhibition in the mTOR and Akt pathways [91]. There have also been clinical trials with bevacizumab, including a phase 2 trial of bevacizumab and trastuzumab that showed the combination was highly effective in patients with HER2-overexpressing metastatic breast cancer who had failed previous therapies [92]. The development of new agents offers the chance for additional treatment in patients who have failed other therapy. While newer agents are generally used first in patients with metastatic treatment who have failed standard therapy, their use should also be explored in the neoadjuvant setting.

ASSESSMENT OF RESPONSE

Evaluation of response of both primary tumor and tumor-bearing lymph nodes is an integral aspect of neoadjuvant therapy for breast cancer. Goals of this assessment include documenting sensitivity of the tumor to the chosen regimen, assessing host toxicity, and facilitating surgical planning. To avoid unnecessary toxicity without potential benefit from treatment, early response evaluation should be performed. The time of response evaluation depends on the particular treatment regimen but should be performed at 6 to 9 weeks from the start of treatment. In patients with insufficient early response and progressive disease, switching the regimen should be considered. In patients who have no response or progressive disease, the goal should be to minimize toxicity, given there is little benefit to be gained if the tumor is resistant to the selected therapy.

Assessment of tumor response involves a combination of physical examination and imaging with mammogram, ultrasound, or magnetic resonance imaging (MRI). Evaluating neoadjuvant therapy with imaging can be difficult, and there appears to be poor correlation between pathologic response and imaging response [93]. In a study at the authors' institution, radiologic images (ultrasonography and mammography) overestimated the amount of residual disease perhaps because the distinction between tumor-free fibrotic tissue and tissue that contains persistent cancer is difficult [94]. The agreement of pathologic residual tumor size with mammography and sonography is moderate, especially in lobular invasive tumors [93,94]. One study compared physical examination and imaging with ultrasound and mammography in 189 patients treated with NAC [93]. When these methods of evaluation were compared with respect to pathologic outcome, the false-positive and false-negative rates ranged from 20% to 65% and 10% to 57% for ultrasound and mammogram, respectively [93].

Due to the inaccuracy of conventional breast imaging in assessing response to NAC, other imaging methods have been explored, namely MRI. In fact, some studies have shown MRI to be superior to mammography, ultrasound, and clinical examination in evaluating the extent of tumor [95]. Multiple studies have suggested that findings on MRI strongly correlate with pathologic response [96–100]. Moreover, MRI has demonstrated greater agreement with the extent of residual disease than that achieved with physical examination or other conventional imaging [96–100]. One of these studies examined MRI, physical examination, ultrasound, and mammography in patients treated with neoadjuvant therapy. The extent of residual disease was correctly predicted by MRI in 63% of cases, physical examination in 52%, mammography in 38%, and ultrasound in 43% of cases [97]. Quantitative tumor size before the start of chemotherapy and subsequent response to chemotherapy as measured by MRI may be helpful in predicting outcome. MRI may also be more helpful in accurately identifying residual disease at the time of surgery. However, false-negative rates are still high enough with MRI that surgery remains an important part of treatment for all patients, including those with no evidence of disease on posttreatment MRI.

In this manner, MRI will not necessarily improve surgical decision making after neoadjuvant therapy [101]. The standard of care will continue to involve clinical documentation of tumor regression and attempts at breast conservation therapy with intraoperative assessment of margins.

Other imaging modalities have been explored for predicting response to agents given in the neoadjuvant setting [102–108]. Fluorodeoxyglucose positron emission tomography (FDG-PET) has been shown to predict response at 2 to 3 months. Combining FDG-PET with MRI was shown to predict response better than either modality alone [104]. Although changes in traditional imaging usually manifest later than changes in underlying tumor viability, functional studies can provide quantitative measurements of the microtumor environment that may allow for earlier assessment of response. Finally, ongoing studies using new techniques such as proton magnetic resonance spectroscopy, diffusion weighted imaging, interstitial fluid pressure, and Doppler ultrasound are under investigation [106–108].

SURGICAL MANAGEMENT OF THE BREAST FOLLOWING NEOADJUVANT CHEMOTHERAPY FOR BREAST CANCER

Application of neoadjuvant therapy has improved breast conservation rates for patients who would otherwise require mastectomy. Breast conservation rates range from 40% to 70% and local recurrence following BCS for downstaged tumors is acceptably low (see Tables 1 and 2). Principles of surgical therapy are the same following NAC as for primary surgery, namely tumor excision with negative margins leaving a cosmetically acceptable residual breast. To achieve this goal, the site of the primary tumor should be marked with titanium clips before initiation of NAC and the dimensions of the tumor recoded by both imaging and the surgeon's physical examination. During the course of NAC, the surgeon should be involved in assessment of tumor response. A decision for attempted BCS following NAC must weigh tumor response, both original and posttreatment tumor size, and breast size.

IS SURGERY NEEDED FOR PATIENTS WHO ACHIEVE A COMPLETE RESPONSE TO NEOADJUVANT CHEMOTHERAPY?

For patients who achieve complete clinical and radiologic responses to NAC, most authorities still recommend surgery to the primary tumor site and axillary lymph nodes. For patients who ultimately have complete pathologic responses it is reasonable to question whether these patients derive benefit from resection and could be adequately treated by radiation alone. A precedent for this approach may be found in the treatment of occult breast cancer, where radiation therapy alone may be considered if examination and imaging are negative. However, in NSABP B18, patients who had a clinical complete response by physical examination and standard imaging had a pCR only 38% of the time [4,39]. This result suggests that improvements in detection of minimal residual disease are required before a nonoperative approach can be endorsed. Addition of MRI and/or PET holds promise to improve the assessment of response to neoadjuvant therapy and is an important component of the I-SPY clinical trial (http://tr.nci.nih.gov/iSpy).

SURGICAL MANAGEMENT OF THE AXILLA FOLLOWING NEOADJUVANT CHEMOTHERAPY FOR BREAST CANCER

The role of axillary surgery in patients who receive NAC mirrors that for patients who have surgery first: to provide prognostic information, improve local control, and possibly impart a benefit in overall survival. Current debate centers on the appropriateness and timing of sentinel lymph node (SLN) biopsy in relation to NAC, the role of surgical clearance of positive nodal basins following NAC with complete imaging and clinical response, and the addition of radiation to surgery in patients with involved nodal basins.

SURGICAL STAGING WITH SENTINEL LYMPH NODE BIOPSY IN PATIENTS RECEIVING NEOADJUVANT CHEMOTHERAPY

Since the early 1990s, SLN mapping and biopsy have increasingly been used in the surgical management of breast cancer for axillary staging. Sentinel node biopsy (SNB) decreases the morbidity associated with breast cancer staging in women by reducing the need for axillary lymph node dissection (ALND) and avoiding the associated morbidity of an axillary node dissection [109]. Accurate staging of the axilla is crucial, as the status of axillary lymph nodes is one of the most important determinants of prognosis for breast cancer patients. Furthermore, the presence of regional metastases in the axillary basin reduces a patients' 5-year survival by approximately 28% to 40% [110]. Many studies have demonstrated the accuracy of SLN mapping in the staging of early breast cancer. In patients who have not received chemotherapy, identification rates range from 84% to 100% and false-negative rates range from 0% to 13% [111,112]. The proportion of successful mappings was significantly higher and the false-negative rate was significantly lower in studies in which a radiolabeled colloid was used for mapping [113]. SNB is now currently recommended as an appropriate initial alternative to routine staging ALND for patients with early-stage breast cancer with clinically negative axillary nodes [113].

NAC has been shown to downstage axillary lymph nodes in a large proportion (30%–40%) of patients [114]. The use of SLN mapping and biopsy after preoperative chemotherapy has also been explored in an effort to spare node-negative patients the morbidity of ALND. Multiple studies have examined the success and accuracy of sentinel node mapping and biopsy in patients with early-stage breast cancer after NAC. One of the largest studies conducted as part of the National Surgical Adjuvant Breast and Bowel Project, trial B-27, retrospectively examined 428 patients who underwent SNB after neoadjuvant therapy [115]. The success rate for the identification and removal of a sentinel node was 84.8%. Of the 218 patients with negative sentinel nodes, nonsentinel nodes were positive in 15 (false-negative rate, 10.7%; 15 of 140 patients). Of importance, there were no significant differences in false-negative rate according to breast tumor response to chemotherapy. This study was criticized for using different methods of SLN identification and had a heterogeneous patient population. More recently, a prospective multi-institutional study to address the feasibility and accuracy of SNB after neoadjuvant therapy was reported [116]. The detection rate was 90% and the false-negative rate was 11.5% in 195 study patients. This study did show that patients with clinical N0 disease had the best detection rate as compared with patients with clinical N1 disease, but there was no difference in false-negative rates [116]. There have also been 2 large meta-analyses of SNB after neoadjuvant therapy [114,117]. A recent systematic meta-analysis [114] reviewed 24 trials and 1799 subjects. Successful lymph node mapping was defined as successful identification rate and false-negative rate. The successful identification rate was 90% and the false-negative rate was 8%. The detection and false-negative rates thus do not appear to differ from those obtained in cases of early breast cancer without neoadjuvant therapy. Taken together, the data suggest that SNB after neoadjuvant therapy is a feasible strategy with the potential to further minimize morbidity associated with the surgical treatment of breast cancer [118]. The ACOSOG has recently initiated a study of the role of SLN biopsy following NAC (ACOSOG Z1072) (www.acosog.org/studies/number/Z1071). The primary aim of this trial is to ascertain the false-negative rate of SLN biopsy after NAC. Secondary aims include the evaluation of axillary ultrasound in evaluating the axilla after NAC.

ADVANTAGES OF SENTINEL LYMPH NODE BIOPSY AFTER NEOADJUVANT CHEMOTHERAPY

Proponents of SLN after NAC state the benefits of the approach are that it requires a single operative procedure as opposed to separate procedures; in addition, NAC has resulted in the eradication of nodal disease in up to 40% of patients [119,120]. Thus, many patients could potentially be spared complete ALND. When the use of NAC has resulted in complete response in the regional nodes, there is no benefit to removing uninvolved nodes. Patients who do have residual nodal disease in the axilla after NAC should benefit from ALND. A recent study from M.D. Anderson Cancer Center found a reduced need for ALND in patients with T2 or T3 disease after chemotherapy as a result of lower incidence or positive SLN biopsies performed after NAC [121]. In that study, patients undergoing SLN biopsy after NAC had fewer positive SLNs than patients who underwent SLN biopsy before chemotherapy for each T stage. As neoadjuvant regimens continue to improve the clinical and pathologic response rates, it may be possible to avoid ALND in more than 50% of patients who have initial clinically node-negative disease [119,121].

ADVANTAGES OF SENTINEL LYMPH NODE BIOPSY BEFORE NEOADJUVANT CHEMOTHERAPY

Some have proposed that patients who are considered candidates for NAC should have an SNB performed before rather than after NAC. The proponents of this approach argue that information on the status of the axillary nodes can be obtained without the potential confounding effects of prior NAC. Specifically, there is some concern that tumor response to chemotherapy may cause lymphatic scarring and fibrosis that could affect drainage patterns. Neoadjuvant treatment has been hypothesized to lower the SLN identification rate, possibly due to fibrosis within the axilla, and has been found in some single-center studies to increase the false-negative rate (from 22% to 33%) [122–124]. SLN biopsy before chemotherapy could give a more accurate evaluation of axillary status, unaffected by any previous therapeutic intervention. Proponents of the pretherapy SNB also argue that sentinel node–negative patients should not require completion axillary dissection after NAC. However, pretherapy SNB does not take advantage of the downstaging effect of NAC in the axillary nodes. Patients with a positive sentinel node pre-NAC will generally require an axillary node dissection either before or after NAC.

SHOULD AXILLARY STAGING BE DONE BEFORE OR AFTER NEOADJUVANT THERAPY?

If the accuracy of SNB after neoadjuvant therapy can be validated, a proportion of initially node-positive patients could eventually be spared axillary dissections if their involved sentinel nodes become uninvolved after the administration of NAC. A pre-NAC SNB approach also commits the patient to 2 surgical procedures irrespective of the status of the sentinel node; women with involved SLNs will experience 2 separate axillary procedures, before and after neoadjuvant therapy. Whether or not the sentinel node is positive also contributes minimally to the decision to use NAC, because this decision is usually made based on clinical patient and tumor characteristics and not on the pathologic status of the axillary nodes. In addition, knowing what the status of the sentinel node is before NAC is of minimal value relative to the subsequent decision to administer additional adjuvant chemotherapy or adjuvant locoregional radiotherapy. Although SNB was initially not recommended for axillary staging of patients receiving NAC [113] mainly due to concerns about the potential for higher false-negative rates, newer data suggest SNB is reliable and feasible after neoadjuvant therapy. Although the authors believe SLN biopsy is accurate after neoadjuvant therapy, knowing the nodal status before chemotherapy is also helpful, especially because the authors routinely administer postmastectomy radiation therapy for any patient with positive nodes at presentation. An approach to axillary lymph nodes in NAC is outlined in Fig. 1.

RADIATION THERAPY AFTER NEOADJUVANT CHEMOTHERAPY AND SURGERY

As with patients treated with surgery first, for patients who have BCS following NAC, radiation to the breast is indicated to substantially reduce the risk of locoregional relapse. This approach is especially relevant in high-risk patients who are young, have large tumors at presentation, and who have true conversion from needing mastectomy to having breast-conserving therapy. In the NAC setting, the radiation dose and fields to treat the breast remain the same. However, because the number of positive nodes often dictates the addition of a supraclavicular or high axillary field, there may be ambiguity in treatment planning after axillary downstaging by NAC. At present there are no clear data to suggest whether additional fields should be added following

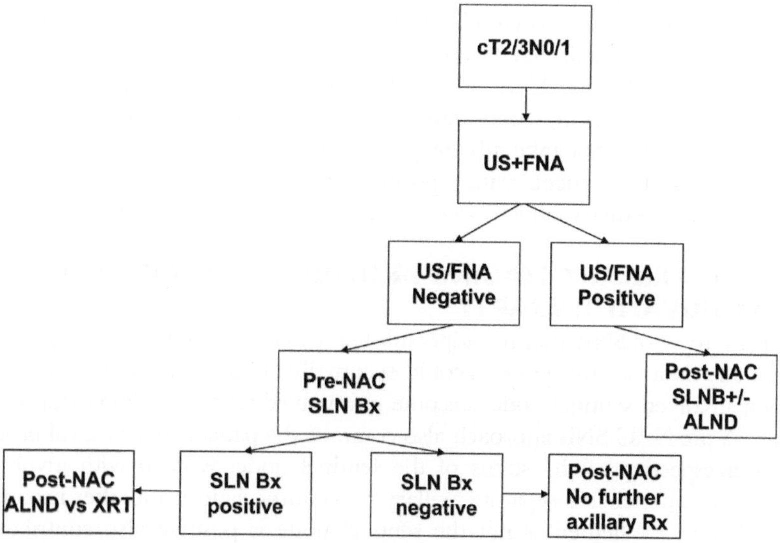

Fig. 1. Approach to axillary lymph nodes in NAC.

NAC [125]. An approach to radiotherapy for patients receiving NAC is outlined in Fig. 2.

The addition of radiation to mastectomy in patients who have surgery before chemotherapy improved local-regional control by 17% at 5 years and reduced breast cancer mortality by 5.4% at 15 years [59,126]. The selection of patients for postmastectomy radiation in conjunction with adjuvant chemotherapy is generally made based on pathologic information concerning the extent of disease burden at presentation; postmastectomy radiation is usually indicated for those with positive axillary lymph nodes and for those with large T2 (>4 cm) and T3 tumors, and clinical stage III or T3 tumors [59,127].

In contrast, the role of postmastectomy radiotherapy in patients who have had NAC, require mastectomy, and have either N0 or N1 disease after NAC remains to be determined. Given that preoperative chemotherapy can achieve pathologic response rates in up to 80% of patients, indications for radiation may be different in these downstaged patients. Assessing the risk of locoregional recurrence after NAC and surgery without radiation is important in determining which patients should undergo radiation. Data from the NSABP-18 and B-27 trials demonstrated the risk of locoregional recurrence after NAC, and mastectomy was 15% for 447 patients who had residual positive lymph nodes after NAC. By contrast, patients in those trials with clinical stage II disease who had negative lymph nodes after NAC had an 8-year risk of locoregional recurrence of less than 10%. In the NSABP trials, postmastectomy radiation was not allowed per protocol. In 150 patients who had mastectomy after NAC, Buchholz (2002) and colleagues [128] showed that the risk of locoregional recurrences for any pathologic tumor size is higher

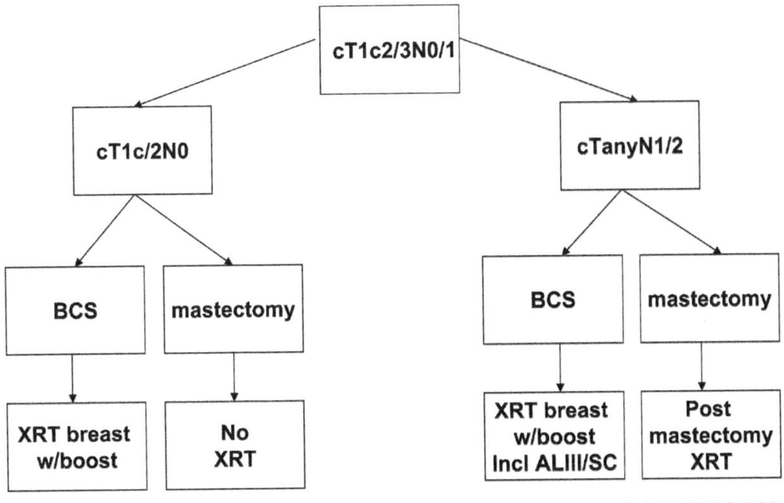

Fig. 2. Approach to radiotherapy in NAC.

for patients treated with initial chemotherapy than for patients treated with initial surgery [129]. These investigators suggested radiotherapy should be offered to all patients with 4 or more positive lymph nodes, tumor size greater than 5 cm, or clinical stage IIIA or greater disease, regardless of whether they receive neoadjuvant or postoperative chemotherapy [129]. While these data are useful in determining who might benefit from radiation, the use of postmastectomy radiation was not assessed.

The use of postmastectomy radiation in patients treated with NAC has been examined retrospectively in several publications. In a retrospective analysis of 542 patients treated with NAC at M.D. Anderson Cancer Center, the combination of mastectomy and radiation was found to benefit both local control and survival in patients who presented with clinical T3 tumors or stage II to stage IV disease, and in patients with 4 or more positive nodes after chemotherapy compared with patients who received NAC and mastectomy alone [130]. Of note, in that same study, for patients presenting with early stage I to stage II disease who achieved a pathologic complete response, no difference in locoregional recurrence rates was observed ($P = .22$). In addition, in the subset of patients with clinical stage II disease with 1 to 3 positive lymph nodes after NAC, no difference in locoregional recurrence rates was observed ($P = .79$). Recently, these same investigators examined the effect of postmastectomy radiation in 106 patients who achieved complete pathologic response and had mastectomy [131]. For patients who presented initially with stage I and stage II disease, there was no locoregional recurrence in either radiated or nonirradiated patients. Patients who presented with stage III disease had an absolute reduction in actuarial local-regional recurrence of 26% (7.3% with radiation vs 33.3% without radiation). This difference was significant and was associated with a reduction in breast cancer mortality. At present, additional prospective randomized studies evaluating the use of radiation after NAC and mastectomy are needed. Although there is currently no consensus, clearly there are subsets of patients who will benefit from postmastectomy radiation.

NEW ISSUES: NEOADJUVANT THERAPY IN THE ERA OF COMPLEX BIOMARKERS

Despite high response rates to NAC, a small proportion of patients fail to respond or even progress during therapy and thereby the surgeon may lose a window of opportunity to obtain durable locoregional control of disease. Alternative treatment options can be implemented with early identification of nonresponders. It is important that the response to NAC in vivo could provide a useful prediction of prognosis and help define strategies for an individual patient's future treatment with an appropriately selected agent. The discovery of predictive markers for tumor response to NAC through the analysis of DNA microarrays and proteomics may help to individualize chemotherapy. Advances in high-throughput data collection and analysis including gene expression, microarray, genomic sequencing, and quantitative multiplex polymerase chain reaction have afforded cancer researchers an unprecedented opportunity to examine tumor biology. Identification and use of predictive biomarkers may help improve survival in patients with breast cancer with a poor prognosis. Biologic markers that can reliably predict clinical or pathologic response early during the course of treatment have considerable clinical potential.

Specific tumor type may be important in determining which patients will respond to chemotherapy. Mathieu and colleagues [132] reported that invasive lobular carcinoma was an independent predictor of a poor clinical response ($P = .02$) and ineligibility for BCS ($P = .03$) in 457 patients who underwent NAC. Another study reported significantly less overall response rates (50% vs 75%; $P = .0151$) and pCR (0% vs 15%; $P = .0066$) for invasive lobular carcinoma compared with invasive ductal carcinoma [133]. Thus lobular carcinoma may be associated with lower response rates to NAC. Other pathologic characteristics such as poor differentiation, tumor necrosis, and lymphatic invasion have been shown to be important in predicting response to NAC [134].

The ER/PR status of a tumor has been identified as an independent variable that is significantly associated with the likelihood of achieving pCR. The European Cooperative Trial in Operable breast cancer (ECTO) discussed previously reported that 42% of patients with ER-negative tumors had a pathologic complete response versus 12% in the ER-positive group. In multivariate analysis, ER status emerged as the only independent variable significantly associated with likelihood of achieving a clinically complete response (odds ratio, 2.1), and most importantly a pCR (odds ratio, 5.77; $P < .0001$). In a retrospective analysis of 1731 patients treated with various neoadjuvant regimens, pCR rates were 24% in patients with ER-negative tumors and 8% in patients with ER-positive tumors ($P < .001$) regardless of the treatment regimens [135]. This finding has been confirmed in multiple other prospective NAC trials [21,120]. Thus ER-negative tumors generally respond better to chemotherapy and can be used to help predict which patients may fail or progress with NAC.

In addition to ER/PR status, molecularly targeted approaches in the neoadjuvant setting may also provide insight into predicting which patients will respond to NAC. Of 42 patients in the randomized phase 2 trial of HER2-positive disease, a higher pathologic complete response rate was seen with the addition of trastuzumab. The pathologic complete response rates were 67% for the combination arm and 25% for the chemotherapy-alone arm ($P < .02$) [85]. In terms of HER2 status and response to NAC, HER2 overexpression may show a poorer response than that with HER2 normal expression for low-dose anthracycline-containing chemotherapy [128,136]. HER2 status can also be used as a predictor of response for both NAC and molecular targeted therapy.

Several other biomarkers with potential to predict which patients might respond to chemotherapy have been explored. In addition to tumor type, ER/PR status, and HER2 expression, expression of topoisomerase-IIa, Ki-67 expression, and the expression of apoptosis-related genes such as p53 and

Bcl-2 have been explored. In addition to specific biomarkers, the application of gene expression signatures to guide NAC is currently an area of active research. Gianni and colleagues [137] examined 89 patients with locally advanced breast cancer who received neoadjuvant paclitaxel and doxorubicin. RNA was extracted from the pretreatment formalin-fixed paraffin-embedded core biopsies, and gene expression was obtained using DNA microarrays. Eighty-six genes correlated with pCR (unadjusted $P<.05$); pCR was more likely with higher expression of proliferation-related genes and immune-related genes, and with lower expression of ER-related genes [137]. Another study examined gene expression signatures in 133 patients with stages I to III breast cancer who all received preoperative weekly paclitaxel and 5-fluorouracil, doxorubicin, and cyclophosphamide (T/FAC) chemotherapy [138,139]. The first 82 cases were used to develop a 30-gene molecular predictor of pathologic complete response and the remaining 52 cases were used to assess the accuracy of the predictor. The test correctly identified all but one of the patients who achieved pCR (12 of 13) and all but one of those who had residual cancer (27 of 28) in the validation set. It showed significantly higher sensitivity than a clinical variable-based predictor including age, grade, and ER status (92% vs 61%) [138]. These early studies have provided powerful information that should allow for better tailoring of treatment, specifically neoadjuvant therapy regimens, in the next few years. A second generation of gene signature studies is currently underway and should provide additional valuable information that could optimize individual treatment in patients with breast cancer.

The new appreciation for breast cancer subtypes and the role of complex biomarkers has implications for the neoadjuvant treatment of breast cancer [140,141]. On the simplest level, the awareness of luminal subtypes and in particular luminal A subtype (approximated by ER-positive, HER2-negative, low Ki-67) and the lack of response of low Oncotype RS score tumor to chemotherapy has led to the suggestion that patients with these tumors could best be treated with endocrine therapy in the neoadjuvant setting. Further work in this area will help define the optimal selection of patients for a specific neoadjuvant regimen.

SUMMARY

Neoadjuvant treatment of breast cancer is currently being used in patients with advanced disease as well as with increasing application in those that present with initially operable breast cancer. The current clinical benefits of the use of NAC include: NAC increases the possibility of the use of BCS, the safety of NAC is comparable with that of adjuvant chemotherapy, and pCR may be predictive of overall survival. Although there are still unresolved clinical questions regarding the use of neoadjuvant therapy in initially operable breast cancer, there appears to be equivalent survival to the standard of care. Future research should be aimed at tailoring treatment to individual patients using specific tumor characteristics that may predict response to different types of chemotherapy, molecular targeted therapy, and endocrine therapy.

References

[1] De Lena M, Zucati R, Viganotti G, et al. Combined chemotherapy-radiotherapy approach in locally advanced (T3b-T4) breast cancer. Cancer Chemother Pharmacol 1978;1(1): 53–9.

[2] Singletary SE, Allred C, Ashley P, et al. Revision of the American Joint Committee on Cancer staging system for breast cancer. J Clin Oncol 2002;20:3628–36.

[3] National Cancer Institute, DCCPS, Surveillance Research Program, Cancer Statistics Branch. SEER Program public use data tapes 1973–1998, November 2000 Submission. Issued: April 2001.

[4] Fisher B, Brown A, Mamounas E, et al. Effect of preoperative chemotherapy on local-regional disease in women with operable breast cancer: findings from National Surgical Adjuvant Breast and Bowel Project B-18. J Clin Oncol 1997;15:2483–93.

[5] Fisher B, Bryant J, Wolmark N, et al. Effect of preoperative chemotherapy on the outcome of women with operable breast cancer. J Clin Oncol 1998;16:2672–85.

[6] Chia S, Swain SM, Byrd DR, et al. Locally advanced and inflammatory breast cancer. J Clin Oncol 2008;26:786–90.

[7] Valagussa P, Zambetti M, Bonadonna G, et al. Prognostic factors in locally advanced noninflammatory breast cancer. Long-term results following primary chemotherapy. Breast Cancer Res Treat 1990;15:137–47.

[8] Gralow JR, Burstein HJ, Wood W, et al. Preoperative therapy in invasive breast cancer: pathologic assessment and systemic therapy issues in operable disease. J Clin Oncol 2008;26:814–9.

[9] Bonadonna G, Valagussa P, Brambilla C, et al. Primary chemotherapy in operable breast cancer: eight year experience of the Milan Cancer Institute. J Clin Oncol 1998;16: 93–100.

[10] Gianni L, Baselga J, Eiermann W, et al. Feasibility and tolerability of sequential doxorubicin/paclitaxel followed by cyclophosphamide, methotrexate, and fluorouracil and its effects on tumor response as preoperative therapy. Clin Cancer Res 2005;11:8715–21.

[11] Wolmark N, Wang J, Mamounas E, et al. Preoperative chemotherapy in patients with operable breast cancer: nine-year results from National Surgical Adjuvant Breast and Bowel Project B-18. J Natl Cancer Inst Monogr 2001;30:96–102.

[12] van der Hage JA, van de Velde CJH, Julien J-P, et al. Preoperative chemotherapy in primary operable breast cancer: Results from the European Organization for Research and Treatment of Cancer Trial 10902. J Clin Oncol 2001;19:4224–37.

[13] Mathew J, Asgeirsson KS, Cheung KL, et al. Neoadjuvant chemotherapy for locally advanced breast cancer: a review of the literature and future directions. Eur J Surg Oncol 2009;35:113–22.

[14] Belembaogo E, Feillel V, Chollet P, et al. Neoadjuvant chemotherapy in 126 operable breast cancers. Eur J Cancer 1992;28:896–900.

[15] Scholl SM, Fourquet A, Asselain B, et al. Neoadjuvant versus adjuvant chemotherapy in premenopausal patients with tumours considered too large for breast conserving surgery: preliminary results of a randomised trial: S6. Eur J Cancer 1994;30:645–52.

[16] Smith IE, Jones AL, O'Brien ME, et al. Primary medical (neo-adjuvant) chemotherapy for operable breast cancer. Eur J Cancer 1993;29:1796–9.

[17] Singletary SE, McNeese MD, Hortobagyi GN. Feasibility of breast-conservation surgery after induction chemotherapy for locally advanced breast carcinoma. Cancer 1992;69: 2849–52.

[18] Chen AM, Meric-Bernstam F, Hunt KK, et al. Breast conserving therapy after neoadjuvant chemotherapy: the M.D. Anderson cancer Center experience. J Clin Oncol 2004;22: 2303–12.

[19] Buchholz TA, Lehman CD, Harris JR, et al. Statement of science concerning locoregional treatments after preoperative chemotherapy for breast cancer: a National Cancer Institute conference. J Clin Oncol 2008;26:791–7.

[20] Mauri D, Pavlidis N, Ionnidis JP, et al. Neoadjuvant versus adjuvant systemic treatment in breast cancer: a meta-analysis. J Natl Cancer Inst 2005;97:188–94.
[21] Makris A, Powles TJ, Ashley SE, et al. A reduction in the requirements for mastectomy in a randomized trial of neoadjuvant chemoendocrine therapy in primary breast cancer. Ann Oncol 1998;9:1179–84.
[22] Chen AM, Meric-Bernstam F, Hunt KK. Breast conservation after neoadjuvant chemotherapy. Cancer 2005;103(4):689–95.
[23] Veronesi U, Bonadonna G, Zurrida S, et al. Conservation surgery after primary chemotherapy in large carcinomas of the breast. Ann Surg 1995;222:612–8.
[24] Gunduz N, Fisher B, Saffer E. Effect of surgical removal on the growth and kinetics of residual tumor. Cancer Res 1979;39:3861–5.
[25] Fisher B, Gebhardt M, Saffer E. Further observations on the inhibition of tumor growth by *C. parvum* with cyclophosphamide: VII. Effect of treatment prior to primary tumor removal on the growth of distant tumor. Cancer 1979;43:451–8.
[26] Fisher B, Gunduz N, Saffer E. Influence of the interval between primary tumor removal and chemotherapy on kinetics and growth metastases. Cancer Res 1983;43:1488–92.
[27] Fisher B, Gunduz N, Coyle J, et al. Presence of a growth-stimulating factor in serum following primary tumor removal in mice. Cancer Res 1989;49:1996–2001.
[28] Fisher B, Saffer E, Rudock C, et al. Effect of local or systemic treatment prior to primary tumor removal on the production and response to a serum growth-stimulating factor in mice. Cancer Res 1989;49:2002–4.
[29] Bear HD, Anderson S, Smith RE, et al. Sequential preoperative or postoperative docetaxel added to preoperative doxorubicin plus cyclophosphamide for operable breast cancer: National Surgical Adjuvant Breast and Bowel Project Protocol B-27. J Clin Oncol 2006;24:2019–27.
[30] Von Minckwitz G, Raab G, Caputo A, et al. Doxorubicin with cyclophosphamide followed by docetaxel every 21 days compared with doxorubicin and docetaxel every 14 days as preoperative treatment in operable breast cancer: the GEPARDUO study of the German Breast Group. J Clin Oncol 2005;23:2676–85.
[31] Buzdar AU, Singletary SE, Theriault RL, et al. Prospective evaluation of paclitaxel versus combination chemotherapy with fluorouracil, doxorubicin, and cyclophosphamide as neoadjuvant therapy in patients with operable breast cancer. J Clin Oncol 1999;17:3412–7.
[32] Schwartz GF, Birchansky CA, Komarnicky LT, et al. Induction chemotherapy followed by breast conservation for locally advanced carcinoma of the breast. Cancer 1994;73:362–9.
[33] Mauriac L, Durand M, Avril A, et al. Effects of primary chemotherapy in conservative treatment of breast cancer patients with operable tumors larger than 3 cm. Ann Oncol 1991;2:347–54.
[34] Mauriac L, MacGrogan G, Avril A, et al. Neoadjuvant chemotherapy for operable breast carcinoma larger than 3 cm: a unicentre randomized trial with a 124-month median follow-up. Ann Oncol 1999;10:47–52.
[35] Scholl SM, Asselain B, Palangie T, et al. Neoadjuvant chemotherapy in operable breast cancer. Eur J Cancer 1991;27:1668–71.
[36] Scholl SM, Pierga JY, Asselain B, et al. Breast tumor response to primary chemotherapy predicts local and distant control as well as survival. Eur J Cancer 1995;31:1969–75.
[37] Broët P, Shcoll SM, De la Rochefordiere A, et al. Short and long term effects on survival in breast cancer patients treated by primary chemotherapy: an updated analysis of a randomized trial. Breast Cancer Res Treat 1999;58:151–6.
[38] Rastogi P, Anderson SJ, Bear HD. Preoperative chemotherapy: updates of National Surgical Adjuvant Breast and Bowel Project Protocols B-18 and B-27. J Clin Oncol 2008;26:778–85.
[39] Kling KM, Ostrzega N, Schmit P. Breast conservation after induction chemotherapy for locally advanced breast cancer. Am Surg 1997;63:861–4.

[40] Asha J, Traish AM. Estrogen and progesterone receptor concentrations and prevalence of tumor hormonal phenotypes in older breast cancer patients. Cancer Detect Prev 1999;23: 238–44.
[41] Colleoni M, Bonetti M, Coates AS, et al. Early start of adjuvant chemotherapy may improve treatment outcome for premenopausal breast cancer patients with tumors not expressing estrogen receptors: the International Breast Cancer Study Group. J Clin Oncol 2000;18:584–90.
[42] Berry DA, Cirrincione C, Henderson IC, et al. Estrogen-receptor status and outcomes of modern chemotherapy for patients with node-positive breast cancer. JAMA 2006;295: 1658–67.
[43] Colleoni M, Minchella I, Mazzarol G, et al. Response to primary chemotherapy in breast cancer patients with tumors not expressing estrogen and progesterone receptors. Ann Oncol 2000;11:1057–9.
[44] Colleoni M, Viale G, Zahrieh D, et al. Chemotherapy is more effective in patients with breast cancer not expressing steroid hormone receptors: a study of preoperative treatment. Clin Cancer Res 2004;10:6622–8.
[45] Aas T, Geisler S, Eide GE, et al. Predictive value of tumour cell proliferation in locally advanced breast cancer treated with neoadjuvant chemotherapy. Eur J Cancer 2003;39:438–46.
[46] Ellis PA, Smith IE, McCarthy K, et al. Preoperative chemotherapy induces apoptosis in early breast cancer. Lancet 1997;349:849.
[47] Shao ZM, Li J, Wu J, et al. Neo-adjuvant chemotherapy for operable breast cancer induces apoptosis. Breast Cancer Res Treat 1999;53:263–9.
[48] Eltahir A, Heys SD, Hutcheon AW, et al. Treatment of large and locally advanced breast cancers using neo-adjuvant chemotherapy: recurrence and survival. Am J Surg 1998;175:127–32.
[49] Piccart-Gebhart MJ, Burzykowski T, Buyse M. Taxanes alone or in combination with anthracyclines as first-line therapy of patients with metastatic breast cancer. J Clin Oncol 2008;12:1980–6.
[50] Henderson IC, Berry DA, Cirrincione C, et al. Improved outcomes from adding sequential paclitaxel but not escalating doxorubicin dose in an adjuvant chemotherapy regimen for patients with node positive primary cancer. J Clin Oncol 2003;21:976–83.
[51] Dieras V, Fumoleau P, Romieu G, et al. A randomized, parallel study of doxorubicin/Taxol (paclitaxel) (AT) and doxorubicin/cyclophosphamide (AC) as neoadjuvant treatment of breast cancer [abstract 25]. Breast Cancer Res Treat 1998;50:233.
[52] Wenzel C, Bartsch R, Locker GJ, et al. Preoperative chemotherapy with epidoxorubicin, docetaxel and capecitabine plus pegfilgrastim in patients with primary breast cancer. Anticancer Drugs 2005;16:441–5.
[53] Schmid P, Krocker J, Schulz CO, et al. Primary chemotherapy with gemcitabine, liposomal doxorubicin, docetaxel in patients with locally advanced breast cancer: results of a phase I trial. Anticancer Drugs 2005;16:21–9.
[54] Schneeweiss A, Bastert G, Huober J, et al. Neoadjuvant therapy with gemcitabine in breast cancer. Oncology 2004;18:27–31.
[55] von Minckwitz G, Bohmner JJ, Loehr A, et al. Comparison of docetaxel/doxorubicin/cyclophosphamide (TAC) versus vinorelbine/capecitabine (NX) in patients non-responding to cycles of neoadjuvant TAC chemotherapy: First results of a phase III GEPARTRIO-study by the German Breast Group [abstract 38]. Breast Cancer Res Treat 2005;94:S19.
[56] von Minckwitz G, Costa SD, Eirmann W, et al. Maximized reduction of primary breast tumor size using preoperative chemotherapy with doxorubicin and docetaxel. J Clin Oncol 1999;17:1999–2005.
[57] Smith IC, Heys SD, Hutcheon AW, et al. Neoadjuvant chemotherapy in breast cancer: significantly enhanced response with docetaxel. J Clin Oncol 2002;20:1456–66.

[58] Ma CX, Ellis MJ. Neoadjuvant endocrine therapy for locally advanced breast cancer. Semin Oncol 2006;33:650–6.
[59] Smith IE, Dowsett M, Ebbs SR, et al. Neoadjuvant treatment of postmenopausal breast cancer with anastrozole, tamoxifen, or both in combination: the Immediate Preoperative Anastrozole, Tamoxifen, or Combined with Tamoxifen (IMPACT) multicenter double-blind randomized trial. J Clin Oncol 2005;23(22):4842–4.
[60] Benson JR, Jatoi I, Keisch M. Early breast cancer. Lancet 2009;373:1463–79.
[61] Marchionni L, Wilson RF, Wolff AC, et al. Systematic review: gene expression profiling assays in early stage breast cancer. Ann Intern Med 2008;148:358–69.
[62] Early Breast Cancer Trialists Collaborative Group. Tamoxifen for early breast cancer: an overview of randomized trials. Lancet 1998;351:1451–61.
[63] Coates AS, Keshaviah A, Thurlimann B, et al. Five years of letrozole compared with tamoxifen as initial therapy for postmenopausal women with endocrine responsive early breast cancer: update of study BIG 1-98. J Clin Oncol 2007;25:486–92.
[64] Hayes DF, Thor AD, Dressler LG, et al. HER2 and response to paclitaxel in node positive breast cancer. N Engl J Med 2008;21:976–83.
[65] Pritchard KI, Messersmith H, Elavathil L, et al. HER2 and topoisomerase II as predictors of response to chemotherapy. J Clin Oncol 2008;26:736–44.
[66] Slamon DJ, Clark GM, Wong SG, et al. Human breast cancer: correlation of relapse and survival with amplification of the HER2/neu oncogene. Science 1987;235:177–82.
[67] Wolff AC, Hammond ME, Schartz JN, et al. American Society of Clinical Oncology/College of American Pathologists guideline recommendations for human epidermal growth factor receptor 2 testing in breast cancer. J Clin Oncol 2007;25:118–45.
[68] Early Breast Cancer Trialists' Collaborative Group (EBCTCG). Effects of chemotherapy and hormonal therapy for early breast cancer on recurrence and 15-year survival: an overview of the randomised trials. Lancet 2005;365(9472):1687–717.
[69] Barnes DM, Millis RR, Gillett CE, et al. The interaction of oestrogen receptor status and pathological features with adjuvant treatment in relation to survival in patients with operable breast cancer: a retrospective study of 2660 patients. Endocr Relat Cancer 2004;11:85–96.
[70] Eiermann W, Paepke S, Appfelstaedt J, et al. Preoperative treatment of postmenopausal breast cancer patients with letrozole: a randomized double-blind multicenter study. Ann Oncol 2001;12:1527–32.
[71] Dixon JM, Renshaw L, Bellamy C, et al. The effects of neoadjuvant anastrozole (Arimidex) on tumor volume in postmenopausal women with breast cancer: a randomized, double-blind, single-center study. Clin Cancer Res 2000;6:2229–35.
[72] Cataliotti L, Buzdar AU, Noguchi S, et al. Comparison of anastrozole versus tamoxifen as preoperative therapy in postmenopausal women with hormone receptor-positive breast cancer: the pre-operative "Arimidex" compared to Tamoxifen (PROACT) trial. Cancer 2006;106:2095–103.
[73] Semiglazov VF, Amiglozoz V, Ivanov V, et al. The relative efficacy of neoadjuvant endocrine therapy versus chemotherapy in postmenopausal women with ER-positive breast cancer [abstract 519]. J Clin Oncol 2004;23:7s.
[74] Semiglazov VF, Semigloazov VV, Dashyan GA, et al. Phase 2 randomized trial of primary endocrine therapy versus chemotherapy in postmenopausal patients with estrogen receptor-positive breast cancer. Cancer 2007;110:244–54.
[75] Olson JA, Budd GT, Carey LA. Improved surgical outcomes for breast cancer patients receiving aromatase inhibitor therapy: results from a multi-center phase II trial. J Am Coll Surg 2009;208:906–14.
[76] Torrisi R, Colleoni M, Mani E, et al. Endocrine and chemoendocrine primary therapy in premenopausal women with endocrine responsive breast cancer: a feasibility study [abstract 2101]. Breast Cancer Res Treat 2004;88.

[77] Macaskill EJ, Dixon JM. Neoadjuvant use of endocrine therapy in breast cancer. Breast J 2007;13:243–50.
[78] Ellis MJ, Coop A, Singh B, et al. Letrozole is more effective neoadjuvant endocrine therapy than tamoxifen for ErbB-1 and/or ErbB-2-positive, estrogen receptor-positive primary breast cancer: Evidence from a Phase III randomized trial. J Clin Oncol 2001;19: 3808–16.
[79] Dowsett M, Smith IE, Ebbs SR, et al. Short term changes in Ki-67 during neoadjuvant treatment of primary breast cancer with anastrozole or tamoxifen alone or combined correlate with recurrence-free survival. Clin Cancer Res 2005;11:951–8.
[80] Ellis MJ, Tao Y, Luo J, et al. Outcome prediction for estrogen receptor-positive breast cancer based on postneoadjuvant endocrine therapy tumor characteristics. J Natl Cancer Inst 2008;100:1380–8.
[81] Bates T, Riley DL, Houghton J, et al. Breast cancer in elderly women: a Cancer Research Campaign trial comparing treatment with tamoxifen and optimal surgery with tamoxifen alone. Br J Surg 1991;78:591–4.
[82] Romond EH, Perez EA, Bryant J, et al. Trastuzumab plus adjuvant chemotherapy for operable HER2 positive breast cancer. N Engl J Med 2005;353:1673–84.
[83] Smith I, Procter M, Gelber RD, et al. 2-year follow-up of trastuzumab after adjuvant chemotherapy in HER2-positive breast cancer: a randomised controlled trial. Lancet 2007;369: 29–36.
[84] Perez EA, Suman VJ, Davidson NE, et al. Cardiac safety analysis of doxorubicin and cyclophosphamide followed by paclitaxel with or without trastuzumab in the North Central Cancer Treatment Group N9831 adjuvant breast cancer trial. J Clin Oncol 2008;26: 1231–8.
[85] Buzdar AU, Ibrahim NK, Francis D, et al. Significantly higher pathologic complete remission rate after neoadjuvant therapy with trastuzumab, paclitaxel, and epirubicin chemotherapy: results of a randomized trial in human epidermal growth factor receptor 2-positive operable breast cancer. J Clin Oncol 2005;23:3676–85.
[86] Buzdar AU, Valero V, Ibrahim NK, et al. Neoadjuvant therapy with paclitaxel followed by 5-fluorouracil, epirubicin, and cyclophosphamide chemotherapy and concurrent trastuzumab in human epidermal growth factor receptor 2 positive operable breast cancer: an update of the initial randomized study population and data of additional patients treated with the same regimen. Clin Cancer Res 2007;13:228–33.
[87] Gianni L, Semiglazov V, Manikhas GM, et al. Neoadjuvant trastuzumab plus doxorubicin, paclitaxel, and CMF in locally advanced breast cancer (NOAH trial): feasibility, safety, and anti-tumor effects [abstract 532]. Proc Am Soc Clin Oncol 2007;10S, Breast Cancer Symposium.
[88] Friedrich MJ. Cardiotoxicity concerns prompt data review in breast cancer trial. J Natl Cancer Inst 2002;94:650–1.
[89] Nahta R, Hung MC, Esteva FJ. The HER2 targeting antibodies trastuzumab and pertuzumab synergistically inhibit the survival of breast cancer cells. Cancer Res 2004;64:2343–6.
[90] Geyer CE, Foster J, Lindquist D, et al. Lapatinib plus capecitibine for HER2 positive advanced breast cancer. N Engl J Med 2006;355:2733–43.
[91] O'Reilly KE, Rojo F, She QB, et al. mTOR inhibition induces upstream receptor tyrosine kinase signaling and activates Akt. Cancer Res 2006;66:1500–8.
[92] Pegram M, Chan D, Cichmann RA, et al. Phase II combined biological therapy targeting the HER2 proto-oncogene and the vascular endothelial growth factor (VEGF) using trastuzumab and bevacizumab as first-line treatment of HER2 amplified breast cancer [abstract 201]. Breast Cancer Res Treat 2006;100.
[93] Chagpar AB, Middleton LP, Sahin AA, et al. Accuracy of physical exam ultrasonography, and mammography in predicting residual pathologic tumor size in patients treated with neoadjuvant chemotherapy. Ann Surg 2006;243:257–64.

[94] Peintinger F, Kuerer HM, Anderson K, et al. Accuracy of the combination of mammography and sonography in predicting tumor response and breast cancer patients after neoadjuvant chemotherapy. Ann Surg Oncol 2006;13:1443–9.
[95] Essermann L, Hylton N, Yassa I, et al. Utility of magnetic resonance imaging in the management of breast cancer: evidence for improved preoperative staging. J Clin Oncol 1999;17:110–9.
[96] Balu-Maestro C, Chapellier C, Bleuse A, et al. Imaging in evaluation of response to neoadjuvant breast cancer treatment benefits of MRI. Breast Cancer Res Treat 2002;72:145–52.
[97] Rosen EL, Blackwell KL, Baker JA, et al. Accuracy of MRI in the detection of residual breast cancer after neoadjuvant chemotherapy. AJR Am J Roentgenol 2003;181:1275–82.
[98] Weatherall PT, Evans GF, Metzger GJ, et al. MRI vs histologic measurement of breast cancer following chemotherapy: comparison with x-ray mammography and palpation. J Magn Reson Imaging 2001;13:868–75.
[99] Yeh E, Slanetz P, Kopans DB, et al. Prospective comparison of mammography, sonography, and MRI in patients undergoing neoadjuvant chemotherapy for palpable breast cancer. AJR Am J Roentgenol 2005;184:868–77.
[100] Partridge SC, Gibbs JE, Lu Y, et al. Accuracy of MR imaging for revealing residual breast cancer in patients who have undergone neoadjuvant chemotherapy. AJR Am J Roentgenol 2002;179:1193–9.
[101] Berg WA, Gutierrez L, NessAiver ME, et al. Diagnostic accuracy of mammography, clinical examinations, US, and MR imaging in preoperative assessment of breast cancer. Radiology 2004;233:830–49.
[102] Zangheri B, Messa C, Picchio M, et al. PET/CT and breast cancer. Eur J Nucl Med Mol Imaging 2004;31(Suppl 1):S135–42.
[103] Mankoff DA, Dunnwald LK. Changes in glucose metabolism and blood flow following chemotherapy for breast cancer. PET Clin 2005;1:71–82.
[104] Rousseau C, Devillers A, Sagan C, et al. Monitoring of early response to neoadjuvant chemotherapy in stage ii and iii breast cancer by [^{18}F] fluorodeoxyglucose positron emission tomography. J Clin Oncol 2006;24:5366–72.
[105] Chen X, Moore MO, Lehman CD, et al. Combined use of MRI and PET to monitor response and assess residual disease for locally advanced breast cancer treated with neoadjuvant chemotherapy. Acad Radiol 2004;11:1115–24.
[106] Wasser K, Klein SK, Fink C, et al. Evaluation of neoadjuvant chemotherapeutic response of breast cancer using dynamic MRI with high temporal resolution. Eur Radiol 2003;13:80–7.
[107] Mardor Y, Pfeffer R, Spiegelmann R, et al. Early detection of response to radiation therapy in patients with brain malignancies using conventional and high b-value diffusion-weighted magnetic resonance imaging. J Clin Oncol 2003;15:1094–100.
[108] Taghian AG, bi-Raad R, Assaad SI, et al. Paclitaxel decreases the interstitial fluid pressure and improves oxygenation in breast cancers in patients treated with neoadjuvant chemotherapy: clinical implications. J Clin Oncol 2005;23:1951–61.
[109] Veronesi U, Paganelli G, Viale G, et al. A randomized comparison of sentinel-node biopsy with routine axillary dissection in breast cancer. N Engl J Med 2003;349:546–53.
[110] Nemoto T, Vana J, Bedwani RN, et al. Management and survival of female breast cancer: results of a national survey by the American College of Surgeons. Cancer 1980;45: 2917–24.
[111] Mittenberg DM, Miller C, Karamlou TB, et al. Meta-analysis of sentinel lymph node biopsy in breast cancer. J Surg Res 1999;84:138–42.
[112] Gurleyik G, Aker F, Sekmen U, et al. Accuracy of sentinel lymph node biopsy for the assessment of axillary status in patients with early (T1) breast carcinoma. J Coll Physicians Surg Pak 2005;15:697–700.
[113] Lyman GH, Giuliano AE, Somerfield MR. American Society of Clinical Oncology guideline recommendations for sentinel lymph node biopsy in early-stage breast cancer. J Clin Oncol 2005;23:7703–20.

[114] Kelly AM, Dwamena B, Cronin P, et al. Breast cancer: sentinel node identification and classification after neoadjuvant chemotherapy—systematic review and meta analysis. Acad Radiol 2009;16:551–63.
[115] Mamounas EP, Brown A, Anderson S, et al. Sentinel node biopsy after neoadjuvant chemotherapy in breast cancer: results from National Surgical Adjuvant Breast and Bowel Project Protocol B-27. J Clin Oncol 2005;23:2694–702.
[116] Classe JM, Bordes VB, Campion L. Sentinel lymph node biopsy after neoadjuvant chemotherapy for breast cancer: results of Ganglion Sentinelle et Chimiotherapie Neoadjuvante, a French prospective multicentric study. J Clin Oncol 2009;27:726–32.
[117] Xing Y, Foy M, Cox DD, et al. Meta-analysis of sentinel lymph node biopsy after pre-operative chemotherapy in patients with breast cancer. Br J Surg 2006;93:539–46.
[118] Mamounas EP. Sentinel lymph node biopsy after neoadjuvant systemic therapy. Surg Clin North Am 2003;83:931–42.
[119] Kuerer HM, Sahin AA, Hunt KK, et al. Incidence and impact of documented eradication of breast cancer axillary lymph node metastases before surgery in patients treated with neoadjuvant therapy. Ann Surg 1999;230:72–8.
[120] Bear HD, Anderson S, Brown A, et al. The effect on tumor response of adding sequential preoperative docetaxel to preoperative doxorubicin and cyclophosphamide: preliminary results from National Surgical Adjuvant Breast and Bowel Project B-27. J Clin Oncol 2003;21:4165–74.
[121] Hunt KK, Yi M, Mittendorf EA. Sentinel lymph node surgery after neoadjuvant chemotherapy is accurate and reduces the need for axillary dissection in breast cancer patients. Ann Surg 2009;250:1–7.
[122] Papa MZ, Zippel D, Kaufman B, et al. Timing of sentinel lymph node biopsy in patients receiving neoadjuvant chemotherapy for breast cancer. J Surg Oncol 2008;98(6):403–6.
[123] Nason KS, Anderson BO, Byrd DR, et al. Increased false negative sentinel node biopsy after preoperative chemotherapy for invasive breast carcinoma. Cancer 2000;89:2187–94.
[124] Shen J, Gilcrease MZ, Babiera GV, et al. Feasibility and accuracy of sentinel lymph node biopsy after preoperative chemotherapy in breast cancer patients with documented axillary metastases. Cancer 2007;109:1255–63.
[125] Whelan TJ, Julian J, Wright J, et al. Does local-regional radiation therapy improve survival in breast cancer? A meta-analysis. J Clin Oncol 2000;18:1220–9.
[126] Huang EH, Tucker SL, Strom EA, et al. Postmastectomy radiation improved locoregional control and survival for selected patients with locally advanced breast cancer treated with neoadjuvant chemotherapy and mastectomy. J Clin Oncol 2004;22:4691–9.
[127] Guarneri V, Broglio K, Kau SW, et al. Prognostic value of pathologic complete response after primary chemotherapy in relation to hormone receptor status and other factors. J Clin Oncol 2006;24:1037–44.
[128] Buchholz TA, Katz A, Strom EA. Pathologic tumor size and lymph node status predict for different rates of locoregional recurrence after mastectomy for breast cancer patients treated with neoadjuvant versus adjuvant chemotherapy. Int J Radiat Oncol Biol Phys 2002;53(4):880–8.
[129] Recht A, Edge SB, Solin LJ, et al. Post-mastectomy radiation: guidelines of the American Society of Clinical Oncology. J Clin Oncol 2001;19:1539–69.
[130] Gusterson BA, Gelber RD, Goldhirsch A, et al. Prognostic importance of c-erb-2 expression in breast cancer. International (Ludwig) Breast Cancer Study Group. J Clin Oncol 1992;10:1049–56.
[131] Petit T, Borel C, Ghnassia J-P, et al. Chemotherapy response of breast cancer depends on HER-2 status and anthracycline dose intensity in the neoadjuvant setting. Clin Cancer Res 2001;7:1577–81.
[132] Mathieu MC, Rouzier R, Llombart-Cussac A, et al. The poor responsiveness of infiltrating lobular breast carcinomas to neoadjuvant chemotherapy can be explained by their biological profile. Eur J Cancer 2004;40:342–51.

[133] Cocquyt VF, Blondeel PN, Depypere HT, et al. Different responses to preoperative chemotherapy for invasive lobular and invasive ductal breast carcinoma. Eur J Surg Oncol 2003;29:361–7.
[134] Tewari M, Krishnamurthy A, Shukla H. Predictive markers of response to neoadjuvant chemotherapy in breast cancer. Surg Oncol 2008;17:301–11.
[135] Gianni L, Zambetti M, Clark K, et al. Gene expression profiles in paraffin-embedded core biopsy tissue predict response to chemotherapy in women with locally advanced breast cancer. J Clin Oncol 2005;23:7265–77.
[136] Hess KR, Anderson K, Symmans W, et al. Pharmacogenomic predictor of sensitivity to preoperative chemotherapy with paclitaxel and fluorouracil, doxorubicin, and cyclophosphamide in breast cancer. J Clin Oncol 2006;24:4236–44.
[137] Buchholz TA, Hunt KK, Whitman GJ, et al. Neoadjuvant chemotherapy for breast carcinoma: multidisciplinary considerations of benefits and risks. Cancer 2003;98(6):1150–60.
[138] Clarke M, Collins R, Darby S, et al. Effects of radiotherapy and of differences in the extent of surgery for early breast cancer on local recurrence and 15-year survival: an overview of the randomised trials. Lancet 2005;366(9503):2087–106.
[139] McGuire SE, Gonzalez-Angulo AM, Huang EH, et al. Postmastectomy radiation improves the outcome of patients with locally advanced breast cancer who achieve a pathologic complete response to neoadjuvant chemotherapy. Int J Radiat Oncol Biol Phys 2007;68(4):1004–9.
[140] Perou CM, Sorlie T, Eisen MB, et al. Molecular portraits of human breast tumours. Nature 2000;406:747–52.
[141] Sorlie T, Perou CM, Tibshirani R, et al. Gene expression patterns of breast carcinomas distinguish tumor subclasses with clinical implications. Proc Natl Acad Sci U S A 2001;98:10869–74.

ELSEVIER
MOSBY
Advances in Surgery 44 (2010) 229–249
ADVANCES IN SURGERY

The Impact of Frailty in the Elderly on the Outcome of Surgery in the Aged

Nefertiti A. Brown, MD*, Michael E. Zenilman, MD
Department of Surgery, SUNY Downstate Medical Center, 450 Clarkson Avenue, Box 40, Brooklyn, NY 11203, USA

With the advances of modern medicine, society has enjoyed a better quality of life where the current average life expectancy in the United States is 78 years of age; it is expected by 2030 that the elderly will represent approximately 20% of the US population [1,2]. As the population continues to expand, the definition of what is elderly, as well as the breadth and scope of its pathophysiology, continues to evolve. This is especially demonstrated within the health care system where a large portion of patient care is directed toward the elderly who, in addition to the basic decline in physiologic reserve (the hallmark of aging), often have multiple comorbidities. Historically, comorbidities encompass cardiac, pulmonary, and renal disease as well as disability, but real aging, as measured by frailty, is only a recent addition. The challenge lies in the ability to screen, assess, and stratify risk in these patients using these measures. A sound preoperative assessment of geriatric patients should, therefore, include evaluation of surgical candidacy, the tailoring of surgical intervention, and the expected result of postoperative care.

The goal of this article is to explore the role of the emerging concept of frailty in the development of specific age-related changes and its role in the preoperative assessment and postoperative course of aged patients. It also identifies frailty's contribution to the morbidity of aging and highlights strategies to use its recognition to improve quality of care and patient safety.

WHAT IS FRAILTY?

Frailty is often described as a syndrome in aged patients where there is increased vulnerability due to decreased biologic reserve and the inability of the body to compensate in response to increased stress [3]. Not at all related to a single disease process, frailty is characterized by a decline in overall health as evidenced by a mass of impairments, such as symptoms, signs, disease, or disability. Despite the recognition of this entity, there is no uniform consensus on its definition or criteria, so it does not even have a designated *International*

*Corresponding author. *E-mail address*: Nefertiti.Brown@downstate.edu.

0065-3411/10/$ – see front matter
doi:10.1016/j.yasu.2010.05.014

Classification of Diseases, Ninth Edition code. Despite this, it is clear that age plays a role and is directly proportional to an increased risk of frailty [4]. The prevalence of frailty is approximately 20% to 30% in persons over 75 years of age, and it is projected that most persons by the age of 85 are frail [5]. With this continuous decline, the rates of morbidity and mortality in individuals with frailty are increased. Some studies cite the mortality rate as high as 18% versus only 4% in the nonfrail elderly [6,7].

The major components of frailty have been defined in the Cardiovascular Heath Study done by Fried and colleagues [8] as the presence of three out of five of the following: unintentional weight loss (more than 4.55 kg in a year), slow walking speed, self-reported exhaustion, low physical activity, and weakness (grip strength). Widely used within the geriatric community, these criteria are felt to contribute to the cyclic nature of the syndrome (Fig. 1). Outside of Fried's criteria, other factors that are also taken into consideration when evaluating for frailty are evidence of cognitive decline (memory loss and loss of verbal fluency) and the presence of psychiatric illness, such as depression and delirium. Patients identified as frail are at an increased risk of adverse events, such as falls, hospitalizations, disability, and death [3,8–10]. They are also recognized as having increased risk for surgery–more so than chronologic age or standard comorbidities.

RISK FACTORS FOR FRAILTY

Dimensions of frailty are determined by its predisposing factors, which fall into the one of the following categories: physiologic, pathologic (medical illness/comorbidities), psychological (cognitive), and functional (disability). The largest

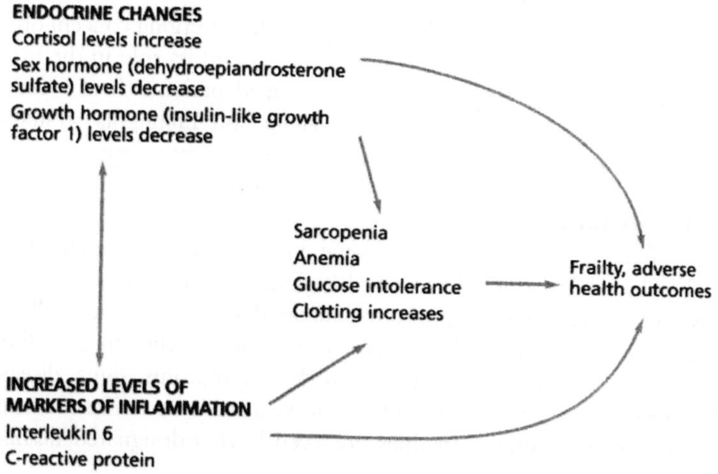

Fig. 1. The physiology of frailty. (*From* Espinoza S, Walston J. Frailty in older adults: insights and interventions. Cleve Clin J Med 2005;72(12):1105–12 [image on page 1108]; with permission.)

clinical study performed to evaluate the risk factors for frailty was done by Woods and colleagues [11] who prospectively evaluated 40,657 women (aged 65–79) from 40 US medical centers as part of the Women Health Initiative Observational Study. Components of frailty included self-reported muscle weakness/impaired walking, exhaustion, low physical activity, and unintended weight loss between baseline and 3 years of follow-up. Death, hip fractures, activities of daily living (ADL) disability, and hospitalizations were ascertained during an average of 5.9 years of follow-up. The investigators concluded that baseline frailty was the strongest predictor of hip fracture, ADL, disability, risk of repeated hospitalizations, and death [11]. The importance of assessing the presence of frailty in this population cannot be overestimated.

THE PHYSIOLOGY OF FRAILTY

Because frailty deals with the physiology of aging, it relates to the inherent decline of various organ systems with age. These may become more apparent with reduction in functional reserve and, as such, clinically significant when performing the preoperative assessment. These changes include sarcopenia, endocrine and immune dysfunction with an increase in inflammatory markers, hypercoagulable state, and anemia (see Fig. 1).

Weakness and fatigue are two of the major components of frailty that directly contribute to declining physical function. Sarcopenia is defined as a low level of muscle mass resulting from muscle loss that is common in adults and increases with age, particularly in people greater than 65 years of age [12,13]. Multifactorial in etiology, it has been strongly linked to alterations at the cellular and hormonal level, which act in tandem to promote a catabolic state leading to muscle breakdown.

Increases in inflammatory markers, such as interleukin (IL)-6 and C-reactive protein (CRP), with age have been linked to the development of sarcopenia. Schaap and colleagues [14] found increased serum levels of IL-6 and CRP as well as tumor necrosis factor (TNF)-α in elderly individuals studied over a period of 5 years. Specifically, reductions in TNF-α were associated with a decline in thigh muscle area as measured by CT and grip strength through clinical examination [14]. Accordingly, Hubbard and colleagues [15], using the frailty criteria as set by Fried and colleagues [8], studied 110 patients (average age 83.9 years) and discovered that with increasing patient frailty, TNF-α ($r = 0.379$, $P<.01$), IL-6 ($r = 0.369$, $P<.01$), and CRP ($r = 0.221$, $P<.05$), increased significantly with a corresponding decrease in albumin ($r = -0.545$, $P<.01$) in the frailest subjects [15].

It is well known that sex hormone levels decline with age, especially in women with the onset of menopause. These hormones play a role not only in sexual differentiation and reproduction but also in bone differentiation, muscle mass, and strength. On the cellular level, sex-binding hormone globulin (SBHG) has been linked to frailty. In a population-based prospective cohort study done over a 9-year period, 646 men, aged 50 to 86, classified by their degree of frailty, were measured in terms of hormone levels of total and free testosterone as well as SBHG levels. Although the study supported that the prevalence of frailty increased with age, it also reflected than men classified as frail had significantly lower free testosterone and higher SBHG levels than intermediate or nonfrail men with no change in total testosterone. After adjusting all groups for confounders, only elevated levels of SBHG were associated with key components of frailty (weight loss, low physical activity, and exhaustion) whereas decreases in total testosterone levels resulted in decreased grip strength [16]. Studies have reflected an inverse relationship between total testosterone levels and SBHG as men age, so high SBHG may be an important indicator of frailty [17,18]. Low testosterone levels have been associated with decreases in muscle mass, strength, and bone density, comparable with men with hypogonadism [19]. Despite this, there is controversy regarding the efficacy and safety of testosterone replacement in men [20,21].

Estrogen receptors have been localized to human skeletal muscle cells and have been found to influence metabolic and myogenic gene expression [22]. Consequently, with the loss of estrogen in menopause, changes in muscle strength are seen. Samson and colleagues [23] measured muscle strength and power in cross section of 74 healthy woman (ages 20–90, mean 49) and 81 healthy men (aged 20–90, mean 51) and observed that in women, muscle strength decreases dramatically after the age of 55. Compared with women 20 to 55 years of age, women 55 to 80 years of age experienced a 40.2% decrease in knee strength and a 28% decrease in handgrip strength (vs 10.3% and 8.2% in the younger group, respectively). Men showed more gradual declines with age.

In addition, estrogen is thought to play an indirect role in the decreasing the synthesis of parathyroid hormone in rat models [24]. So, low levels of estrogen can predispose women to elevated levels of parathyroid hormone leading to vitamin D deficiency. In the setting of vitamin D deficiency, muscle function and strength are reduced [25,26]. Bischoff and colleagues [27] also showed that vitamin D deficiency leads to decline of muscle strength in the elderly. Twelve percent of female (aged 65–86) and 18% of male (aged 66–95) subjects had 25-hydroxyvitamin D values below threshold. Strength, as measured by leg extension power, was lower in women and this correlated with decreased levels of vitamin D [27]. Because this deficiency is easily detected, its correction has shown physical benefits in terms of muscle strength gains and mobility [28,29], but to date, estrogen replacement (or hormone replacement therapy) is not recommended in frail women.

Further declines in endocrine function with aging (endocrine senescence) include decreases in growth hormone and insulinlike growth factor 1. These changes result in promotion of a catabolic state resulting in the perpetuation of sarcopenia with muscle breakdown and reduction in strength [30,31]. This is even more apparent in postmenopausal women because cortisol levels also increase as they enter this period [32]. A well-known catabolic hormone, its role in the propagation of sarcopenia is not surprising.

The cytokine, IL-6, has a major role in the frailty phenotype. Activation of the inflammatory cascade via IL-6 can affect the coagulation pathway through stimulation of thrombopoietin. Because thrombopoietin is responsible for platelet production, its activation by IL-6 results in a reactive thrombocytosis and hypercoagulability [33]. Additionally, IL-6 is intimately involved in the synthesis and release of fibrinogen [34]. These factors, in concert with the increase of D-dimer and factor VIII levels already associated with aging [35], promote a prothrombotic state. This dual effect places the elderly at increased risk for the development of deep venous thrombosis and pulmonary embolus. These risks are supported by data that age-related elevations in D-dimer and IL-6 levels are associated with a decline in function and increased mortality [36].

Chronic anemia is associated with frailty and ultimately poorer outcomes in older persons [37]. Multifactorial in etiology, anemia can be due to iron, folate, or vitamin B_{12} deficiency, all resulting in decreased hemoglobin levels [38]. This prevalence of anemia has also been linked to decreased erythropoietin function in the elderly stemming from age-related reduced functional reserve of the kidney [39]. Even anemia has been correlated with elevations in IL-6 levels in frail persons via an effect on myelosuppression. Compared with nonfrail persons, it is now believed that the main determinant in frail people is the presence of a chronic inflammatory state as marked by increased IL-6 production [40].

ILLNESS, COMORBIDITY, AND FRAILTY

One of the major pitfalls clinicians face is mistaking frailty for comorbidity. Frailty has been associated with age-related organ dysfunction in many studies. The best example is cardiovascular disease, in which increased cardiac dysfunction is associated with increased likelihood of frailty [11,38,41]. Woods and colleagues [11] identified other chronic diseases, such as stroke, diabetes, hypertension, arthritis, cancer, and chronic obstructive pulmonary disease, that could be used to predict frailty risk (Table 1). In the Cardiovascular Health Study, Fried and colleagues [8] reported that at least 25% of frail persons had at least one chronic disease, with 56% of these patients having arthritis, 25% hypertension, 8% diabetes, and less than 5% each of angina, congestive heart failure, cancer, and pulmonary disease. Despite excluding patients with Mini-Mental State Examination (MMSE) scores less than 18, they found lower cognition and greater depressive symptoms were associated with frailty. In both studies, self-reported health was also a good indicator of frailty, with the probability of frailty increasing from very good, good, fair, to poor impressions of general health.

BODY MASS AND FRAILTY

The sarcopenia of aging, although it does have physiologic bearing, also relates to the nutritional status. Signs of malnutrition, such as body mass index less than 18.5 or unintentional weight loss greater than 4.55 kg over a year and

Table 1
Baseline health characteristics with frailty in elderly men and women at baseline

Study	Factor	Nonfrail (%)	Intermediate (%)	Frail (%)
Cardiovascular Health Initiative (n = 5317)	Age at screening			
	65–74	76.1	62.9	38
	75–84	22.6	32.7	48.9
	85+	1.3	4.5	13
	Sex			
	Female	56.4	56.7	68.5
	Male	43.6	42.3	31.5
	Subjective view of general health			
	Excellent	19.5	10.7	3.5
	Very good	31.1	21.3	11.4
	Good	36.1	39.4	28.3
	Fair	12.6	24.4	40.3
	Poor	0.7	4.1	16.4
	Chronic disease at baseline			
	Hypertension	38.8	45.9	50.8
	MI	7.3	10.3	13.3
	Angina	14.5	21	28.8
	Heart failure	2	4.5	13.6
	Diabetes	12.1	18.2	25
	PVD	1.5	2.7	3.8
	COPD[a]	5.8	8.8	14.1
	Cancer	14.2	14.7	15.8
	Number of chronic diseases			
	0	23.2	15.4	7.3
	1	36.8	31	24.7
	2	24	27	26.9
	3–4	14.5	23.2	32.9
	= 5	1.5	3.5	8.2

Abbreviations: COPD, chronic obstructive pulmonary disease; MI, myocardial infarction; PVD, peripheral vascular disease.

[a]Chronic emphysema, bronchitis, or asthma.

Adapted from Fried LP, Tangen CM, Walston J, et al. Cardiovascular Health Study Collaborative Research Group. Frailty in older adults: evidence for a phenotype. J Gerontol A Biol Sci Med Sci 2001;56(3):M146–56.

poor appetite with food intake, are common in frailty [5,8,11]. Most studies surrounding nutrition relate to vitamin deficiency because it is common in the elderly. In one study, serum vitamins A, D, E, B_6, and B_{12}, carotenoids, folate, zinc, and selenium were measured at baseline and followed over 3 years in women 65 years and older of age (n = 766). At the beginning of the study, 32.6% of women (n = 250) were classified as frail versus 67.4% (n = 516) who were not frail. At the end of the 3 years, 31.9% of the nonfrail group became frail, and there was an association between deficiencies of vitamins D and E and carotenoids and frailer subjects [42]. Despite current ideology that weight loss and low body mass index are markers of frailty, however, "sarcopenic obesity," a disparity between muscle loss and fat gain caused by metabolic abnormalities, is a new entity becoming recognized as a possible sign of malnutrition derived frailty [8,11,43,44].

BONE DENSITY AND FRAILTY

Patients with a history of fracture or osteoporosis are also prone to frailty. The diminution of bone and bone density with age influences mobility and inclines toward fracture [45,46]. Fractures in elderly people are associated with a higher morbidity and mortality [47,48]. Nguyen and colleagues [49], using the Dubbo Osteoporosis Epidemiology Study, longitudinally characterized the residual lifetime risk of fracture in men and women 60 years of age and older (n = 2216) as 25% and 44%, respectively. When adjusted for bone mineral density, those with dual energy x-ray absorptiometry (DEXA) scores less than or equal to −2.5 had a risk of 42% (men) and 66% (women) of developing any fracture type. The most common fractures were those of the hip and vertebrae [49]. Hence, prevention of the progression of osteoporosis and fracture [50] is key to preventing the physical disability associated with the cycle of frailty in elderly subjects.

POLYPHARMACY AND FRAILTY

With the age-related development of illness, multiple medications are often required for daily maintenance and physiologic functioning. Despite the efficacy of these medications, the reduced hepatic and renal reserve associated with aging places the elderly at an increased risk of adverse drug reaction. This phenomenon, described as polypharmacy, is important to assess not only to document patients' comorbidities but also in anticipation of anesthesia administration as part of the surgical plan to predict and prevent adverse drug reactions/drug-drug interactions. Commonly prescribed agents, such as cardiovascular agents (aspirin, antihypertensive medications, and statins) and anticoagulants, have been linked to a higher likelihood of drug interactions when used concurrently and in conjunction with over-the-counter medications [51]. Qato and colleagues [51] examined medication usage in men and women aged 57 to 85 years (n = 3005) and found that 81% used at least one prescribed medication; 29% of respondents used at least 5 medications simultaneously, the majority of whom were between 75 and 85 years of age. The use of over-the-counter medications by those taking prescription medications correlated with a 4% risk of adverse drug reaction (Table 2). The highest risk was with anticoagulants. In all, the investigators calculated that 1 in 25 persons were at risk for an adverse drug reaction [51].

A recent review of more than 30,000 Medicare recipients receiving care in a clinical ambulatory setting detected 1523 adverse drug events over 1 year, 24.6% of which were preventable. Thirty-eight percent of these events were classified as life threatening or fatal, with the overall rate of adverse drug events 50.1 per 1000 person-years, with a rate of 13.8 preventable adverse drug events per 1000 person-years [52]. Unequivocal data such as these mandate that the

Table 2
Potential major medication interactions

Medication interaction type	Drugs	Potential effects
Prescription-prescription	Albuterol-Atenolol	Decreased effectiveness
Prescription-prescription	Albuterol-Metoprolol	Decreased effectiveness
Prescription-prescription	Clopidogrel-Warfarin	Increased risk of bleeding
Prescription-prescription	Lisinopril-Potassium	Increased risk of hyperkalemia
Prescription-prescription	Warfarin-Simvastatin	Increased risk of bleeding/ rhabdomyolysis
Nonprescription-prescription	Aspirin-Warfarin	Increased risk of bleeding
Nonprescription-prescription	Garlic-Warfarin	Increased risk of bleeding
Nonprescription-prescription	Niacin-Simvastatin	Increased risk of myopathy or rhabdomyolysis
Nonprescription-nonprescription	Ginkgo-aspirin	Increased risk of bleeding

Adapted from Qato DM, Alexander GC, Conti RM, et al. Use of prescription and over-the-counter medications and dietary supplements among older adults in the United States. JAMA 2008;300(24):2867–78.

surgical community address the issue of polypharmacy before, during, and after surgery.

COGNITION AND FRAILTY

Age-related declines in cognitive function have been well documented and are associated with increased disability and poor health outcomes [53]. Therefore, it is important to assess aging patients for these deficits. Although originally it was believed that cognitive decline contributed to the cycle of frailty through decreased food intake leading to weight loss and sarcopenia [54], studies show progressive central nervous system structural changes from chronic cerebrovascular disease [41]. Here, too, IL-6 has been found to play a role in age-related cognitive decline, specifically in mouse models, through a decrease in γ-aminobutyric interneurons. This decreases the ability of the hippocampus and cerebral cortex to retrieve, process, and encode information [55]. In addition, age-associated insulin resistance and insulin receptor dysfunction relate to decreased executive functioning in the elderly due to defects in glucose metabolism in the brain [56]. Decreased cognition and dementia as measured by the MMSE show that of the 7% of persons considered frail, 22% had evidence of significant impairment (discussed later). So, frail persons had higher incidence and overall risk of hospitalization, disability, dementia, and death [57].

From a psychiatric standpoint, depression and symptoms related to delirium and dementia have been strongly linked to frailty [8,11,58]. Changes in levels of cytokines like IL-6 are associated with central nervous system changes associated with aging that predispose frail persons to the development of neuropsychiatric syndromes [44,59]. A total of 165 brain autopsies and medical records from elderly subjects with known frailty were studied. Anatomically, more than half of the frail patients were found to have Alzheimer disease pathology. After controlling for age, gender, and education, Alzheimer disease was associated with a 2-fold increase in frailty [60]. Additional studies reinforce that along with depression, psychiatric illness in general had a higher frailty index in nondemented persons [61] and, in particular, the presence of depressive symptoms increased risk of hospitalization and mortality at 1 year [62]. All of these elements explain the high incidence and prevalence of falls, fracture, and mortality [63] in this population that follow overall decline in executive functioning and reduced insight.

DISABILITY AND FRAILTY

Defined by the Americans with Disabilities Act of 1990, disability is "a condition which limits a person's ability to function in major life activities–including communication, walking, and self-care (such as feeding and dressing oneself)–which may last indefinitely." A total of 41.3 million Americans are classified as disabled, 41% of them over the age of 65 [64]. The assessment of disability in the aging population involves ADL and instrumental ADL. In particular, the inability to perform ADL is highly predictive of frailty [8,11]. Fried and colleagues [8] predicted that frailty led to an increased incidence of disability, falls, hospitalization, and death over 3 years. Conversely, a history of frequent falls, presence of an ADL disability, and the baseline intermediate frailty all were allied with a greater frailty and hospitalization risk [11]. Recent studies support that prefrail and frail statuses are associated with an increased risk of ADL disability over a 10-year follow-up period in subjects not disabled at baseline [65].

FRAILTY IN SURGERY

It is estimated that approximately 46 million surgeries are performed annually in the United States, with a lifetime chance of a person over age 65 having at least one surgical procedure being one-third [66,67]. Although age is an independent risk factor of perioperative mortality, it is augmented in the setting of multiple comorbidities [68,69]. A prospective cohort study of patients over 50 years of age showed that regardless of undergoing cardiac or noncardiac surgery, patients 70 years of age or older had greater perioperative complications, longer length of inpatient stay, and in-hospital mortality [70].

Frailty, an age-related entity, has been linked to surgical risk. Recent studies show that increasing frailty is correlated with more postoperative complications, longer length of stay in the hospital, and decreased likelihood of being discharged home [71]. Robinson and colleagues [4] were the first to elucidate the relationship between frailty and 6-month postoperative mortality and identified that components of frailty, such as increased comorbidities, anemia, lower albumin, impaired cognition, recent fall, and reduced functional status, were key preoperative risk factors for postoperative mortality and postdischarge institutionalization. Additionally, any level of functional dependence was the strongest predictor of mortality [4]. Functional disability, with impaired cognition and depressive symptoms, has been linked to a higher likelihood of developing delirium in the postoperative period [72,73]. Similarly, Fukuse and colleagues [74] found that in elderly thoracic surgery patients, malnutrition, inability to perform ADL, and dementia were connected to a 7-fold incidence of prolonged air leak ($P = .0013$) and development of delirium postoperatively ($P = .0003$). Given the risk of vulnerable elderly to surgery, McGory and colleagues [75] outlined perioperative quality indicators for elderly patients undergoing surgery. Eight major domains were cited as necessary in evaluating surgical candidacy, addressing the appropriateness of the surgical plan and directing postoperative care. They include comorbidity assessment, elderly issues, medication use, patient-provider discussions, intraoperative care, postoperative management, discharge planning, and ambulatory surgery.

ASSESSMENT OF THE GERIATRIC PATIENT

Below is a straightforward algorithm to guide the care of elderly patients. This is best in conjunction with a geriatric consultation.

Preoperative assessment

1. History and physical examination
2. Past medical history

   Medication history

   Beers criteria, first described by Beers and colleagues in 1981, were created to address inappropriate medication use (where the risks outweigh the benefits of use) in elderly people. Most recently updated in 2002, the Beers criteria classifies medications to account for the illnesses dependent and independent of the patient's comorbidities (Table 3) [76]. Medications are clearly identified along with their potential issues and severity rating. Use of these criteria by the surgeon and the anesthesiologist in the tailoring of drug therapy will curtail drug-related complications in perioperative and postoperative period.

   Osteoporosis screening

   The American College of Preventive Medicine [77] recommends that all patients aged 50 years or older of age be evaluated for osteoporotic risk factors. Formal screening guidelines include bone mineral density testing in women aged 65 years or older and in men aged 70 years or older. Younger postmenopausal women and men aged 50 to 69 years should undergo screening if they have at least one major or two minor risk factors [78] for osteoporosis.

   Assessing comorbidities-comorbidity index (Charlson comorbidity index and the chronic illness rating scale)

   The Charlson comorbidity index is the most widely used method of classifying morbidity and estimating risk of death by predicting the 1-year mortality for patients who may have a range of comorbid conditions, such as heart disease, diabetes, or cancer [79]. Conditions are rated

Table 3
2002 Beers criteria for potentially inappropriate medication usage in older adults

Drug	Concerns	Severity rating (high or low)
Short-acting benzodiazepines (Ativan, Xanax)	Increased sensitivity in elderly patients Smaller doses may be effective and safer Total daily doses should not exceed maximum recommended doses	High
Long-acting benzodiazepines (Librium, Valium)	Long half-life in elderly patients (days) producing prolonged sedation/respiratory depression with risk of falls and fractures	High
Digoxin	Decreased renal clearance may lead to increased Toxic effects	Low
Anticholinergics/antihistamines (Benadryl, Atarax)	May cause confusion and sedation. Use in the smallest possible dose	High
Demerol	May cause confusion and has a higher side-effect profile than other narcotic drugs	High
Toradol	Immediate and long-term should be avoided Increased risk of renal and GI dysfunction	High
Non-COX selective NSAIDS (Aleve, Naproxen)	Increased risk of GI bleeding, renal failure, hypertension, and heart failure	High
NSAIDs and aspirin	Risk of GI ulceration with bleeding, platelet dysfunction with increased bleeding	High
Plavix, Coumadin	May prolong clotting time and elevate INR, resulting in increased bleeding risk	High
Long-term use of stimulant laxatives (Dulcolax, Cascara)	May exacerbate bowel dysfunction	High
Amiodarone	Associated with QT interval problems and torsades de pointes	High
Prozac	Long half-life with risk of increasing agitation and sleep disturbance. Safer alternatives exist	High
Clonidine	Orthostatic hypotension and central nervous system adverse effects	Low

Abbreviations: COX, cyclooxygenase; INR, international normalized ratio.
Adapted from Fick DM, Cooper JW, Wade WE, et al. Updating the Beers criteria for potentially inappropriate medication use in older adults. Arch Intern Med 2003;163:2716–24.

Table 4
Charlson comorbidity index

Comorbid condition	Weight
Myocardial infarct	1
Congestive heart failure	1
Peripheral vascular disease	1
Cerebrovascular disease	1
Dementia	1
Chronic pulmonary disease	1
Connective tissue disease	1
Ulcer disease	1
Diabetes	1
Hemiplegia	2
Moderate or severe renal disease	2
Diabetes with end-organ dysfunction	2
Any tumor	2
Leukemia	2
Lymphoma	2
Moderate or severe liver disease	3
Metastatic solid tumor	6
AIDS	6

Adapted from Charlson ME, Pompei P, Ales KL, et al. A new method of classifying prognostic comorbidity in longitudinal studies: development and validation. J Chronic Dis 1987;40(5):373–83.

on a scale (1, 2, 3, 6), depending on the risk of dying associated with the condition [80]. Nineteen predefined morbidities are listed in Table 4.

3. Preoperative tests
   - Blood: complete blood count, complete metabolic panel (serum electrolytes renal function, liver function tests), coagulation profile, type and screen (if indicated)
   - Cardiac evaluation (as indicated based on comorbidities)
     - Electrocardiogram, echocardiogram, carotid ultrasound (if extreme flexion/extension of the neck is likely or for patients undergoing cardiothoracic surgery)
     - Exercise testing, thallium stress testing, Holter monitoring
   - Pulmonary evaluation (as indicated [81])
     - Chest radiograph, arterial blood gas, pulmonary function testing
4. Assessing functional reserve
   - American Society of Anesthesiologists physical status classification system [82]—indicates degree of organ dysfunction and functional impairment and acts as predictor of morbidity and mortality in surgical patients
   - Physiologic and Operative Severity Score for the enUmeration of Mortality and Morbidity (POSSUM) [83]—has been shown to be highly predictive and compares morbidity and mortality of surgical procedures using physiologic and operative variables
5. Sarcopenia/nutritional status—mininutritional assessment
6. Cognition/mood—MMSE (Table 5), geriatric depression scale, assessing postoperative delirium risk (Box 1)

Table 5
Mini-mental state examination

Score	Item	Score	Item
5	*Orientation*	3	*Recall*
5	(Year) (Season)	2	Recall 3 objects above
3	(Date) (Day)	1	*Language*
5	(Month)	3	Name a pencil and a watch
	(State)	1	Repeat "no ifs, ands, or buts"
	(Country)	1	Follow a 3-step command (take this
	(Town)	1	paper, fold in half, and place on the
	(Building)		floor)
	(Floor)		Read and obey "close your eyes"
	Registration		Write a sentence
	Name three objects		Copy intersecting pentagons
	Record number of trials to learn		
	Attention & Calculation		
	Serial 7's (stop after 5 answers)		
	or spell "WORLD" backward		

Total possible score = 30

Scoring:
A score of 20 or less has a LR of 14.5 for dementia
A score between 21 and 25 has a LR of 2.2 for dementia (less conclusive)
A score of 26 or more has a LR of 0.1 for dementia

Abbreviation: LR, lattice reduction.

Adapted from Folstein MF, Folstein SE, McHugh PR. "Mini-mental state". A practical method for grading the cognitive state of patients for the clinician. J Psychiatr Res 1975;12(3):189–98.

7. Disability
   Osteoporosis screening (described previously)
   ADL—to assess baseline function and degree of independence in daily tasks (eg, feeding and bathing): Barthel index or the functional independence measure.

Postoperative management

Postoperative management of frail patients is similar to that of nonfrail patients. Postoperative care begins with a thorough preoperative assessment (discussed previously) and quality perioperative care. During the recovery period, special attention should be paid to the following:

Airway

Because most patients are extubated within 24 hours of surgery, it is important to ensure continued patency of the airway and that patients are able to competently protect it. Ambulation along with aggressive pulmonary toilet (chest physiotherapy and deep breathing/coughing) with incentive spirometry has been shown to be of great benefit in preventing pulmonary complications [84]. Additionally, patients should be monitored with pulse oximetry and given supportive oxygen therapy as needed. If there are signs of respiratory instability, intubation with mechanical ventilatory support in indicated.

Box 1: Major risk factors for postoperative delirium

Demographics
- Age >65
- Male gender

Comorbidities
- Multiple chronic illnesses
- Chronic kidney or liver disease
- History of stroke/neurologic disease
- Metabolic derangements
- HIV infection
- Fracture or trauma
- Severe illness
- Terminal illness

Decreased oral intake
- Malnutrition, dehydration

Drugs
- Polypharmacy
- Alcohol abuse

Functional status
- Requires assistance to perform ADL
- Low physical activity
- Immobility
- History of falls

Cognitive status
- History of delirium
- Depression
- Dementia
- Cognitive impairment

Adapted from Brown TM, Boyle MF. Delirium. BMJ 2002;325(7365):644–7.

Pain

Because elderly patients often have multiple medical problems managed with several medications, treatment of postoperative pain can be difficult. Pain management should involve communication between the patient, surgeon, and anesthesia and pharmacy teams to ensure efficacy as well as safety of the proposed treatment. In this group, it is recommended that opioids be administered at 25% to 50% of the adult dose and titrated accordingly until pain is specified as mild by patient report on the pain scale [85]. If there is no history of renal impairment or gastrointestinal (GI) bleed, nonsteroidal anti-inflammatory drugs (NSAIDs) can be used for breakthrough pain and to reduce the dose of opioids given. NSAIDS lower side-effect profile also allows it to be used alone and is significant, as opioid use as described in Beers criteria [76]. For example, Demerol use in the elderly is a well-known risk factor for the development of delirium [86].

Cognition

Frail patients are highly predisposed to the development of delirium in the postoperative period (see Box 1) and, as such, require constant mental status evaluations. Current recommendations for delirium prevention include correction of electrolyte and fluid imbalances, early mobilization, maintenance of appropriate oxygenation, and avoidance of certain drugs (Box 2) [87]. Treatment of delirium should be focused on the key factors of delirium: visual and hearing impairment, cognitive impairment, sleep deprivation, immobility, and dehydration [88]. Keeping patients constantly oriented to their surroundings along with other cognitive and physical exercises helps with delirium in addition to assistance with feeds and hydration as needed. Nonpharmacologic sleep aids (relaxation and massage) should be used if at all possible. For refractory symptoms, haloperidol (Haldol) is the drug of choice in this patient population [89]. Collaboration with geriatricians may also prove helpful [90].

Functional status and nutrition

Increases in D-dimer and factor VIII increase with age and with IL-6 stimulation of thrombopoietin might contribute to a prothrombotic state in frailty [33–35]. This, paired with decreased functionality or mobility, increases the risk of thromboembolic events [91]. Prophylaxis for deep venous thrombosis should begin from the time of admission or, alternatively, after surgery with low-dose unfractionated (5000 U twice a day) or low molecular weight heparin ($\leq$3400 U daily) for mild to moderate risk groups. For higher risk patients, low-dose unfractionated (5000 U 3 times a day) or low molecular weight heparin (>3400 U daily) is recommended [92]. Also, intermittent pneumatic compression should be added supplementally until patients are ambulatory.

Sarcopenia is a concern as loss of muscle mass leads to decrease mobility and strength [12,13], which is increased in the postoperative period if patients are on prolonged bed rest. Therefore, early mobilization is essential to recovery and patients should be encouraged to sit up, transfer to chair, stand, and exercise as often as possible. If assistance is required, inpatient rehabilitation services should work along with the surgical team to assist in recovery of mobility. To aid in the development of muscle mass and aid in wound healing, oral intake with a balanced diet containing essential vitamins and minerals is recommended. Whether or not patients

Box 2: Steps to preventing delirium in elderly subjects

Delirium prevention

Preoperative assessment

- Detailed history of medications
- Review of past medical history
- Mental preparation before surgery
- Neuropsychologic testing
- Neurologic examination to detect sensory or perceptual deficits
- Anesthesiology assessment

Intraoperative

- Adequate oxygenation and perfusion
- Correct electrolyte imbalances
- Adjust drug dosing
- Minimize the variety of drugs used
- Avoid anticholinergics, benzodiazepines

Postoperatively

- Environmental support
  Well-lit, cheerful room
  Quiet surroundings
  Keep patient oriented
  Encourage visits by friends and family
- Treat pain
- Identify risk-associated drugs
  Anticholinergics
  Depressants
  H_2 antagonists
  Digoxin, lidocaine
- Reassure patient and family

Adapted from Parikh SS, Chung F. Postoperative delirium in the elderly. Anesth Analg 1995;80(6):1223–32.

are at risk for malnutrition should be guided by the mininutritional assessment as well as albumin levels, because protein energy malnutrition is directly related to hypoabuminemia [93]. If oral intake is insufficient or patients are unable to eat by mouth, supplemental tube feeds or parenteral feeds are indicated. Current research involves use of anabolic agents in concert with enteral nutrition to restore body mass, strength, and promote wound healing [94].

SUMMARY

As the population continues to age, we will continue to encounter issues involving aging and the elderly. Despite these issues, knowledge is expanding and evolving with new solutions to ongoing problems. Mechanistically, frailty at its root is a symptom of growing old, with cascades and circuitous feedback between organ systems at all levels. Clinically, frailty is as equally dynamic and its multifactorial nature represents a unique challenge to the surgical community and warrants the integration of geriatric assessment into clinical practice. Integration within clinical practice includes using an interdisciplinary approach, where surgeons work with anesthesiologists, geriatricians, nursing, rehabilitation, nutritionists, and other support staff to provide holistic assessment, efficient delivery, and higher quality of care. This in hand, recognition of frailty can occur in a timely fashion to initiate treatment, decreasing the risk of morbidity and mortality for improved surgical outcomes.

References

[1] The statistical abstract of the United States. The U.S. Census Bureau 2009.
[2] Kulminski A, Yashin A, Akushevich S, et al. Frailty index as a major indicator of aging processes and mortality in the elderly. J Am Geriatr Soc 2007;55(6):935–40.
[3] Gallucci M, Ongaro F, Amici GP, et al. Frailty, disability and survival in the elderly over the age of seventy: evidence from "The Treviso Longeva (TRELONG) Study". Arch Gerontol Geriatr 2009;48(3):281–3.
[4] Robinson TN, Eiseman B, Wallace JI, et al. Redefining geriatric preoperative assessment using frailty, disability and co-morbidity. Ann Surg 2009;250(3):449–55.
[5] Topinkova E. Aging, disability and frailty. Ann Nutr Metab 2008;52(Suppl 1):6–11.
[6] Avila-Funes JA, Helmer C, Amieva H, et al. Frailty among community-dwelling elderly people in France: the three-city study. J Gerontol A Biol Sci Med Sci 2008;63(10): 1089–96.
[7] Puts MT, Lips P, Deeg DJ. Sex differences in the risk of frailty for mortality independent of disability and chronic diseases. J Am Geriatr Soc 2005;53(1):40–7.
[8] Fried LP, Tangen CM, Walston J, et al. Cardiovascular Health Study Collaborative Research Group. Frailty in older adults: evidence for a phenotype. J Gerontol A Biol Sci Med Sci 2001;56(3):M146–56.
[9] Boyd CM, Ricks M, Fried LP, et al. Functional decline and recovery of activities of daily living in hospitalized, disabled older women: the Women's Health and Aging Study I. J Am Geriatr Soc 2009;57(10):1757–66.
[10] Suh TT, Lyles KW. Osteoporosis considerations in the frail elderly. Curr Opin Rheumatol 2003;15(4):481–6.
[11] Woods NF, LaCroix AZ, Gray SL, et al. Women's Health Initiative. Frailty: emergence and consequences in women aged 65 and older in the Women's Health Initiative Observational Study. J Am Geriatr Soc 2005;53(8):1321–30.
[12] Lang T, Streeper T, Cawthon P, et al. Sarcopenia: etiology, clinical consequences, intervention, and assessment. Osteoporos Int 2009;21(4):543–59.
[13] Iannuzzi-Sucich M, Prestwood KM, Kenny AM. Prevalence of sarcopenia and predictors of skeletal muscle mass in healthy, older men and women. J Gerontol A Biol Sci Med Sci 2005;57:M772–7.
[14] Schaap LA, Pluijm SM, Deeg DJ, et al. Higher inflammatory marker levels in older persons: associations with 5-year change in muscle mass and muscle strength. J Gerontol A Biol Sci Med Sci 2009;64(11):1183–9.
[15] Hubbard RE, O'Mahony MS, Savva GM, et al. Inflammation and frailty measures in older people. J Cell Mol Med 2009;13(9B):3103–9.

[16] Mohr BA, Bhasin S, Kupelian V, et al. Testosterone, sex hormone-binding globulin, and frailty in older men. J Am Geriatr Soc 2007;55(4):548–55.
[17] Feldman HA, Longcope C, Derby CA, et al. Age trends in the level of serum testosterone and other hormones in middle-aged men: longitudinal results from the Massachusetts male aging study. Clin Endocrinol Metab 2002;87(2):589–98.
[18] Liu PY, Beilin J, Meier C, et al. Age-related changes in serum testosterone and sex hormone binding globulin in Australian men: longitudinal analyses of two geographically separate regional cohorts. J Clin Endocrinol Metab 2007;92(9):3599–603.
[19] Snyder PJ, Peachey H, Berlin JA, et al. Effects of testosterone replacement in hypogonadal men. J Clin Endocrinol Metab 2000;85(8):2670–7.
[20] Anawalt BD, Merriam GR. Neuroendocrine aging in men. Andropause and somatopause. Endocrinol Metab Clin North Am 2001;30(3):647–69.
[21] Gooren L. Androgen deficiency in the aging male: benefits and risks of androgen supplementation. J Steroid Biochem Mol Biol 2003;85(2–5):349–55.
[22] Dieli-Conwright CM, Spektor TM, Rice JC, et al. Oestradiol and SERM treatments influence oestrogen receptor coregulator gene expression in human skeletal muscle cells. Acta Physiol (Oxf) 2009;197(3):187–96.
[23] Samson MM, Meeuwsen IB, Crowe A, et al. Relationships between physical performance measures, age, height and body weight in healthy adults. Age Ageing 2000;29(3):235–42.
[24] Carrillo-López N, Román-García P, Rodríguez-Rebollar A, et al. Indirect regulation of PTH by estrogens may require FGF23. J Am Soc Nephrol 2009;20(9):2009–17.
[25] Pedrosa MA, Castro ML. Role of vitamin D in the neuro-muscular function. Arq Bras Endocrinol Metabol 2005;49(4):495–502.
[26] Mowé M, Haug E, Bøhmer T. Low serum calcidiol concentration in older adults with reduced muscular function. J Am Geriatr Soc 1999;47(2):220–6.
[27] Bischoff HA, Stahelin HB, Urscheler N, et al. Muscle strength in the elderly: its relation to vitamin D metabolites. Arch Phys Med Rehabil 1999;80(1):54–8.
[28] Moreira-Pfrimer LD, Pedrosa MA, Teixeira L, et al. Treatment of vitamin D deficiency increases lower limb muscle strength in institutionalized older people independently of regular physical activity: a randomized double-blind controlled trial. Ann Nutr Metab 2009;54(4):291–300.
[29] Songpatanasilp T, Chailurkit LO, Nichachotsalid A, et al. Combination of alfacalcidol with calcium can improve quadriceps muscle strength in elderly ambulatory Thai women who have hypovitaminosis D: a randomized controlled trial. J Med Assoc Thai 2009;92(Suppl 5):S30–41.
[30] Johannsson G, Svensson J, Bengtsson BA. Growth hormone and ageing. Growth Horm IGF Res 2000;10(Suppl B):S25–30.
[31] Lissett CA, Shalet SM. Effects of growth hormone on bone and muscle. Growth Horm IGF Res 2000;10(Suppl B):S95–101.
[32] Gusenoff JA, Harman SM, Veldhuis JD, et al. Cortisol and GH secretory dynamics, and their interrelationships, in healthy aged women and men. Am J Physiol Endocrinol Metab 2001;280(4):E616–25.
[33] Kaser A, Brandacher G, Steurer W, et al. Interleukin-6 stimulates thrombopoiesis through thrombopoietin: role in inflammatory thrombocytosis. Blood 2001;98(9):2720–5.
[34] Castell JV, Gómez-Lechón MJ, David M, et al. Interleukin-6 is the major regulator of acute phase protein synthesis in adult human hepatocytes. FEBS Lett 1989;242(2):237–9.
[35] Tracy RP, Bovill EG, Fried LP, et al. The distribution of coagulation factors VII and VIII and fibrinogen in adults over 65 years. Results from the Cardiovascular Health Study. Ann Epidemiol 1992;2(4):509–19.
[36] Cohen HJ, Harris T, Pieper CF. Coagulation and activation of inflammatory pathways in the development of functional decline and mortality in the elderly. Am J Med 2003;114(3):180–7.
[37] Penninx BW, Guralnik JM, Onder G, et al. Anemia and decline in physical performance among older persons. Am J Med 2003;115:104–10.

[38] Chaves PH, Semba RD, Leng SX, et al. Impact of anemia and cardiovascular disease on frailty status of community-dwelling older women: the Women's Health and Aging Studies I and II. J Gerontol A Biol Sci Med Sci 2005;60(6):729–35.
[39] Nafziger J, Pailla K, Luciani L, et al. Decreased erythropoietin responsiveness to iron deficiency anemia in the elderly. Am J Hematol 1993;43(3):172–6.
[40] Leng S, Chaves P, Koenig K, et al. Serum interleukin-6 and hemoglobin as physiological correlates in the geriatric syndrome of frailty: a pilot study. J Am Geriatr Soc 2002;50(7): 1268–71.
[41] Newman AB, Gottdiener JS, Mcburnie MA, et al. Cardiovascular Health Study Research Group. Associations of subclinical cardiovascular disease with frailty. J Gerontol A Biol Sci Med Sci 2001;56(3):M158–66.
[42] Semba RD, Bartali B, Zhou J, et al. Low serum micronutrient concentrations predict frailty among older women living in the community. J Gerontol A Biol Sci Med Sci 2006;61(6):594–9.
[43] Stenholm S, Harris TB, Rantanen T, et al. Sarcopenic obesity: definition, cause and consequences. Curr Opin Clin Nutr Metab Care 2008;11(6):693–700.
[44] Blaum CS, Xue QL, Michelon E, et al. The association between obesity and the frailty syndrome in older women: The Women's Health and Aging Study. J Am Geriatr Soc 2005;53:927–34.
[45] Ma SL, Oyler J, Glavin S, et al. Self-reported frailty is associated with low calcaneal bone mineral density in a multiracial population of community-dwelling elderly. Osteoporos Int 2009;20(11):1837–46.
[46] Rolland Y, Abellan van Kan G, Bénétos A, et al. Frailty, osteoporosis and hip fracture: causes, consequences and therapeutic perspectives. J Nutr Health Aging 2008;12(5):335–46.
[47] Ioannidis G, Papaioannou A, Hopman WM, et al. Relation between fractures and mortality: results from the Canadian Multicentre Osteoporosis Study. CMAJ 2009;181(5):265–71.
[48] Jalava T, Sarna S, Pylkkänen L, et al. Association between vertebral fracture and increased mortality in osteoporotic patients. J Bone Miner Res 2003;18(7):1254–60.
[49] Nguyen ND, Ahlborg HG, Center JR, et al. Residual lifetime risk of fractures in women and men. J Bone Miner Res 2007;22(6):781–8.
[50] Qaseem A, Snow V, Shekelle P, et al. Clinical Efficacy Assessment Subcommittee of the American College of Physicians. Pharmacologic treatment of low bone density or osteoporosis to prevent fractures: a clinical practice guideline from the American College of Physicians. Ann Intern Med 2008;149(6):404–15.
[51] Qato DM, Alexander GC, Conti RM, et al. Use of prescription and over-the-counter medications and dietary supplements among older adults in the United States. JAMA 2008;300(24):2867–78.
[52] Gurwitz JH, Field TS, Harrold LR, et al. Incidence and preventability of adverse drug events among older persons in the ambulatory setting. JAMA 2003;289(9):1107–16.
[53] Gill TM, Williams CS, Richardson ED, et al. Impairments in physical performance and cognitive status as predisposing factors for functional dependence among nondisabled older persons. J Gerontol A Biol Sci Med Sci 1996;51:M283–8.
[54] Morley JE, Perry HM 3rd, Miller DK. Editorial: something about frailty. J Gerontol A Biol Sci Med Sci 2002;57(11):M698–704.
[55] Dugan LL, Ali SS, Shekhtman G, et al. IL-6 mediated degeneration of forebrain GABAergic interneurons and cognitive impairment in aged mice through activation of neuronal NADPH oxidase. PLoS One 2009;4(5):e5518.
[56] Abbatecola AM, Paolisso G, Lamponi M, et al. Insulin resistance and executive dysfunction in older persons. J Am Geriatr Soc 2004;52(10):1713–8.
[57] Avila-Funes JA, Amieva H, Barberger-Gateau P, et al. Cognitive impairment improves the predictive validity of the phenotype of frailty for adverse health outcomes: the three-city study. J Am Geriatr Soc 2009;57(3):453–61.
[58] Marcantonio ER, Flacker JM, Michaels M, et al. Delirium is independently associated with poor functional recovery after hip fracture. J Am Geriatr Soc 2000;48(6):618–24.

[59] Hickie I, Lloyd A. Are cytokines associated with neuropsychiatric syndromes in humans? Int J Immunopharmacol 1995;17(8):677–83.
[60] Buchman AS, Schneider JA, Leurgans S, et al. Physical frailty in older persons is associated with Alzheimer disease pathology. Neurology 2008;71(7):499–504.
[61] Andrew MK, Rockwood K. Psychiatric illness in relation to frailty in community-dwelling elderly people without dementia: a report from the Canadian Study of Health and Aging. Can J Aging 2007;26(1):33–8.
[62] Lupón J, González B, Santaeugenia S, et al. Prognostic implication of frailty and depressive symptoms in an outpatient population with heart failure. Rev Esp Cardiol 2008;61(8): 835–42.
[63] van Iersel MB, Verbeek AL, Bloem BR, et al. Frail elderly patients with dementia go too fast. J Neurol Neurosurg Psychiatry 2006;77(7):874–6.
[64] American Community Survery Data. The U.S. Census Bureau 2008.
[65] Al Snih S, Graham JE, Ray LA, et al. Frailty and incidence of activities of daily living disability among older Mexican Americans. J Rehabil Med 2009;41(11):892–7.
[66] National Center for Health Statistics. 2006 National Hospital Discharge Survey. Atlanta (GA): Centers for Disease Control and Prevention; 2009.
[67] Khuri SF, Henderson WG, Daley J, et al. Successful implementation of the Department of Veterans Affairs' National Surgical Quality Improvement Program in the private sector: the Patient Safety in Surgery study. Ann Surg 2008;248(2):329–36.
[68] Lausen M, Kirchner R, Schöffel U, et al. [Is advanced age by itself a risk factor in large abdominal surgical interventions]. Langenbecks Arch Chir Suppl II Verh Dtsch Ges Chir 1990;1321–4 [in German].
[69] Berry AJ, Smith RB 3rd, Weintraub WS, et al. Age versus comorbidities as risk factors for complications after elective abdominal aortic reconstructive surgery. J Vasc Surg 2001;33(2):345–52.
[70] Polanczyk CA, Marcantonio E, Goldman L, et al. Impact of age on perioperative complications and length of stay in patients undergoing noncardiac surgery. Ann Intern Med 2001;134(8):637–43.
[71] Dasgupta M, Rolfson DB, Stolee P, et al. Frailty is associated with postoperative complications in older adults with medical problems. Arch Gerontol Geriatr 2009;48(1):78–83.
[72] Litaker D, Locala J, Franco K, et al. Preoperative risk factors for postoperative delirium. Gen Hosp Psychiatry 2001;23(2):84–9.
[73] Greene NH, Attix DK, Weldon BC, et al. Measures of executive function and depression identify patients at risk for postoperative delirium. Anesthesiology 2009;110(4): 788–95.
[74] Fukuse T, Satoda N, Hijiya K, et al. Importance of a comprehensive geriatric assessment in prediction of complications following thoracic surgery in elderly patients. Chest 2005;127(3):886–91.
[75] McGory ML, Kao KK, Shekelle PG, et al. Developing quality indicators for elderly surgical patients. Ann Surg 2009;250(2):338–47.
[76] Fick DM, Cooper JW, Wade WE, et al. Updating the beers criteria for potentially inappropriate medication use in older adults. Arch Intern Med 2003;163:2716–24.
[77] Lim LS, Hoeksema LJ, Sherin K, et al. Screening for osteoporosis in the adult U.S. population: ACPM position statement on preventive practice. Am J Prev Med 2009;36(4):366–75.
[78] Brown JP, Josse RG. Scientific Advisory Council of the Osteoporosis Society of Canada. 2002 clinical practice guidelines for the diagnosis and management of osteoporosis in Canada. Am J Prev Med 2009;36(4):366–75.
[79] De Groot V, Beckerman H, Lankhorst GJ, et al. How to measure comorbidity: a critical review of available methods. J Clin Epidemiol 2003;56(3):221–9.
[80] Charlson ME, Pompei P, Ales KL, et al. A new method of classifying prognostic comorbidity in longitudinal studies: development and validation. J Chronic Dis 1987;40(5): 373–83.

[81] Barnard NA, Williams RW, Spencer EM. Preoperative patient assessment: a review of the literature and recommendations. Ann R Coll Surg Engl 1994;76:293–7.
[82] The American Society of Anesthesiologists. ASA relative value guide 2009.
[83] Copeland GP, Jones D, Walters M. POSSUM: a scoring system for surgical audit. Br J Surg 1991;78(3):355–60.
[84] Thomas JA, McIntosh JM. Are incentive spirometry, intermittent positive pressure breathing, and deep breathing exercises effective in the prevention of postoperative pulmonary complications after upper abdominal surgery? A systematic overview and meta-analysis. Phys Ther 1994;74(1):3–10.
[85] McDonald D. Postoperative pain management for the aging patient. Geriatr Aging 2006;9(6):395–8.
[86] Skrobik Y. Delirium prevention and treatment. Crit Care Clin 2009;25(3):585–91.
[87] Parikh SS, Chung F. Postoperative delirium in the elderly. Anesth Analg 1995;80(6): 1223–32.
[88] Inouye SK, Bogardus ST, Charpentier PA, et al. A mutlicompartment intervention to prevent delirium in hospitalized older patients. N Engl J Med 1999;340:669–76.
[89] Deiner S, Silverstein JH. Postoperative delirium and cognitive dysfunction. Br J Anaesth 2009;103(Suppl 1):i41–6.
[90] Marcantonio ER, Flacker JM, Wright RJ, et al. Reducing delirium after hip fracture: a randomized trial. J Am Geriatr Soc 2001;49:516–22.
[91] Sellier E, Labarere J, Sevestre MA, et al. Association pour la Promotion de l'Angiologie Hospitalière. Risk factors for deep vein thrombosis in older patients: a multicenter study with systematic compression ultrasonography in postacute care facilities in France. J Am Geriatr Soc 2008;56(2):224–30.
[92] Geerts WH, Pineo GF, Heit JA, et al. Prevention of venous thromboembolism: the Seventh ACCP Conference on Antithrombotic and Thrombolytic Therapy. Chest 2004;126(3 Suppl):338S–400S.
[93] Rosenthal RA. Nutritional concerns in the surgical patient. J Am Coll Surg 2004;199:785.
[94] Collins N. Protein-energy malnutrition and involuntary weight loss: nutritional and pharmacological strategies to enhance wound healing. Expert Opin Pharmacother 2003;4(7): 1121–40.

Advances in Surgery 44 (2010) 251–267

ADVANCES IN SURGERY

Quality Improvement in Surgery: the American College of Surgeons National Surgical Quality Improvement Program Approach

Angela M. Ingraham, MD[a,b,*], Karen E. Richards, BS[a], Bruce L. Hall, MD, PhD, MBA[c,d,e], Clifford Y. Ko, MD, MS, MSHS[a,f,g]

[a]Division of Research and Optimal Patient Care, American College of Surgeons, 633 North Saint Clair Street, Floor 22NE, Chicago, IL 60611, USA
[b]Department of Surgery, University of Cincinnati College of Medicine, Cincinnati, 231 Albert Sabin Way, Room 1586, Cincinnati, OH 45267, USA
[c]Washington University and St Louis, University Schools of Medicine, 915 North Grand Boulevard, St Louis, MO 63106, USA
[d]Section of Endocrine and Oncology Surgery, Campus Box 8109, 6605 Euclid Avenue, St Louis, MO 63130, USA
[e]Center for Health Policy, Olin Business School at Washington University in St Louis, Campus Box 113, One Brookings Drive, St Louis, MO 63130, USA
[f]Department of Surgery, University of California, Los Angeles (UCLA), Los Angeles, 72-215 CHS, 10833 Le Conte Avenue, CA 90095, USA
[g]Department of Surgery, VA Greater Los Angeles Healthcare System, 11301 West Wilshire Boulevard, University of California, Los Angeles (UCLA), Los Angeles, CA 90073, USA

SURGICAL QUALITY: MEANING AND ASSESSMENT

The Donabedian model consists of 3 components for measuring the quality of health care: structure, process, and outcome. Structural measures evaluate the patient care resources afforded by a hospital. Process measures assess the treatments health care professionals provide, often in terms of compliance with recommended guidelines. Outcome measures quantify patients' health status and related parameters, such as morbidity, mortality, length of stay, and costs of care [1–3]. As patients, providers, and payors focus on improving surgical care, renewed efforts have been directed toward identifying optimal measures

Financial Disclosures: Dr Ingraham is supported by the Clinical Scholar in Residence Program at the American College of Surgeons. Dr Hall is supported by the Center for Health Policy, Washington University St Louis.

*Corresponding author. Division of Research and Optimal Patient Care, American College of Surgeons, 633 North Saint Clair Street, Floor 22NE, Chicago, IL 60611. *E-mail address:* aingraham@facs.org.

0065-3411/10/$ – see front matter
doi:10.1016/j.yasu.2010.05.003

of health care quality [4,5]. The National Surgical Quality Improvement Program (NSQIP), which was initiated through the Department of Veterans Affairs and has continued through the American College of Surgeons (ACS), has sought to improve the quality of surgical care for approximately 20 years by providing hospitals with risk-adjusted outcomes allowing for external benchmarking. This article discusses the evolution of the program, key elements to quality improvement, the success of the ACS NSQIP, as well as cost and health policy considerations for future quality improvement endeavors. The means through which the ACS NSQIP is adapting to meet the needs of the participating hospitals and health care providers in the pursuit of high-quality surgical care are also discussed.

THE NSQIP: INITIATION IN THE VETERANS AFFAIRS HEALTH SYSTEM AND EXPANSION TO THE PRIVATE SECTOR

After it was noticed that the rates of postoperative morbidity and mortality in the Veterans Affairs (VA) Health System were high, the Department of Veterans Affairs was mandated in 1985 (Public Law 99–166) by the United States Congress to periodically compare its risk-adjusted surgical outcomes to those of the private sector. At the time, no registries were available to provide risk-adjusted surgical outcomes for the VA or the private sector. Thus, the National VA Surgical Risk Study (NVASRS) prospectively collected data on major operations at 44 of the largest VA hospitals between October 1, 1991, and December 31, 1993 [6–9]. From these data, predictive models for determining risk-adjusted 30-day morbidity and mortality outcomes in 8 surgical subspecialties (general surgery, vascular surgery, noncardiac thoracic surgery, orthopedic surgery, urology, plastic surgery, otolaryngology, and neurosurgery) were constructed. With the NVASRS, the VA showed that a system for the prospective collection of postoperative outcomes and subsequent comparative assessment of risk-adjusted hospital performance had been successfully developed and implemented.

Based on the results of the NVASRS, the NSQIP was initiated at the 132 VA hospitals performing major surgery in 1994 [10]. The NSQIP provided annual reports to chiefs of surgery departments detailing the characteristics of their patient populations and their risk-adjusted outcomes. Peers conducted site visits at centers having worse-than-expected outcomes. The Institute of Medicine's Leadership by Example report identified the VA NSQIP as "one of the most highly regarded VHA (Veterans Health Administration) initiatives employing performance measures" [11]. From 1991 to 2006, 30-day postoperative morbidity in the VA was reduced by 43% and mortality by 47% [12].

Expansion of the NSQIP into the private sector began with 3 sites (University of Michigan, Emory University, and University of Kentucky at Lexington) participating in the NSQIP on a pilot basis beginning in 1998. This α testing was limited to general and vascular surgery and showed that the risk-adjustment models developed from data within the VA were applicable to the 3 private sector hospitals [13]. The Reporting System to Improve Patient Safety in Surgery was a patient safety grant submitted through the ACS and funded by the Agency for Health care Research and Quality (AHRQ) for the period of October 1, 2001, to September 30, 2004 (#5U18HS11913-03). The Patient Safety in Surgery Study involved 14 private sector hospitals funded by the AHRQ as well as 4 community hospitals funded by the Partners HealthCare Corporation of Massachusetts and studied major general and vascular surgery [14]. Within the AHRQ-funded hospitals, statistically significant reductions were seen in overall postoperative morbidity (8.7%, $P = .002$), surgical site infections (9.1%, $P = .02$), and renal complications (23.7%, $P = .004$) [15]. Before the Patient Safety in Surgery Study, no risk-adjusted surgical outcomes for the private sector were available. The results of The Patient Safety in Surgery Study, as well as the positive feedback of the 14 participating hospitals, prompted the ACS to establish the ACS NSQIP. At the end of 2004, the ACS NSQIP became an open subscription program.

As described in further detail later, the ACS NSQIP is among the first national, validated, multispecialty programs for measuring risk-adjusted surgical outcomes and improving the quality of surgical care [16]. From medical records and personal communication with patients, comprehensive clinical data regarding patient demographics, preoperative risk factors and laboratory values, operative information, as well as perioperative and postoperative outcomes within 30 days of the index operation are collected by Surgical Clinical Reviewers (SCRs). The ACS NSQIP uses a systematic sampling strategy designed to select broad mixtures of general and vascular surgeries, or surgeries among a larger set of specialties. The sampling procedure is influenced by hospital surgical volume and subject to several sampling limits. For instance, the number of inguinal herniorrhaphies, breast lumpectomies, and laparoscopic cholecystectomies are restricted because of the low incidence of associated morbidity and mortality and to avoid inefficient use of data-collection resources. Intensive training, continuing education, and on-site audit programs standardize data collection, ensuring consistency and reliability [17].

Logistic regression models are used to construct patient-level predicted probabilities of the outcomes of interest across all hospitals. These probabilities are summed for each hospital to estimate each hospital's risk-adjusted probability of the outcomes of interest. For each hospital, the observed number of events (O) is divided by the risk-adjusted expected number events (E) to produce an observed/expected (O/E) ratio (Fig. 1). An O/E ratio of 1.0 indicates that the number of observed events equals the number of expected events. O/E ratios less than 1.0 indicate better than expected outcomes; ratios greater than 1.0 indicate worse than expected outcomes. Confidence intervals are also calculated. If the confidence interval of the O/E ratio for morbidity or mortality does not include 1.0, then the risk-adjusted outcome is deemed statistically significant, and the hospital is designated as an outlier. Through reviews of unadjusted rates of complications, as well as risk-adjusted performance (including outlier status), the ACS NSQIP affords hospitals the ability to conduct in-depth, blinded quality comparisons with the other participants [12].

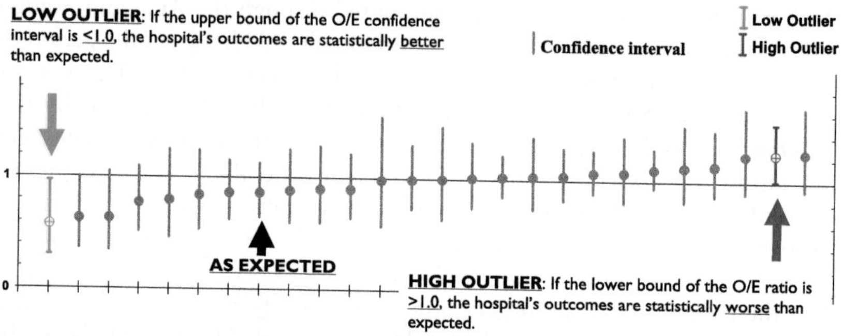

Fig. 1. Depiction of O/E ratios and identification of outlier status as determined by the ACS NSQIP.

Benefit from participating in the ACS NSQIP was documented in a recent study showing that, on average, the outcomes of all hospitals participating in the ACS NSQIP improved over time [16]. Data from 3 years were analyzed, with improvement defined as a reduction in risk-adjusted O/E ratios over time, with risk-adjustment held constant. Of the 118 hospitals participating in the final 2 years of this period, the risk-adjusted mortality was improved for 66%, and the risk-adjusted complication rate was improved for 82%. Improvement was seen for hospitals that initially had high O/E ratios (worse outcomes) as well as those that initially had low O/E ratios (better outcomes), although those with worse initial outcomes had a tendency toward greater improvement. Further analyses estimated that, for a large hospital participating during this period, by the end of the period, participation in ACS NSQIP may have resulted in the avoidance, on average, of more than 200 complications and 12 to 36 deaths (all results statistically significant) [16]. A separate study examined the performance of 12 of the longest-participating hospitals in the ACS NSQIP in the 6 year period 2002 to 2007 (Bruce L. Hall and colleagues, St Louis, MO, submitted, November 2009). This study confirmed the finding of quality improvement over time: on average, the participating hospitals improved mortality by 4.8% per year, and morbidity by 6.1% per year (all results statistically significant by end of period). These data support the success of the ACS NSQIP within the private sector as an effective tool for achieving significant gains in surgical quality.

VITAL LESSONS IN SURGICAL QUALITY IMPROVEMENT: QUALITY DATA, COLLABORATIVES, BEST PRACTICES GUIDELINES AND CASE STUDIES, AND SURGEON CHAMPION CONFERENCE CALLS

Although the foundation of the ACS NSQIP is its high-quality clinical data, simply providing feedback to hospitals on their risk-adjusted outcomes does not translate into quality improvement. Quality improvement professionals and health care providers must scrutinize their data, identify areas for improvement, implement quality improvement initiatives, and monitor the success of such endeavors. Such undertakings can be challenging, especially for institutions without significant quality improvement resources. Therefore, in addition to high-quality data, the ACS NSQIP provides resources to assist participants in the identification of targeted areas for improvement and development of quality initiatives.

Quality data

Quality improvement programs can be based on clinical or administrative data [15,18,19]. Administrative data are often readily available but are usually collected with financial motivations and represent only the billable events that occur within the hospital; adverse events and otherwise. These administrative data can be driven by 2 incentives: (1) the desire to capture maximal resources for events and services, and (2) the desire to avoid accusations of fraud. The first incentive could lead to overreporting, whereas the second could lead to underreporting, with the result being variable levels of bias. Thus, the patient's health status can potentially be inaccurately represented, limiting the usefulness of pure administrative data for hospital benchmarking [20–24]. Clinical data are more difficult and expensive to collect but are abstracted by health care professionals with a focused intent and explicit guidelines, providing more granular information for quality improvement initiatives [15]. The ACS NSQIP also follows patients and assesses outcomes until 30 days after the index operation [25]. The ACS NSQIP program collects comprehensive and reliable clinical data from medical records and personal communication with patients.

The ACS NSQIP achieves robust, high-quality clinical data based on precise definitions and collection by trained and audited data abstractors (SCRs). The ACS NSQIP uses the following methods to ensure high-quality data: (1) dedicated SCRs, (2) initial SCR training, (3) ongoing online SCR training and examination, (4) continuous SCR support, (5) creation and ongoing review of data definitions, (6) dilemma resolution, (7) checks for data integrity, (8) interrater reliability audits, and (9) the ACS NSQIP SCR coordination team support [17]. Before collecting data for the hospital, SCRs must complete a 2-day training session, which includes a program overview and details on data collection, including the sampling methods and specific information on variables and definitions. SCRs must achieve a minimum of 90% on the post-test administered after completion of the training. SCR certification also requires successful completion (a minimum score of 80% on each) of 6 online training modules. After initial certification, the ACS NSQIP supports SCRs through conference calls, online resources, and the ACS NSQIP annual conference. Whenever possible, the ACS NSQIP Data Definitions Committee generates rigorous definitions of variables that are adapted from definitions developed by regulatory agencies. Data integrity checks include, but are not limited to, monitoring for illogical entries and comparisons against similar sites and national benchmarks for a variety of items related to case ascertainment and transmission. Interrater reliability audits are conducted through information collected by on-site reviews. Site reviewers examine operative logs to ensure correct sampling of cases as well as data collected from a sample of charts that are randomly selected and specifically identified to detect potential reporting errors. A disagreement rate greater than 5% for the individual site's audit of variables collected or an individual variable within the overall program generates corrective action. A recent analysis of interrater reliability of variables in the ACS NSQIP found that the reliability of the data was high from the inception and has only improved over time (3.15% disagreement in 2005 vs 1.56% disagreement in 2008). Furthermore, the disagreement rates for variables identified as needing corrective action have improved over time, with the number of variables with disagreement rates greater than 5% falling from 26 variables in 2005 to 2 variables in 2008 [17].

In addition to being of high quality, the data used by the ACS NSQIP includes outcomes that occur 30 days after the index operation. Patients are followed for postoperative outcomes for 30 days after the index operation irrespective of whether the patient is an inpatient, has been discharged to their home or another facility, or has been readmitted to another hospital. In a recent analysis using data from the ACS NSQIP (2006–2007), postdischarge complications accounted for 32.9% of all complications [26]. In addition, certain complications occurred frequently after discharge, including surgical site infections (66.0%), urinary tract infections (39.4%), pulmonary emboli (42.2%), and deep venous thromboses (34.5%). Furthermore, of all patients experiencing complications, 39.7% had only postdischarge complications. Of the 5827 postoperative deaths, 23.6% occurred after discharge. The exclusion of postdischarge data from the ACS NSQIP would greatly influence the perceived outcomes at the level of the patient. Similarly, the exclusion or inclusion of postdischarge complications also affects hospital-level performance comparisons. Hospital quality rankings changed when postdischarge outcomes were excluded versus included for morbidity (median hospital rank change: 16 ranks; IQR, 7–36) and mortality (median hospital rank change: 14 ranks; IQR, 6–29). There was some disagreement in outlier status designations depending on whether postdischarge events were included. These data support the inclusion of postoperative complications and deaths that occur after discharge but within 30 days of the operation when assessing the quality of surgical care. An important aspect of the value of strict 30-day outcomes is not just that they are typically longer than inpatient-only outcomes but also that they are fixed in time and not variable from case to case based on discharge. This 30-day time horizon requires an investment of time and effort, but it provides valuable and worthwhile information.

Although high-quality data are essential to quality improvement initiatives, feedback of data alone does not translate into improved outcomes. Quality improvement occurs at the local level and requires hospitals and health care providers to share their experiences of providing high-quality care and the initiatives they have undertaken to improve their outcomes [27].

The essential elements to improving surgical care beyond the data were outlined in a recent article featuring the ACS NSQIP experience at Henry Ford Hospital [28]. The investigators identified 12 critical steps to achieving success in implementing the ACS NSQIP at the local level. The steps are:

1. Developing infrastructure: selecting 1 or more surgeon champions (SCs), hiring an SCR, and identifying an administrative location from which to operate
2. Gaining multiarea leadership support: securing support from leadership at the system, hospital, and department of surgery levels
3. Building a committed surgical quality improvement team: incorporating SCs, SCRs, and other quality improvement personnel
4. Obtaining surgeon buy-in: promoting data transparency and encouraging participation in quality initiatives through sharing of individual surgeon data with selected individuals
5. Understanding the patient's surgical experience: developing a conceptual framework of the steps and health care providers involved in a patient's care
6. Understanding where problems lie: examining the potential for inappropriate selection of patients or operative procedures, noncompliance with accepted processes of care, delayed identification of complications, and so forth
7. Using data review and analysis to select targets for improvement: identifying areas of poor performance
8. Communicating the target of quality improvement: detailing actual rates of adverse events, reviewing the literature on the associated incidence, causative factors, and treatment, and seeking proposals for improvement
9. Continually engaging hospital administration: communicating with hospital administration to facilitate support when policy changes or financial resources are needed to implement quality improvement initiatives
10. Embracing additional support: participating in a collaborative
11. Communicating and celebrating success: sharing results of quality improvement initiatives with all stakeholders
12. Understanding the need to engage other specialties in the process: expanding surgical quality improvement beyond surgeons, involving anesthesiology as well as ancillary staff

The ACS NSQIP facilitates quality improvement beyond feedback of data through several mechanisms, including collaboratives, Best Practices Guidelines, and Best Practices Case Studies.

Collaboratives

An early example of the collaborative approach to quality improvement was implemented by health care providers in cardiovascular surgery. The Northern New England Cardiovascular Consortium developed a multi-institutional collaborative of hospitals performing coronary artery bypass grafting, leading to a 24% reduction in hospital mortality [29]. Similarly, the Blue Cross/Blue Shield Cardiovascular Consortium of Michigan reduced its hospital mortality by 25% during the first 4 years [30]. The Keystone Collaborative has been established to target quality improvement within the intensive care unit, focusing on the prevention of bloodstream-associated infections [31].

The ACS NSQIP is actively supporting the development of collaboratives among participating hospitals. The ACS NSQIP hospitals participating in collaboratives discuss best practices, share quality improvement initiatives, or compare their surgical outcomes in a positive learning environment. Collaboratives focus on procedures or outcomes that the members have identified as areas of interest or concern. Through the use of custom data fields, collaboratives collect information on variables necessary for their unique quality improvement initiatives but not included in the standard ACS NSQIP data collection. If desired, collaborative benchmarking reports can be generated to compare the results of each site with the collaborative as a whole as well as comparing the collaborative as a whole with all participating sites nationwide.

Within the ACS NSQIP, a collaborative can range from being highly organized with formal data-sharing agreements, payor support, group oversight, and specialized reporting to being an informal group of hospitals that discuss their quality improvement experiences. Currently, there are more than 20 ACS NSQIP collaborative groups in existence or in development. (Table 1) The collaboratives range from small system-wide groups, such as Kaiser Permanente Northern California and the Mayo Clinic, to large regional groups such as the Michigan Surgical Quality Collaborative (MSQC) and the Tennessee Surgical Quality Collaborative (TSQC). Collaboratives receive support and guidance from the ACS NSQIP staff in developing data-sharing strategies, designing specialized reports, and publicizing the group's efforts. The collaborative determines which data are shared with the group and who has access to the data. The ACS staff provide data-sharing templates and assistance in creating data-sharing language. The ACS NSQIP is also creating procedure-specific and outcome-specific virtual collaboratives, allowing all participating and interested hospitals to work together remotely via Web conference, teleconference, and e-mail toward a common quality improvement goal. Collaboratives focusing on colectomy procedures and perioperative glucose control will be the first virtual collaboratives to be developed.

Best practices initiatives: guidelines and case studies

In addition to collaboratives, the ACS NSQIP has facilitated the dissemination of quality improvement strategies through its best practices initiatives. The initiatives consist of the ACS NSQIP Best Practices Guidelines and the ACS NSQIP Best Practices Case Studies. (Fig. 2) The ACS NSQIP Best Practices Guidelines provide health care professionals with evidence-based recommendations regarding the prevention, diagnosis, or treatment of urinary tract infection, venous thromboembolism, catheter related bloodstream infection, and surgical site infection. The information contained within the Best Practices Guidelines is evidence-based and has been assembled through reviews of the current literature and consultation with expert panels. The ACS NSQIP Best Practices Case Studies showcase how participating hospitals have

Table 1
Comparison of type, number of participating sites, and payor involvement for current and developing ACS NSQIP collaboratives

Group	Type	Number of sites	Payor involvement
Florida Surgical Care Initiative (FSCI)	Regional	TBD	None at this time
Illinois Surgical Quality Improvement Collaborative (ISQIC)	Regional	10	None at this time
Michigan Surgical Quality Collaborative (MSQC)	Regional	34	Blue Cross Blue Shield Michigan
Nebraska Collaborative	Regional	4	Pending
Oregon NSQIP Consortia (ONC)	Regional	7	None at this time
Pennsylvania Collaborative	Regional	10	None at this time
Tennessee Surgical Quality Collaborative (TSQC)	Regional	10	Blue Cross Blue Shield of Tennessee Health Foundation
Upstate New York Surgical Quality Initiative (UNYSQI)	Regional	6	Excellus
Virginia Collaborative	Regional	5	None at this time
Clarian Health System	System-wide	2	Clarian Health System
Department of Defense/ TRICARE	System-wide	16	Department of Defense/ TRICARE
Fraser Health-Canada	System-wide	3	Fraser Health Authority
Kaiser Permanente Southern California	System-wide	4	Kaiser Permanente Southern California
Kaiser Permanente Northern California (KPNC)	System-wide	6	Kaiser Permanente Northern California
Mayo Clinic Surgical Quality Collaborative (MCSQC)	System-wide	4	Mayo Clinic
Partners HealthCare	System-wide	5	Blue Cross Blue Shield Massachusetts
ACS NSQIP Colectomy Collaborative	Virtual	TBD	None at this time
ACS NSQIP Glucose Control Collaborative	Virtual	TBD	None at this time

Abbreviation: TBD, to be determined.

analyzed ACS NSQIP data and implemented quality improvement initiatives to improve their performance and outcomes. The case studies outline the planning, development, and troubleshooting process of initiating the hospital's quality improvement efforts, from getting buy-in of the appropriate parties to monitoring the initiative's success. Each case study was developed as a collaborative effort between ACS and the participating hospital's SCR, SC, or other surgical and quality improvement professionals. The initial volume of the ACS NSQIP Best Practices Case Studies presents information from hospitals on the detection and follow-up of postoperative stroke, improvements in coding and referrals to risk management, the reduction of urinary tract

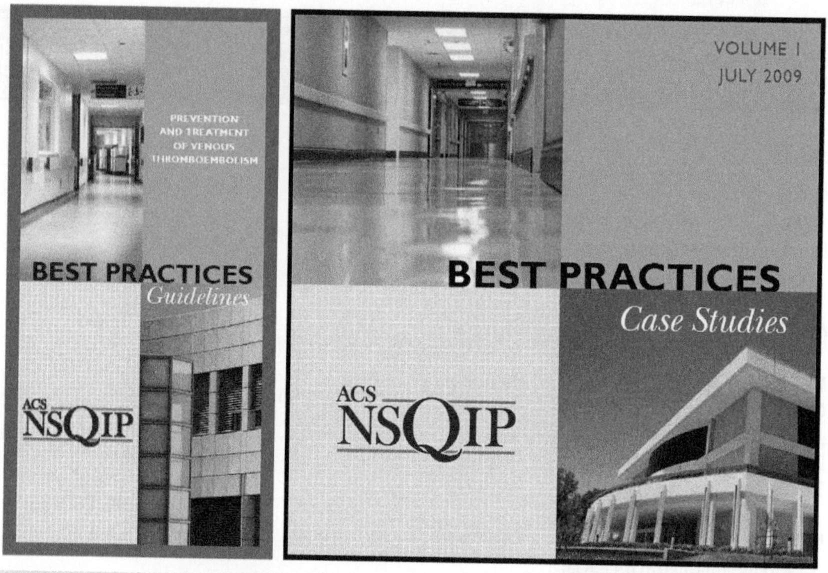

Fig. 2. Covers of ACS NSQIP resource materials.

infections and deep vein thromboses, and the development and use of a preoperative pulmonary conditioning program. The ACS NSQIP Best Practices Guidelines and Case Studies are available to participating hospitals through a secure Web site.

SC conference calls

The ACS NSQIP provides support through monthly SC conference calls. Hospitals participating in the ACS NSQIP identify surgeons to be SCs; SCs not only serve as liaisons between the hospitals and the ACS NSQIP but are charged with fostering quality improvement at the local level. SCs are invited to present their quality improvement initiatives, often highlighting the mechanisms through which they achieved colleague and administration buy-in and the financial benefits afforded to the institution through participation in the ACS NSQIP.

HEALTH CARE FINANCE AND HEALTH POLICY REFORM

Prompted in part by a landmark Institute of Medicine report, government and private groups have developed programs to measure and improve health care quality [13,32–37]. Variation in health care quality has stimulated renewed interest in research to address the consumption and delivery of health care. This development is highlighted by the recent American Recovery and Reinvestment Act of 2009, which allocated a 1.1 billion down payment to support clinical outcomes, comparative effectiveness, and appropriateness research concerning the use of drugs, devices, surgical procedures, and treatments [38].

Thus, any discussion of health care quality must address the financial and health policy challenges to providing high-quality surgical care.

Hospitals and health care providers need to provide high-quality care at the lowest feasible cost. Central to achieving this goal are quality improvement initiatives to reduce the number of complications following surgeries. Most of the costs of adverse surgical events are absorbed by the hospital [39–41]. Furthermore, this amount is increasing as the Centers for Medicare and Medicaid Services and other payors adopt financial policies that no longer cover payments for hospital-acquired conditions and other unacceptable outcomes [42]. The costs of complications are significant. Examples of estimated costs include: $18,310 for thromboembolic complications [39]; $7789 for cardiovascular complications [39]; $1398 to $4901 for infectious complications [39,43]; $18,414 to $25,219 for acute renal failure [39–44]; $18,852 to $33,471 for septicemia [39–44]; $9573 for myocardial infarction [39]; $7777 for pulmonary failure [39]; and $10,019 to $57,158 for ventilator-associated pneumonia [45–47].

Quality improvement initiatives have been associated with significant cost savings. For instance, Memorial Hermann Hospital in Houston initiated a performance improvement initiative to decrease ventilator-associated pneumonia that involved in-service education and monitoring of daily compliance with a ventilator bundle, with weekly feedback. This initiative translated into a cost saving of $428,685 per 100 admissions [45]. Perhaps the most compelling accounts of how hospital quality improvement initiatives can translate into financial savings for the hospital come from efforts initiated after review of ACS NSQIP data. In 2009, the SC and SCR from Surrey Memorial Hospital in British Columbia conducted an extensive cost analysis based on data from the ACS NSQIP. Based on their analysis, using cost estimates for procedures and outcomes from the Canadian Institute of Health Information, Surrey Memorial Hospital experienced a cost avoidance estimated at $180,000 in 2008 through initiatives to reduce surgical site infections after breast procedures. Surrey also avoided an estimated $380,000 in costs in a 4-month period by implementing initiatives to reduce the rate of urinary tract infection, and an estimated $2,500,000 in costs in a 2-year period by implementing initiatives to reduce the rate of surgical site infections after all surgeries (Angela Tecson, British Columbia, Canada, personal communication, 2009).

Henry Ford Hospital, an ACS NSQIP participant, reduced their length of stay by an average of 1.54 days after reviewing data from all patients who underwent a general, vascular, or colorectal procedure and were subsequently admitted to the hospital, including those not selected by the ACS NSQIP sampling methodology. This translated into an annual savings of $2,000,000 (Jennifer Ritz, Detroit, MI, personal communication, 2009). Participation in the ACS NSQIP also prompted Henry Ford Hospital to review their coding practices [48]. After identifying errors in procedural coding and inadequate concurrent coding. Henry Ford Hospital implemented measures, provided education, and facilitated communication between the appropriate parties to improve the accuracy of coding. Through these and other efforts, Henry

Ford Hospital increased General Surgery professional billing by $2,250,000 over a year (Jennifer Ritz, Detroit, MI, personal communication, 2009).

Health policy: future efforts in surgical quality measurement

As mentioned earlier, the assessment of quality in health care has frequently used the Donabedian model of examining structure, process, or outcome. Process measures are usually evidence-based, nonthreatening to surgeons, controllable, and easy to measure. These advantages have led to certain process measures, such as those developed by the Surgical Care Improvement Project (SCIP), being endorsed by regulatory agencies as means to assess quality of care. Conversely, outcomes are often more difficult to define, expensive to collect, and can be considered threatening to provider reputations. Despite these disadvantages, outcomes might better represent the ultimate goal of quality care and Ernest Codman's end result of the surgical procedure. However, the association between process measures and patient outcomes in surgical patients has not been well defined. Understanding this relationship could facilitate the identification of process measures that are highly correlated with outcomes and guide the use of quality improvement resources. To this end, compliance with the widely adopted SCIP process measures has been compared with ACS NSQIP risk-adjusted outcomes. This work reveals that relationships between ACS NSQIP risk-adjusted outcomes and compliance with SCIP process measures are not as strong as might be hoped, which could have important consequences for the ongoing promotion of processes of care as quality measures (Angela Ingraham, submitted, June 2010).

Recognizing the weak association between compliance with process measures and risk-adjusted outcomes, the ACS NSQIP has been working to develop relevant risk-adjusted, outcomes-based measures for National Quality Forum (NQF) endorsement that may potentially be used in conjunction with, or as an alternative to, the current SCIP measures. One measure has already been endorsed by the NQF to evaluate hospital-specific risk-adjusted mortality or 1 or more of the following major complications: cardiac arrest, myocardial infarction, cerebrovascular accident/stroke, on ventilator for more than 48 hours, acute renal failure requiring dialysis, bleeding/transfusions, graft/prosthesis/flap failure, septic shock, sepsis, and organ space surgical site infection, within 30 days of a lower extremity vascular bypass in patients aged 16 years and older [49].

ONGOING ACS NSQIP ADVANCES

With the ACS NSQIP in its sixth year, feedback from participating programs has led to a variety of ongoing modifications, some of which have already been described [50]. The heterogeneity of hospitals in the private sector has played a strong role in the changes being instituted. A brief summary of some of the more substantial changes follows.

Parsimonious data collection

Given the current environment of increasing requirements for tracking quality and performance metrics, the burden of data collection is continually increasing. In response, the ACS NSQIP has re-evaluated the number and types of variables being collected. The ACS NSQIP has prioritized the collection of variables necessary for quality improvement compared with other research interests. In parallel with decreasing the volume of data collected, the ACS NSQIP has shown the feasibility of constructing statistical models using a parsimonious dataset while maintaining high standards for risk-adjustment.

Targeted procedures

The ACS NSQIP has traditionally instituted a systematic sampling strategy for selection of procedures. This method provides an overall picture of how a hospital is performing and has distinct advantages. However, many hospitals in the current program have discovered that certain procedures, such as those performed in an outpatient setting, tend not to be associated with a high incidence of complications. For many hospitals, outpatient procedures account for a substantial portion of selected cases; however, these cases account for a small number of complications. For such hospitals, it would be more advantageous to collect cases that are more likely associated with complications. In general surgery, the 10 most commonly performed procedures account for more than 60% of complications [51]. In vascular surgery, the 3 to 4 most commonly performed procedures account for more than 75% of complications [52]. For such hospitals, a targeted procedure case-selection strategy is being developed for each of the surgical specialties. Targeted case selection affords a greater opportunity to identify areas for quality improvement and ability to collect all (or nearly all) cases, thus providing more robust statistical analyses based on larger sample sizes.

Small hospital/rural option

The ACS NSQIP has largely been implemented in high-volume hospitals. Smaller and rural hospitals have indicated that changes to the ACS NSQIP are needed to meet their specific needs. Specifically, these centers desire to examine outcomes and identify areas for quality improvement in the context of the resources available to a small/rural hospital. As discussed earlier, parsimony of data collection is essential to this end. In addition, given the smaller numbers of cases being performed, collection of all cases would facilitate the identification of quality improvement opportunities as well as the demonstration of high-quality care. By identifying a small core of necessary variables, such case collection is feasible. Almost 50% of hospitals in the United States that perform surgery have fewer than 100 beds based on an analysis of the Nationwide Inpatient Sample data (Mehul V. Raval, Chicago, IL, personal communication, 2009) and there are more than 1300 critical access hospitals (<25 beds) [53], so the small hospital/rural option will play an important role in evaluating and improving the quality of surgical care in the United States.

Collaborative efforts with individual societies

The need for, and interest in, collecting meaningful, clinical data through surgery registries is increasing. In an effort not to duplicate efforts, the ACS NSQIP is working closely with several surgical societies to identify opportunities for collaboration. With the ACS NSQIP following patients for 30 days after operations, this provides a framework for societies interested in outcomes beyond 30 days as well as a foundation for data collection beyond the parsimonious variable list needed for ACS NSQIP risk-adjusted outcomes. Several surgical societies have identified additional procedure-specific variables to be collected in addition to the parsimonious dataset identified by the ACS NSQIP. Such efforts fulfill the needs of the ACS NSQIP and individual surgical societies while not duplicating efforts and wasting resources.

Risk calculators

Using the ACS NSQIP statistical models, risk calculators are being developed to provide an estimate of the patient's preoperative risk of adverse events following specific surgical procedures [54]. Health care providers can use this tool to provide patients and their families with a more objective, approximate risk associated with the procedure and to enhance the informed consent process.

Individual surgeon data

Although the ACS NSQIP is a facility-based program, many have inquired whether the program will provide measures of individual surgeon performance. Individual participating sites currently have the ability to review unadjusted outcomes for individual surgeons, but individual surgeon performance at a national level currently is not analyzed. Determining individual performance measures poses several practical and intellectual challenges. First, given the potentially small sample sizes and the variation in number of cases performed by an individual, it may be difficult to develop accurate and appropriate statistical models to distinguish individual surgeons. Second, there is the issue of attribution or accountability [55]. Given that a perioperative team, including the anesthesiologist, nurses, surgeons, as well as other providers, cares for a patient, is it appropriate to attribute desirable or untoward outcomes to the individual surgeon alone? Thus, the ACS NSQIP will continue to carefully consider surgeon-specific outcomes.

SUMMARY

The history and development of the NSQIP, from its inception in the Veterans Administration Health System to its implementation within the private sector sponsored by the ACS, documents the growth of a program that has substantially improved the quality of surgical care and has had a considerable influence on the culture of quality improvement in the profession. The success of the ACS NSQIP is the result of providing hospitals with rigorous, clinical data, networking opportunities, and resources to improve their risk-adjusted outcomes. In this manner, the ACS NSQIP challenges its hospitals and health care providers to continually improve the care they provide. In addition to reducing the complications and mortality experienced by patients after surgical procedures, hospitals that participate in the ACS NSQIP have seen the financial rewards of their quality improvement efforts. Continued growth of the ACS NSQIP will facilitate achievement of the primary goal surrounding the current health care reform debate: efficient, high-quality care.

References

[1] Donabedian A. The quality of care. How can it be assessed? JAMA 1988;260(12): 1743–8.
[2] Donabedian A. Evaluating the quality of medical care. Milbank Mem Fund Q 1966;44(3): 166–206.
[3] Bratzler DW, Nsa W, Houck PM. Performance measures for pneumonia: are they valuable, and are process measures adequate? Curr Opin Infect Dis 2007;20(2):182–9.
[4] Birkmeyer JD, Dimick JB, Birkmeyer NJ. Measuring the quality of surgical care: structure, process, or outcomes? J Am Coll Surg 2004;198(4):626–32.
[5] Ko CY, Maggard M, Agustin M. Quality in surgery: current issues for the future. World J Surg 2005;29(10):1204–9.
[6] Khuri SF, Daley J, Henderson W, et al. Risk adjustment of the postoperative mortality rate for the comparative assessment of the quality of surgical care: results of the National Veterans Affairs Surgical Risk Study. J Am Coll Surg 1997;185(4):315–27.
[7] Daley J, Khuri SF, Henderson W, et al. Risk adjustment of the postoperative morbidity rate for the comparative assessment of the quality of surgical care: results of the National Veterans Affairs Surgical Risk Study. J Am Coll Surg 1997;185(4):328–40.
[8] Daley J, Forbes MG, Young GJ, et al. Validating risk-adjusted surgical outcomes: site visit assessment of process and structure. National VA Surgical Risk Study. J Am Coll Surg 1997;185(4):341–51.
[9] Khuri SF, Daley J, Henderson W, et al. The National Veterans Administration Surgical Risk Study: risk adjustment for the comparative assessment of the quality of surgical care. J Am Coll Surg 1995;180(5):519–31.
[10] Khuri SF, Daley J, Henderson W, et al. The Department of Veterans Affairs' NSQIP: the first national, validated, outcome-based, risk-adjusted, and peer-controlled program for the measurement and enhancement of the quality of surgical care. National VA Surgical Quality Improvement Program. Ann Surg 1998;228(4):491–507.
[11] Corrigan JM, Eden J, Smith BM, editors. Leadership by example. Coordinating government roles in improving healthcare quality. Washington, DC: National Academic Press; 2002.
[12] Khuri SF. The NSQIP: a new frontier in surgery. Surgery 2005;138(5):837–43.
[13] Fink AS, Campbell DA Jr, Mentzer RM Jr, et al. The National Surgical Quality Improvement Program in non-veterans administration hospitals: initial demonstration of feasibility. Ann Surg 2002;236(3):344–53 [discussion: 353–4].
[14] Khuri SF, Henderson WG, Daley J, et al. The patient safety in surgery study: background, study design, and patient populations. J Am Coll Surg 2007;204(6):1089–102.
[15] Khuri SF, Henderson WG, Daley J, et al. Successful implementation of the Department of Veterans Affairs' National Surgical Quality Improvement Program in the private sector: the Patient Safety in Surgery study. Ann Surg 2008;248(2):329–36.
[16] Hall BL, Hamilton BH, Richards K, et al. Does surgical quality improve in the American College of Surgeons National Surgical Quality Improvement Program: an evaluation of all participating hospitals. Ann Surg 2009;250(3):363–76.
[17] Shiloach M, Frencher SK, Steeger JE, et al. Toward robust information: data quality and inter-rater reliability in the American College of Surgeons National Surgical Quality Improvement Program. J Am Coll Surg 2010;210(1):6–16.

[18] Guller U, Hervey S, Purves H, et al. Laparoscopic versus open appendectomy: outcomes comparison based on a large administrative database. Ann Surg 2004;239(1):43–52.
[19] Delaney CP, Chang E, Senagore AJ, et al. Clinical outcomes and resource utilization associated with laparoscopic and open colectomy using a large national database. Ann Surg 2008;247(5):819–24.
[20] Shahian DM, Silverstein T, Lovett AF, et al. Comparison of clinical and administrative data sources for hospital coronary artery bypass graft surgery report cards. Circulation 2007;115(12):1518–27.
[21] Krumholz HM, Brindis RG, Brush JE, et al. Standards for statistical models used for public reporting of health outcomes: an American Heart Association Scientific Statement from the Quality of Care and Outcomes Research Interdisciplinary Writing Group: cosponsored by the Council on Epidemiology and Prevention and the Stroke Council. Endorsed by the American College of Cardiology Foundation. Circ J 2006;113(3):456–62.
[22] Parker JP, Li Z, Damberg CL, et al. Administrative versus clinical data for coronary artery bypass graft surgery report cards: the view from California. Med Care 2006;44(7): 687–95.
[23] Best WR, Khuri SF, Phelan M, et al. Identifying patient preoperative risk factors and postoperative adverse events in administrative databases: results from the Department of Veterans Affairs National Surgical Quality Improvement Program. J Am Coll Surg 2002;194(3): 257–66.
[24] Romano PS, Chan BK, Schembri ME, et al. Can administrative data be used to compare postoperative complication rates across hospitals? Med Care 2002;40(10):856–67.
[25] American College of Surgeons. American College of Surgeons National Surgical Quality Improvement Program operations manual; 2007.
[26] Bilimoria KY, Cohen ME, Ingraham AM, et al. Effect of postdischarge morbidity and mortality on comparisons of hospital surgical quality. Ann Surg. (Epub ahead of publication).
[27] Campbell DA Jr. Quality improvement is local. J Am Coll Surg 2009;209(1):141–3.
[28] Velanovich V, Rubinfeld I, Patton JH Jr, et al. Implementation of the National Surgical Quality Improvement Program: critical steps to success for surgeons and hospitals. Am J Med Qual 2009;24(6):474–9.
[29] O'Connor GT, Plume SK, Olmstead EM, et al. A regional intervention to improve the hospital mortality associated with coronary artery bypass graft surgery. The Northern New England Cardiovascular Disease Study Group. JAMA 1996;275(11):841–6.
[30] Moscucci M, Share D, Kline-Rogers E, et al. The Blue Cross Blue Shield of Michigan Cardiovascular Consortium (BMC2) collaborative quality improvement initiative in percutaneous coronary interventions. J Interv Cardiol 2002;15(5):381–6.
[31] Pronovost P, Needham D, Berenholtz S, et al. An intervention to decrease catheter-related bloodstream infections in the ICU. N Engl J Med 2006;355(26):2725–32.
[32] Institute of Medicine. Crossing the quality chasm: a new health system for the twenty-first century. Washington, DC: National Academy Press; 2001.
[33] Pennsylvania Health Care Cost Containment Council. Cardiac surgery in Pennsylvania: 2005–2006. Available at: http://www.phc4.org/reports/cabg/06/default.htm. Accessed February 24, 2009.
[34] New Jersey Department of Health and Senior Services. Cardiac surgery in New Jersey: 2004. Available at: http://www.state.nj.us/health/healthcarequality/documents/cardconsumer04.pdf. Accessed February 24, 2009.
[35] Shroyer AL, Coombs LP, Peterson ED, et al. The Society of Thoracic Surgeons: 30-day operative mortality and morbidity risk models. Ann Thorac Surg 2003;75(6):1856–64 [discussion: 1864–55].
[36] Grover FL, Shroyer AL, Hammermeister K, et al. A decade's experience with quality improvement in cardiac surgery using the Veterans Affairs and Society of Thoracic Surgeons national databases. Ann Surg 2001;234(4):464–72 [discussion: 472–4].

[37] Society for Vascular Surgery. Vascular registry. Available at: http://www.vascularweb.org/professionals/Vascular_Registry/index.html. Accessed May 5, 2009.
[38] United States House of Representatives. H.R.1: Making supplemental appropriations for job preservation and creation, infrastructure investment, energy efficiency and science, assistance to the unemployed, and State and local fiscal stabilization, for fiscal year ending September 30, 2009, and for other purposes; United State House of Representatives Bill; 2009
[39] Dimick JB, Chen SL, Taheri PA, et al. Hospital costs associated with surgical complications: a report from the private-sector National Surgical Quality Improvement Program. J Am Coll Surg 2004;199(4):531–7.
[40] Englesbe MJ, Dimick J, Mathur A, et al. Who pays for biliary complications following liver transplant? A business case for quality improvement. Am J Transplant 2006;6(12): 2978–82.
[41] Dimick JB, Weeks WB, Karia RJ, et al. Who pays for poor surgical quality? Building a business case for quality improvement. J Am Coll Surg 2006;202(6):933–7.
[42] Centers for Medicare and Medicaid. Medicare and Medicaid move aggressively to encourage greater patient safety in hospitals and reduce never events. Available at: http://www.cms.hhs.gov/apps/media/press/release.asp? Accessed May 5, 2009.
[43] Olsen MA, Chu-Ongsakul S, Brandt KE, et al. Hospital-associated costs due to surgical site infection after breast surgery. Arch Surg 2008;143(1):53–60 [discussion: 61].
[44] Pronovost P, Garrett E, Dorman T, et al. Variations in complication rates and opportunities for improvement in quality of care for patients having abdominal aortic surgery. Langenbecks Arch Surg 2001;386(4):249–56.
[45] Cocanour CS, Ostrosky-Zeichner L, Peninger M, et al. Cost of a ventilator-associated pneumonia in a shock trauma intensive care unit. Surg Infect (Larchmt) 2005;6(1):65–72.
[46] Safdar N, Dezfulian C, Collard HR, et al. Clinical and economic consequences of ventilator-associated pneumonia: a systematic review. Crit Care Med 2005;33(10): 2184–93.
[47] Warren DK, Shukla SJ, Olsen MA, et al. Outcome and attributable cost of ventilator-associated pneumonia among intensive care unit patients in a suburban medical center. Crit Care Med 2003;31(5):1312–7.
[48] Patton Jr JH, Ritz J, Rubinfeld I, et al. Revenue opportunities in quality: leveraging data accuracy for improved RVU Yield. American College of Surgeons National Surgical quality improvement program Annual Conference. Boca Raton (FL); 2008.
[49] National Quality Forum. NQF # 0534: hospital specific risk-adjusted measure of mortality or one or more major complications within 30 days of a lower extremity bypass (LEB). Available at: http://www.qualityforum.org/Measures_List.aspx. Accessed June 11, 2009.
[50] Birkmeyer JD, Shahian DM, Dimick JB, et al. Blueprint for a new American College of Surgeons: national surgical quality improvement program. J Am Coll Surg 2008;207(5): 777–82.
[51] Schilling PL, Dimick JB, Birkmeyer JD. Prioritizing quality improvement in general surgery. J Am Coll Surg 2008;207(5):698–704.
[52] Raval MV, Bilimoria KY, Cohen ME, et al. The next generation of quality assessment - developing a specialty and outcome specific American College of Surgeons National Surgical Quality Improvement Program. Chicago (IL): American College of Surgeons Clinical Congress; 2009.
[53] Rural Assistance Center. CAH [Critical Access Hospitals] frequently asked questions. Available at: http://www.raconline.org/info_guides/hospitals/cahfaq.php#howmany. Accessed November 15, 2009.
[54] Cohen ME, Bilimoria KY, Ko CY, et al. Development of an American College of Surgeons National Surgery Quality Improvement Program: morbidity and mortality risk calculator for colorectal surgery. J Am Coll Surg 2009;208(6):1009–16.
[55] Pronovost PJ, Faden RR. Setting priorities for patient safety: ethics, accountability, and public engagement. JAMA 2009;302(8):890–1.

Advances in Surgery 44 (2010) 269–279

ADVANCES IN SURGERY

Management of Disappearing Colorectal Hepatic Metastases

Susanne Carpenter, MD, Yuman Fong, MD*

Department of Surgery, Memorial Sloan-Kettering Cancer Center, 1275 York Avenue, New York, NY 10065, USA

Hepatic resection for patients with metastatic colorectal lesions has become a standard treatment of patients with resectable disease [1–4]. Until recently, patients presenting with unresectable disease had few treatment options and extremely poor prognoses. However, advances in chemotherapy have revolutionized the current management of colorectal hepatic metastases. With downstaging facilitated by neoadjuvant therapy, patients with previously dismal prognoses are now able to undergo hepatic resection, and are thus enjoying survival benefits similar to their initially resectable counterparts [5]. With new neoadjuvant regimens, many lesions previously considered unresectable can now be safely removed with measurable survival benefits (Table 1) [5–7]. Reported rates of conversion from unresectable to resectable are highly variable, ranging from 12.5% to 47.5%, with a variety of different regimens and administration stratagems (see Table 1). Most of the regimens detailing significant success involve 5-fluorouracil (5-FU) and leucovorin, with oxaliplatin or irinotecan.

Several investigators advocate the use of regional administration of chemotherapy for downstaging hepatic metastases. The advantages of first-pass clearance to minimize systemic toxicity of the regional chemotherapy allow concomitant use of systemic chemotherapy at nearly full doses [8–10]. Although there is some debate concerning the effect of hepatic arterial infusion (HAI) on survival, there is no doubt that regional therapies produce a high rate of tumor response in cases of unresectable hepatic metastases [4,9,10].

This review examines the effects of these advances on current and future surgical practice, and addresses several dilemmas that accompany this recent progress.

CORRELATION OF CLINICAL AND PATHOLOGIC RESPONSES

Several investigators have reported complete regression of aggressive disease even before attempted resection. Although the results of effective neoadjuvant therapies are cause for celebration, clinicians are left with several new questions.

*Corresponding author. *E-mail address*: fongy@mskcc.org.

0065-3411/10/$ – see front matter
doi:10.1016/j.yasu.2010.05.001

Table 1
Conversion to resectability with neoadjuvant chemotherapy

Year and journal	Senior author	Number of patients	Chemotherapeutic agent	Number converted to resectable (%)	5-y Survival after resection (%)
1996 Ann Surg	Bismuth [35]	330	5-FU Leucovorin Oxaliplatin	53 (16)	OS: 40 DFS: 36
1999 Ann Oncol	Levi [30]	151	5-FU Leucovorin Oxaliplatin	58 (38)	OS: 50 DFS: 21
2001 Ann Surg Onc	Adam [7]	701	5-FU Leucovorin Oxaliplatin	95 (13.5)	OS: 35 60 large tumors 49 ill-located 34 multinodular disease, 18 extrahepatic disease + resected liver metastases[b] DFS: 22
2004 Ann Surg	Adam [5]	1104	5-FU + oxaliplatin (70) 5-FU + irinotecan (7) 5-FU + both (4)	138 (12.5)	OS: 33 DFS: 22
2009 J Clin Oncol	D'Angelica [9]	49	Floxuridine and dexamethasone[a] Oxaliplatin Irinotecan	23 (47)	(Median follow-up 26 mo) Median OS: 39.8 mo
2007 Ann Oncol	Kemeny [36]	39	Floxuridine and dexamethasone[a] Oxaliplatin Irinotecan	7 (18)	(Median follow-up 19.1 mo) Median OS: 20.1 mo (from HAI)
2005 J Clin Oncol	Donohue [37]	42	5-FU Leucovorin Oxaliplatin (FOLFOX4)	17 (40)	(Median follow-up 22 mo) Median OS (all patients): 26 mo
2007 J Br Canc	Pozzo [38]	40	5-FU Leucovorin Irinotecan	19 (47.5)	Last follow-up (5 y): OS: 62 DFS: 46

Abbreviations: DFS, disease-free survival; OS, overall survival.
[a] Administered via hepatic artery infusion (HAI).
[b] 35% 5-year survival found when all patients were analyzed for extrahepatic disease rather than those for whom extrahepatic metastases was the main cause of nonresectability.

If large portions of hepatic metastases are eliminated, should a surgeon resect areas previously inhabited by tumors? Furthermore, how many of the lesions that have vanished on imaging are now histologically benign? If all of the tumors vanish, what is the next appropriate course of action? To begin to answer these questions, one must first know to what extent a radical radiologic response yields a true pathologic response. The available literature concerning correlation of imaging with pathology of missing metastases is contradictory (Table 2). Several studies have indicated that complete clinical response (defined as postchemotherapy disappearance of lesions that were present before chemotherapy on various imaging modalities) does not always correlate with complete pathologic response [11–14]. However, to what extent this occurs remains a contentious issue.

As indicated in Table 2, Benoist and colleagues [12] included patients with fewer than 10 liver metastases before chemotherapy, with disappearance of at least 1 metastasis on preoperative computed tomography (CT) and ultrasound (US), and with no evidence of extrahepatic disease. Although Benoist and colleagues [12] and Fiorentini and colleagues [14] paint a dismal picture of high local recurrence rates of lesions missing from CT and US, more specific imaging modalities like magnetic resonance imaging (MRI) and positron emission tomography (PET) were not used as routine postchemotherapy staging of these patients. In addition, the more optimistic findings of Elias and colleagues [13] were reached using more stringent imaging evaluation, using US, CT, and MRI, and detailed scan reading by 2 radiologists specializing in liver imaging, in addition to 2 hepatobiliary surgeons. Using strict entrance criteria for the definition of a missing metastasis, the investigators identified 15 of 104 patients with disappearance of at least 1 lesion and excluded 4 of those 15 patients (27%) who exhibited macroscopic disease at laparotomy, discovered via intraoperative US or direct visualization [13]. Of the remaining 11 patients, 8 (73%) are still without evidence of recurrence of the missing lesions [13]. A subset of patients examined by Elias and colleagues [13] had undergone HAI chemotherapy with systemic therapy rather than systemic therapy alone, which was used by the other investigators detailed in Table 2. At our institution, Auer and colleagues [15] reviewed 435 patients over 3 years and included only patients with fewer than 12 hepatic lesions and at least 1 vanished lesion to find that 39 (9%) of the patients had a total of 118 disappearing lesions. Of these, 68 were resected and 50 were followed clinically [15]. Overall, 75 (64%) of the 118 missing lesions were found to be true pathologic (44 lesions) or durable clinical (31) responses [15]. Auer and colleagues further performed multivariate analyses to determine that use of HAI chemotherapy, inability to visualize a missing lesion on MRI, and normalization of serum carcinoembryonic antigen (CEA) were independently associated with a true clinical or pathologic response [15].

Thus, it is clear that between 18% and 64% of lesions that radiologically disappear are true pathologic responses. However, radiologic responses do not always correspond with pathologic responses. Many small lesions seen

Table 2
Correlation of imaging and pathologic tumor response to neoadjuvant chemotherapy

Year and journal	Senior author	Number of patients with disappearance of at least 1 lesion after chemotherapy	Chemotherapy agent	Number with tumor disappearance shown by imaging (%)	Tumor disappearance pathology (%)	Clinical outcomes
2006 J Clin Oncol	Nordlinger [12]	38	5-FU and leucovorin or LV5FU2 and oxaliplatin or LV5FU2 and irinotecan	66 of 183 (36) lesions in 22 of 38 (58) patients CRR of 31 lesions in 14 of 38 (37) patients[a]	11 lesions (18) in 3 of 15 (20) patients 31 old lesion sites left in remnant without biopsy or resection	7 of 15 (47) patients hepatic recurrence within 1 y 23 of 31 (74) lesions left in 11 of 14 (79) patients recurred within 1 y
2004 J Surg Oncol	Ducreux [13]	11	5-FU and oxaliplatin or irinotecan HAI oxaliplatin and systemic therapy	54 of 98 (55) lesions in 11 patients	46 lesions in 5 of 11 (45) patients	27% missing lesions recurred
June 2007 presented to ASCO (currently in press)	D'Angelica	39	CPT-11 and 5-FU with leucovorin or HAI floxuridine with systemic CPT-11	118 of 166 (71) lesions in 39 of 435 (9) patients	102 lesions evaluated in or 68 resected lesions 44 of 68 (65) lesions CPR	17 of 39 (44) patients with hepatic recurrence 17 of 39 (44) disease free at median 40 mo 31 of 50 (62) lesions followed on imaging had DCR Predicted 5-y OS of 65%
2008 Tumori	Cantore [14]	106 lesions	HAI floxuridine	106 lesions	Persistent macroscopic disease observed in or 52 of 106 liver metastases 22/35 (63) tumors on pathology at site of disappeared lesion	19% without recurrence at 2 y

Abbreviations: CRR, complete radiologic response; CPR, complete pathologic response; DCR, durable clinical response; OR, operating room; OS, overall survival.
[a] These disappeared metastases were not visualized intraoperatively and were left in remnant liver after resection without biopsy.

radiologically after chemotherapy are scars that prove to be complete pathologic responses. The choice of imaging modality for restaging of patients after chemotherapy greatly influences the number of lesions found.

HEPATIC IMAGING MODALITIES AFTER CHEMOTHERAPY

Finding the optimal hepatic imaging modality for patients who have undergone chemotherapy can be complicated. US, CT, MR, and PET images are all used, often in concert, in modern evaluation of hepatic metastases. Each of the 4 major modalities used in current practice has its benefits and limitations (Table 3). Chemotherapy also produces changes in liver parenchyma that can greatly exaggerate weaknesses in imaging of cancerous deposits. It is more common after chemotherapy for the radiologic tests to be incorrect in the staging of patients. One such patient is illustrated in Fig. 1. This patient seemed to have a dramatic response to chemotherapy, with the disappearance of 1 hepatic metastasis and significantly diminished size of a second following neoadjuvant therapy. However, on exploration, approximately 50 malignant lesions were discovered. Thus, debate regarding the best imaging modality or combination thereof for analysis of hepatic metastases continues.

Several investigators contend that [^{18}F]fluorodeoxyglucose (FDG)-PET imaging is the most sensitive test for colorectal hepatic metastases [16]. One highly selective meta-analysis stringently evaluated 11 studies to conclude that FDG-PET scans have a 96% sensitivity and a 99% specificity for identification of hepatic recurrences of colorectal malignancy [17]. However, a later meta-analysis pooled 61 studies to find that, although FDG-PET had significantly higher sensitivity on a per-patient basis, on a per-lesion basis it was not superior to other modalities [18]. In addition, sensitivity of FDG-PET for colorectal liver metastases directly relates to tumor size, with smaller size yielding low sensitivity, especially in lesions less than 1 cm in diameter [19,20]. Proponents of PET usage are unable to discern how often a metabolic response to chemotherapy is reflective of actual tumor destruction versus

Table 3
Obstacles for imaging in patients undergoing neoadjuvant therapy

Modality	Obstacle
CT	Chemotherapy-induced steatosis and steatohepatitis decrease contrast between liver and tumor
Sonography	Hyperechoic appearance of fatty liver obscures tumors Poor sensitivity for lesions <1 cm diameter
PET	Chemotherapy impairs glucose uptake in tumors High background of hepatocyte glucose uptake Insensitive for small tumors. Less than 5% of live lesions <1 cm are detected
MRI	Best modality for patients with small liver tumors, particularly in the setting of steatosis

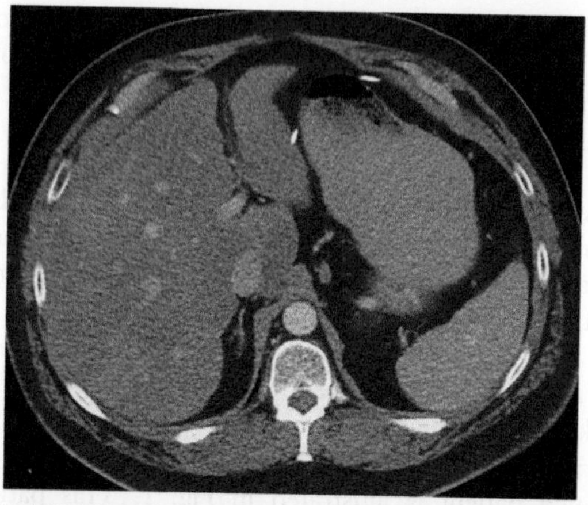

Fig. 1. Fatty liver hiding more than 50 tumors. On CT, no definitive tumors were noted in patient with high CEA. The liver is darker than the spleen, indicating steatosis. Tumors were discovered at exploration, and patient was treated with regional chemotherapy.

chemotherapy-induced impairment of glucose uptake [16]. Akhurst and colleagues [21] analyzed FDG-PET images of chemotherapy-naive patients versus those receiving neoadjuvant chemotherapy before hepatectomy. The study revealed that hepatic lesions have significantly impaired FDG uptake following neoadjuvant chemotherapy in comparison with lesions of chemotherapy-naive patients, and that this was at least partially the result of diminished hexokinase activity [21]. The result is that live liver tumors less than a centimeter in size have only a 3% chance of being seen by PET while a patient is on chemotherapy. Thus, although a positive PET is highly sensitive for live tumor, the likelihood of seeing small liver tumors is low.

Chemotherapy has also caused problems with CT scan interpretation. Chemotherapy-associated steatohepatitis has been associated with 5-FU, irinotecan, and oxaliplatin [22–24]. On CT, such steatohepatitis results in a darker-appearing liver, which, in combination with the hypovascular (and ergo hypoattenuated) lesion on CT [25,26], enables a fatty liver to hide certain residual tumors [27].

Similarly, changes in parenchymal appearance on US hinders detection of liver tumors in patients on chemotherapy. US is commonly used in the staging of patients with metastatic colorectal cancer to the liver, particularly in the operating room. When patients develop steatosis in the liver, the US appearance becomes highly echogenic. In terms of disappearing colorectal metastases, such echogenic appearance of noncancerous liver can obscure cancerous lesions, because they will appear isoechoic to the surrounding hepatic parenchyma [28]. Although there is some evidence that contrast enhancement can dramatically improve sensitivity and specificity of US in the detection of hepatic metastases, such contrast agents are not currently approved in the United States [28].

Of the various imaging modalities, MRI is probably the most useful in patients with chemotherapy-associated steatohepatitis and small lesions. MRI can compensate for the fat content of the liver by using differences between in- and out-of-phase imaging to exploit image characteristics of fat and water [25]. Although there is currently no consensus regarding the most sensitive imaging method for detection of colorectal hepatic metastases, several studies show MRI to be superior to CT. One study prospectively compared the accuracy of CT scan with gadolinium-enhanced MRI and superparamagnetic iron oxide (SPIO)-enhanced MRI in the examinations of 215 lesions in 58 patients with hepatic metastases and correlated imaging with intraoperative findings on US and histology [29]. The study noted that gadolinium and SPIO-enhanced MRI depicted 10% and 19% more lesions measuring less than 1 cm, respectively, compared with CT [29]. Bipat and colleagues [18] performed a large-scale meta-analysis evaluating the roles of CT, MRI, and FDG-PET in colorectal hepatic metastases and found that, on a per lesion basis, helical CT, MRI, and FDG-PET were comparable in accuracy. However, in subgroup analysis, the investigators found that SPIO- and gadolinium-enhanced MRI were significantly more accurate than nonenhanced MRI and helical CT performed with a contrast agent that has less than or equal to 45g of iodine [18]. Although several studies show superior sensitivity and specificity of FDG-PET compared with MRI, PET is unable to provide a surgical map and must therefore always be used in conjunction with MRI or CT in preoperative evaluation. Thus, in our practice, MRI is considered the most accurate and cost-effective means of preoperative hepatic evaluation, and is used in conjunction with other modalities on a case-by-case basis. Patients with disappearing lesions on chemotherapy should have MRI as part of the preoperative staging process.

MANAGEMENT OF COMPLETE CLINICAL RESPONSE

When hepatic lesions exhibit strong, or even complete, responses to neoadjuvant chemotherapy, surgeons are often left with difficult decisions in management. These patients are likely to have a much better prognosis than their counterparts who do not respond to chemotherapy [5,30].

In patients with some lesions disappearing, surgery should be performed after restaging with MRI and PET. All sites seen at any point before or after chemotherapy should be assessed in the operating room for gross residual disease. All lesions seen by PET should be treated. All lesions seen by MRI should be biopsied or treated. Currently, most investigators advocate resection of tumor remnants with uncertain malignant potential and areas previously occupied by lesions that have radiologically disappeared by date of operation [31,32]. Whether ablation of some of these small lesions will be adequate treatment, particularly if it will save a lot of functional parenchyma, is being tested [33].

Several studies have found that a radiologic response is often absent in patients with complete pathologic responses. For example, Adam and colleagues [32] reviewed 767 patients receiving preoperative chemotherapy and hepatectomy, and identified only 2 patients with complete radiologic responses on CT, neither of whom correlated with complete pathologic response. All 29 patients identified with complete pathologic response had partial responses or stabilization of lesions visible on preoperative CT [32]. Tan and colleagues [16] reached similar conclusions using FDG-PET imaging in combination with CT or MRI, noting that, although 7 of 14 patients had complete metabolic responses on PET and complete lesion response on CT, only 1 showed complete pathologic response at resection. In our own practice, we have seen patients with multiple lesions on postchemotherapy preoperative imaging who are found to be pathologically free of malignancy on resection (Fig. 2). New modalities of imaging, such as with tumor-specific antibodies [34], will be necessary to identify completely necrotic lesions after chemotherapy as opposed to residual malignancy. Others are attempting to use cross-sectional imaging characteristics, such as absence of a diffusely infiltrative tumor margin, to predict nonviable hepatic metastases [31]. Such predictions could spare patients unnecessary operations in the future and are worth investigation. However, there are currently not enough data to unilaterally support watchful waiting without tissue confirmation of tumor resolution in patients with residual lesions.

The situation is more difficult for patients with complete resolution of lesions. In general, a surgeon must choose between exploration of each previous site of metastasis via biopsy or resection, and close observation with or without continued chemotherapy. In our practice, management of patients with complete radiologic response involves intensive review of MRI films by a radiologist specializing in hepatic lesions, and a hepatobiliary surgeon. We then have a comprehensive discussion with patients, detailing potential risks and benefits of resection and observation. The decision usually depends in large part on the patient's level of comfort with either option. When

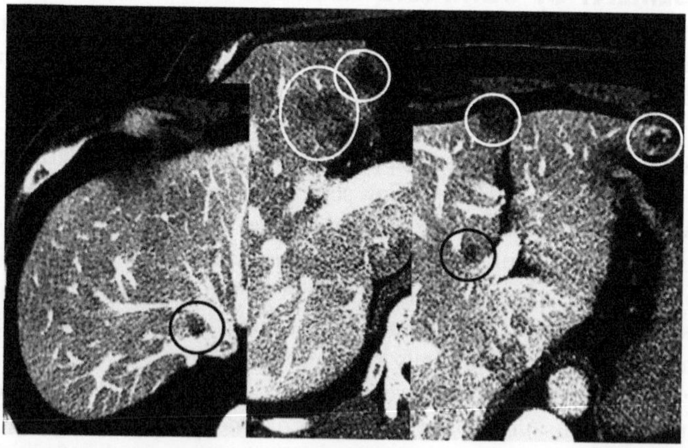

Fig. 2. Patient with multiple lesions seen on CT after neoadjuvant chemotherapy, all of which were benign on final pathology.

observation is chosen, we recommend completion of a 6-month course of chemotherapy, even if lesions disappear early in this course. If CEA remains normal and MRI remains clear after 6 months of chemotherapy, we will recommend cessation of chemotherapy with close follow-up of blood work and repeat MRI every 3 months. For surveillance, we will replace MRI with CT only if patients are free of steatohepatitis. When exploration is chosen to verify pathologic complete response, all areas that had previously been documented to have cancer must be examined. The ultimate goal should be to identify and remove all cancerous lesions.

SUMMARY

Disappearance of liver lesions during neoadjuvant chemotherapy is common and is the basis for the increasing number of patients suitable for potentially curative hepatectomy in patients with hepatic colorectal metastases. Many of the liver lesions disappearing on radiologic evaluation after successful chemotherapy for metastatic colorectal cancer are still present and alive. In patients with only some disappearing lesions, exploration should be undertaken to thoroughly evaluate all sites of previous disease. Because many small residual lesions are scars and complete pathologic responses, treatment should include not only complete treatment of all remaining lesions but also parenchymal conservation techniques such as ablations and limited resections. For patients with completely disappearing lesions, the standard therapy is still exploration and direct intraoperative assessment. However, if the patient chooses observation in the setting of negative CEA, MRI, and PET, close follow-up should be undertaken to avoid missing treatable and resectable recurrences.

References

[1] Nordlinger B, Parc R, Delva E, et al. Hepatic resection for colorectal liver metastases. Ann Surg 1987;205:256–63.

[2] Ewing H, Sali A, Kune GA. Klatskin tumours: a 20 year experience. Aust N Z J Surg 1989;59:25–30.

[3] Butler J, Attiyeh FF, Daly JM. Hepatic resection for metastases of the colon and rectum. Surg Gynecol Obstet 1986;162:109–13.

[4] Morris KT, Song TJ, Fong Y. Recent advancements in diagnosis and treatment of metastatic colorectal cancer to the liver. Surg Oncol 2006;15:129–34.

[5] Adam R, Delvart V, Pascal G, et al. Rescue surgery for unresectable colorectal liver metastases downstaged by chemotherapy: a model to predict long-term survival. Ann Surg 2004;240(4):644–57.

[6] Silverberg E, Boring CC, Squires TS. Cancer statistics 1990. CA Cancer J Clin 1990;40:9.

[7] Adam R, Avisar E, Ariche A, et al. Five-year survival following hepatic resection after neoadjuvant therapy for nonresectable colorectal [liver] metastases. Ann Surg Oncol 2001;8(4):347–53.

[8] Ensminger WD, Rosowsky A, Raso V, et al. A clinical pharmacological evaluation of hepatic arterial infusions of 5-fluoro-2-deoxyuridine and 5-fluorouracil. Cancer Res 1978;38(11): 3784–92.

[9] Kemeny NE, Huitzil Melendez FD, Capanu M, et al. Conversion to resectability using hepatic artery infusion plus systemic chemotherapy for the treatment of unresectable liver metastases from colorectal carcinoma. J Clin Oncol 2009;27:3465–71.

[10] Kemeny N, Jarnagin W, Paty P, et al. Phase I trial of systemic oxaliplatin combination chemotherapy with hepatic arterial infusion in patients with unresectable liver metastases from colorectal cancer. J Clin Oncol 2005;23(22):4888–96.
[11] Kattan MW, Karpeh MS, Mazumdar M, et al. Postoperative nomogram for disease-specific survival after an R0 resection for gastric carcinoma. J Clin Oncol 2003;21(19):3647–50.
[12] Benoist S, Brouquet A, Penna C, et al. Complete response of colorectal liver metastases after chemotherapy: does it mean cure? J Clin Oncol 2006;24(24):3939–45.
[13] Elias D, Youssef O, Sideris L, et al. Evolution of missing colorectal liver metastases following inductive chemotherapy and hepatectomy. J Surg Oncol 2004;86(1):4–9.
[14] Fiorentini G, Del CA, De SM, et al. Complete response of colorectal liver metastases after intra-arterial chemotherapy. Tumori 2008;94(4):489–92.
[15] Auer RC, White RR, Kemeny NE, et al. Predictors of a true complete response among disappearing liver metastases from colorectal cancer after chemotherapy. Cancer 2010;116(6):1502–9.
[16] Tan MC, Linehan DC, Hawkins WG, et al. Chemotherapy-induced normalization of FDG uptake by colorectal liver metastases does not usually indicate complete pathologic response. J Gastrointest Surg 2007;11(9):1112–9.
[17] Huebner RH, Park KC, Shepherd JE, et al. A meta-analysis of the literature for whole-body FDG PET detection of recurrent colorectal cancer. J Nucl Med 2000;41(7):1177–89.
[18] Bipat S, van Leewen MS, Comans EF, et al. Colorectal liver metastases: CT, MR imaging and PET for diagnosis–meta-analysis. Radiology 2005;237(1):123–31.
[19] Fong Y, Saldinger PF, Akhurst T, et al. Utility of 18F-FDG-PET scanning on selection of patients for resection of hepatic colorectal metastases. Am J Surg 1999;178:282–7.
[20] Kelloff GJ, Hoffman JM, Johnson B, et al. Progress and promise of FDG-PET imaging for cancer patient management and oncologic drug development. Clin Cancer Res 2005;11(8):2785–808.
[21] Akhurst T, Kates TJ, Mazumdar M, et al. Recent chemotherapy reduces the sensitivity of [18F]fluorodeoxyglucose positron emission tomography in the detection of colorectal metastases. J Clin Oncol 2005;23(34):8713–6.
[22] Peppercorn PD, Reznek RH, Wilson P, et al. Demonstration of hepatic steatosis by computerized tomography in patients receiving 5-fluorouracil-based therapy for advanced colorectal cancer. Br J Cancer 1998;77(11):2008–11.
[23] Vauthey JN, Pawlik TM, Ribero D, et al. Chemotherapy regimen predicts steatohepatitis and an increase in 90-day mortality after surgery for hepatic colorectal metastases. J Clin Oncol 2006;24(13):2065–72.
[24] Zorzi D, Laurent A, Pawlik TM, et al. Chemotherapy-associated hepatotoxicity and surgery for colorectal liver metastases. Br J Surg 2007;94(3):274–86.
[25] Valls C, Iannacconne R, Alba E, et al. Fat in the liver: diagnosis and characterization. Eur Radiol 2006;16(10):2292–308.
[26] Oliva MR, Mortele KJ, Segatto E, et al. Computed tomography features of nonalcoholic steatohepatitis with histopathologic correlation. J Comput Assist Tomogr 2006;30(1):37–43.
[27] Cho CS, Curran S, Schwartz LH, et al. Preoperative radiographic assessment of hepatic steatosis with histologic correlation. J Am Coll Surg 2008;206(3):480–8.
[28] Albrecht T, Blomley MJ, Burns PN, et al. Improved detection of hepatic metastases with pulse-inversion US during the liver-specific phase of SHU 508A: multicenter study. Radiology 2003;227(2):361–70.
[29] Ward J, Robinson PJ, Guthrie JA, et al. Liver metastases in candidates for hepatic resection: comparison of helical CT and gadolinium- and SPIO-enhanced MR imaging. Radiology 2005;237(1):170–80.
[30] Giacchetti S, Itzhaki M, Gruia G, et al. Long-term survival of patients with unresectable colorectal cancer liver metastases following infusional chemotherapy with 5-fluorouracil, leucovorin, oxaliplatin and surgery. Ann Oncol 1999;10(6):663–9.

[31] Znajda TL, Hayashi S, Horton PJ, et al. Postchemotherapy characteristics of hepatic colorectal metastases: remnants of uncertain malignant potential. J Gastrointest Surg 2006;10(4):483–9.
[32] Adam R, Wicherts DA, de Haas RJ, et al. Complete pathologic response after preoperative chemotherapy for colorectal liver metastases: myth or reality? J Clin Oncol 2008;26(10): 1635–41.
[33] Wong SL, Mangu PB, Choti MA, et al. American Society of Clinical Oncology 2009 clinical evidence review on radiofrequency ablation of hepatic metastases from colorectal cancer. J Clin Oncol 2009;28:493–508.
[34] Pinkas L, Robins PD, Forstrom LA, et al. Clinical experience with radiolabelled monoclonal antibodies in the detection of colorectal and ovarian carcinoma recurrence and review of the literature. Nucl Med Commun 1999;20(8):689–96.
[35] Bismuth H, Adam R, Levi F, et al. Resection of nonresectable liver metastases from colorectal cancer after neoadjuvant chemotherapy. Ann Surg 1996;224(4):509–20.
[36] Gallagher DJ, Capanu M, Raggio G, et al. Hepatic arterial infusion plus systemic irinotecan in patients with unresectable hepatic metastases from colorectal cancer previously treated with systemic oxaliplatin: a retrospective analysis. Ann Oncol 2007;18(12):1995–9.
[37] Alberts SR, Horvath WL, Sternfeld WC, et al. Oxaliplatin, fluorouracil, and leucovorin for patients with unresectable liver-only metastases from colorectal cancer: a North Central Cancer Treatment Group phase II study. J Clin Oncol 2005;23(36):9243–9.
[38] Barone C, Nuzzo G, Cassano A, et al. Final analysis of colorectal cancer patients treated with irinotecan and 5-fluorouracil plus folinic acid neoadjuvant chemotherapy for unresectable liver metastases. Br J Cancer 2007;97(8):1035–9.

Advances in Surgery 44 (2010) 281–292
ADVANCES IN SURGERY

Endovascular Repair of Traumatic Aortic Injuries

David G. Neschis, MD[a], Thomas M. Scalea, MD[a,b,*]

[a]Department of Surgery, University of Maryland School of Medicine, 22 South Greene Street, Baltimore, MD 21201, USA
[b]R Adams Cowley Shock Trauma Center, 22 South Greene Street, Baltimore, MD 21201, USA

Since the first description of endograft repair for traumatic aortic injury in 1997, this less invasive option has become increasingly popular for the treatment of aortic injury [1]. Coincidentally, the same year, the first prospective multicenter study of repair of blunt aortic injury was published by the American Association for the Surgery of Trauma (AAST) [2]. A total of 274 subjects were evaluated from 50 participating centers (AAST1). Overall mortality in subjects who arrived at the hospital alive was 31% with a paraplegia rate of 8.7%.

Just 10 years later, the AAST again published the results of a nonrandomized prospective multicenter study of the treatment of blunt aortic injury (AAST 2) [3]. There are several significant differences between the two studies. After a period of only 10 years, the percentage of subjects treated with an endograft rose from 0% in the initial study to 64.9%. Overall mortality, excluding subjects in extremis, decreased from 22% to 13% [4]. Most notable, however, were the improvements in the incidence of paraplegia. In the open group, the paraplegia rate decreased from 8.7% to 2.9%. This decrease was thought to be caused by the increase in the use of extracorporeal bypass, which increased from 64.7% to 83.8% of open cases. The use of endografts was associated within the even greater drop in the incidence of paraplegia to 0.8%. Mortality in the endograft treatment group was 7.2%.

However, these clear improvements in mortality and paraplegia appeared to have come at the expense of an increased incidence of graft-related failure. Endograft repair was associated with a 14.4% incidence of endoleak of which one-third of these subjects eventually required conversion to open repair. Other device-related complications included iliac injury and stroke. The authors of AAST 2 concluded that there was a major and urgent need for improvement of the available endovascular devices [3].

*Corresponding author. *E-mail address:* tscalea@umm.edu.

0065-3411/10/$ – see front matter
doi:10.1016/j.yasu.2010.05.004

Currently, there are no devices available in the United States with a US Food and Drug Administration indication for repair of blunt aortic injury. Outside of investigational trials, centers in the United States currently use a variety of available thoracic and abdominal aortic endograft components for repair. This article discusses the evaluation and management of patients with blunt aortic injury, focusing on endograft repair.

INITIAL EVALUATION AND IMAGING

The majority of blunt aortic injuries occur as a result of motor vehicle crashes [2]. Other mechanisms include motorcycle crashes, pedestrian versus automobile, light-weight aircraft crashes, and falls [5]. Based on the pioneering work of Parmley in his landmark article in 1958, it is estimated that approximately 85% of patients die at the scene [6]. Of those that survive to the hospital, the majority will die within the next 24 to 48 hours without treatment.

Years ago, all patients suspected of having a blunt aortic injury underwent catheter-based aortography. This study is clearly not ideal because it requires a special team to perform the procedure, which is somewhat invasive. In addition, angiography is less sensitive in detecting blunt aortic injury when compared with contrast-enhanced helical CT scan. With modern CT scanners, sensitivity has improved to 100% as compared with 92% for angiography [7]. Because of the near universal availability of modern CT equipment and the speed in which the study can be performed, CT angiography has become the study of choice for the evaluation of blunt aortic injuries. Other modes of imaging the thoracic aorta include MRI, intravascular ultrasonography, and transesophageal echocardiography. The latter two modalities can be particularly useful in patients with a mechanism of injury, or chest radiograph, that creates a high index of suspicion for a blunt aortic injury that requires emergent operative therapy for the treatment of other life-threatening injuries.

Unfortunately, patients presenting with blunt aortic injury often have other coexisting, potentially life-threatening, injuries. Associated injuries include severe brain injury, pulmonary contusion, abdominal hemorrhage, and multiple long bone fractures [2]. Priority must be given to the most immediately life-threatening injuries, usually severe intra-abdominal or intracranial hemorrhage.

Years ago, immediate operative repair of the blunt aortic injury was the rule. However, numerous studies have reported on the relative safety of delayed repair using inotropic and blood pressure control to prevent rupture before repair. This practice allows operative repair to be delayed until patients are in better condition to tolerate thoracotomy and aortic clamping [7–10].

Although this may improve results in patients undergoing open repair, it creates a dilemma particularly with respect to the treatment of coexisting brain injury. Treatment of patients with brain injuries often centers on optimizing cerebral perfusion pressure, which often requires elevation of the patients' systemic blood pressure. This practice would be contradictory to efforts to reduce systemic pressures in patients with an aortic injury. By avoiding a thoracotomy and cross clamping of the aorta, endograft repair allows treatment of patients with multiple injuries and frailer or elderly patients that would have otherwise been considered too high risk for traditional early open repair.

MINIMAL AORTIC INJURY

When aortic imaging demonstrates a large defect with pseudoaneurysm and mediastinal blood, repair is generally wise. However, approximately 10% of patients with blunt aortic injury have a lesion that could be described as minimal [11]. The proper treatment of minimal aortic injury remains unclear. This lack of clarity is further complicated by the fact that minimal aortic injury is a vague term involving lesions that could range from a tiny intimal defect up to a small pseudoaneurysm without significant associated mediastinal blood. Although endograft repair would likely be successful in excluding these small lesions from the circulation, it is unclear whether they require any procedure. This point is particularly important given the potential long-term complications of an endograft device. However, it has been reported that as many as 50% of minimal aortic injuries, defined as an intimal flap of less than 1 cm with no or minimal periaortic hematoma, develop pseudoaneurysms by 8 weeks after injury [11].

The authors currently follow small lesions, such as small intimal defects and pseudoaneurysms of the aorta of a few millimeters in diameter, until resolution is observed on serial CT scans. More moderate lesions, such as small (but > a few millimeters) pseudoaneurysms, without significant mediastinal blood should be considered for repair. In situations where patients would be good candidates from an anatomic standpoint and the chance of success high, repair probably should be performed. In cases where the anatomy is more unfavorable and carries a higher risk for technical failure observation and serial imaging may be warranted. Anatomic features predictive of success or failure are discussed in detail later in this article.

PREOPERATIVE PLANNING

As with endograft repair of aneurysms, the preoperative planning phase is critical to assure a successful outcome. Evaluation of the entire patient is required to minimize potential pitfalls. Available imaging should be reviewed to determine if there are other sources of bleeding. Common sources include intracranial and intra-abdominal bleeding. Perioperative administration of anticoagulation in such a setting could be particularly hazardous. With respect to patients with brain injuries, the surgeon needs to be clear as to whether patients can be placed in the supine position. Although the authors have performed successful endograft repair in patients who required head elevation, this requires use of a standard operating table as most endovascular suites do not have a table that allows the head and back to be raised.

A complete pulse examination should be performed and the groins examined for determination of access sites. Typically, 1 groin is chosen for the cut down and the other used for percutaneous angiography. The presence of direct injury or associated hematoma from pelvic or femur fractures may steer the surgeon to avoid a particular groin. Alternatively, left brachial access can be used for angiography. This access has the added benefit of allowing wire placement to mark the location of the left subclavian artery (LSCA) origin. Any assessment should be made as to the overall length of the patients' torso, because torso length may affect the introducer length required.

The contrast enhanced CT scan is then carefully reviewed for treatment planning. Key measurements include the diameter of the normal aorta just proximal and just distal to the area of injury. An estimate of the total treatment length is made. Review of reconstructed images is helpful in making an estimate of the degree of angulation of the aortic arch and the relationship of the treatment zone to that area of angulation (Fig. 1). An estimate of distance from the area of injury to the left subclavian artery and to the left common carotid artery is made, as well as a general assessment of the vertebral arterial anatomy. Additionally, the diameter and quality of the access vessels are assessed. The surgeon should be aware, however, that if the CT scan was obtained during a period of relative hypotension, the diameters of the access vessels and even the thoracic aorta may be under estimated [12].

OPERATIVE APPROACH

Patients are taken to the operating suite and anesthesia administered according to treatment team preference. The authors' choice is usually general anesthesia to minimize patient movement and to be able to reliably control respirations. Routine use of spinal drainage is not performed because a short area of the aorta is expected to be covered and these injuries do not typically affect the distal thoracic aorta. Access is usually obtained via a cut down on one groin and a puncture for angiography on the other. Access site choices are made based on considerations previously described.

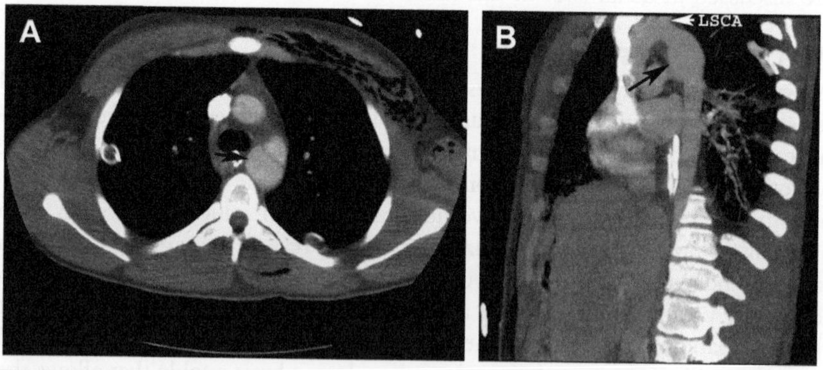

Fig. 1. (*A*) Contrast-enhanced CT demonstrating site of aortic injury with pseudoaneurysm (*arrow*). (*B*) Same study, reconstructed image, better delineating the area of injury (*arrow*) and its relationship to the origin of the left subclavian artery.

An arch angiogram is then usually performed early in the procedure, which is assessed for the presence of vertebral dominance. If the left vertebral artery is significantly larger than the right and the images suggest that the coverage of the left subclavian artery will be required, consideration should be made for preservation of left subclavian artery flow either via a pre-endograft carotid subclavian bypass or plans made for chimney-style stenting of the left subclavian artery at the time of endograft placement. However, CT reconstructions often underestimate the degree of angulation and the anatomic complexity.

The angiogram is then reviewed for the relationship of the area of injury to the angulation of the aortic arch and a final choice of endograft is made. If there appears to be a significant discrepancy in aortic diameter based on the angiogram as compared with the original CT scan, intravascular ultrasound can help make a final determination of the aortic diameter [13].

Access choices are previously described. Often common, femoral vessels in young patients are narrow in diameter and go into spasm with minimal manipulation. Fortunately, however, these vessels are normally healthy and easily dilated to accommodate the required introducer devices. There may be times where length or diameter constraints necessitate a sheathless entry technique.

Unlike patients with aneurysmal disease, the average age of patients with blunt aortic injury is about 44 years [5]. The aortic arches in young patients tend to be considerably smaller and more acutely angulated. The authors have found that the Lunderquist super-stiff wire will become permanently bent in some of these acute angled arches. It has been the authors' experience that the Amplatz wire maintains adequate stiffness, but is also able to negotiate the young aortic arch [14]. In obtaining wire access, it is the authors' practice to form a pigtail in the catheter in the distal thoracic aorta and pass this formed pigtail up past the area of the injury and on into the aortic arch, which is then used to guide the Amplatz wire into the aortic arch. The authors find that this reduces the chance of a wire engaging the injured area and further injuring the torn aorta. The initial pigtail, which was used to obtain angiography, is advanced in similar fashion.

Once access is obtained, a decision is made with respect to heparin anticoagulation. Early in the authors' experience, they were hesitant to perform the procedure without heparin for fear of creating limb thrombosis or stroke. This approach, however, created situations where endovascular repair was delayed for several days in cases of significant head injury or intra-abdominal hemorrhage. Other authors have routinely performed endograft repair of traumatic aortic injury without the use of heparin anticoagulation [15]. Based on this experience, the authors liberalized their approach. Now, in selective cases in which anticoagulation would be potentially hazardous and in which the anatomy was simple, the authors have performed several cases without the use of intraoperative heparin [5]. This approach has allowed timelier repair in patients with ongoing bleeding risk.

Once the device is selected (device specifics discussed subsequently) it is advanced into approximate position. At this point, a predeployment angiogram is obtained. One decision point frequently is whether or not to cover the origin of the left subclavian artery, which is not required in the majority of cases [5]. The potential complications resulting from coverage of the left subclavian artery origin include left upper extremity ischemia and stroke, particularly if the left vertebral artery is dominant. It has been the authors' experience that 21% of cases require partial or complete subclavian artery coverage. There have been no sequelae in those patients that underwent subclavian artery coverage [5].

Although the proximal coverage length of at least 15 mm to 20 mm would be ideal, successful repair can be achieved with coverage lengths as short as 5 mm [5]. In contrast to treatment of aneurysmal disease, the adjacent aorta is normal in aortic injury. Additionally, because there is no aneurysm present there is less likelihood that there will be sufficient space for an endograft to migrate into.

Once proper position is confirmed, the device is deployed (Fig. 2). Additional devices are deployed as needed. On occasion, because CT scanning is more sensitive for the detection of injury than angiography, the area of injury may not be seen on the angiogram [7]. In this situation, the authors' practice is to deploy the endograft to cover the area that corresponds to the area of injury seen on the CT scan. Following deployment, completion angiography is performed to evaluate for patency of the endograft, confirm the patency of the arch vessels, and to confirm successful exclusion of the pseudoaneurysm. Generally, balloon dilatation is not performed unless an endoleak is present, which should be resolved by balloon dilatation.

It has been the authors' experience that, particularly in young patients, the arterial pulsations are hyperdynamic, which can become a particular problem when using devices not designed for placement in the proximal thoracic aorta. A variety of techniques have been described to reduce the arterial pressures

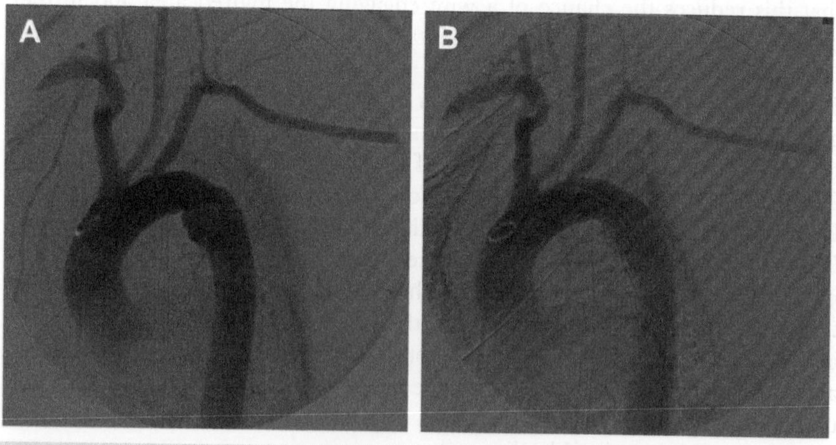

Fig. 2. (*A*) Intraoperative aortogram demonstrating pseudoaneurysm. (*B*) Completion aortogram demonstrating successful exclusion of pseudoaneurysm.

within the aorta at the time of deployment, including use of adenosine to induce hypotension or the use of rapid ventricular pacing [16,17]. The authors have found the use of adenosine to create temporary asystole to be useful and safe in this situation. The authors have used adenosine to augment placement in 51% of patients. An average dose of 20 mg was used, usually as either an 18 mg or 20 mg dose [5].

Following successful deployment of the device, the introducer catheters are removed. The arteriotomy is repaired with interrupted Prolene suture. The percutaneously placed sheath is removed after the heparin effect has worn off. Follow-up CT angiography is generally performed within a week of placement and before patients' discharge. The authors' patients are instructed to return for a follow-up visit within 2 weeks following discharge for evaluation of groin wounds and pulses and to establish a point of contact for future visits. Follow-up CT angiography and frontal and lateral chest radiographs are obtained at 6 months and then yearly thereafter. Because of concerns of radiation exposure from CT scans in young patients, the authors have increased intervals between visits to more than 1 year in selected cases with repairs that appear to be stable [18].

AVAILABLE DEVICES

Currently there are no devices available in the Unites States that are approved specifically for use in traumatic aortic injuries. Currently, the available thoracic endograft devices include the TAG thoracic endovascular device (W.L. Gore and Associates, Newark, DE, USA), Zenith TX2 thoracic endograft (Cook, Bloomington, IN, USA), and the Talent thoracic endograft (Medtronic Vascular, Minneapolis, MN, USA). Other devices that had been used include the Excluder (W.L. Gore and Associates), Zenith (Cook), and AneuRx (Medtronic Vascular) abdominal devices. (Table 1) Each of these devices have their own characteristics, advantages, and pitfalls. Several years ago, the only available thoracic endograft was the Gore TAG device. Its advantages include simplicity of design and ease of deployment; however, covered proximal phalanges and poor apposition in tight aortas limited its usefulness in the treatment of thoracic transections.

The authors have overcome these disadvantages by using the Excluder abdominal cuff. This device has the longest introducer of the abdominal devices and has a flat covered proximal edge, which allows precise placement. However, one disadvantage includes the short device length requiring multiple devices stacked over each other [19]. With the availability of the Talent and Zenith devices, there are more options available. The Talent device comes in a wide range of diameters and can handle the tight aortic arch well. Disadvantages include a 22-French introducer sheath for the smallest device and bare springs proximally, which creates a theoretical concern for aortic wall perforation [20]. This complication, to the authors' knowledge, has not yet been described in the setting of treatment for aortic injury. The Zenith device allows precise placement, however, the length of the individual stent segments can at

Table 1
Characteristics of currently available devices in the United States

Thoracic devices	Diameter (mm)	Covered length (mm)	Introducer diameter	
Talent (Medtronic)	22–46	112–116	22–25 Fr (OD)	—
TAG (Gore)	26–40	100–200	20–24 Fr (ID)	—
Zenith TX2 (Cook)	28–42	108–216	20–22 Fr (ID)	—
Abdominal devices				Introducer length (cm)
AneuRx aortic cuffs (Medtronic)	20.0–28.0	37.5	21 Fr (OD)	55
AneuRx iliac cuffs (Medtronic)	16.0–20.0	55.0–135.0	16 Fr (OD)	55
Zenith aortic cuffs (Cook)	22.0–36.0	39.0	18–20 Fr (ID)	40
Zenith iliac cuffs (Cook)	8.0–24.0	55.0	14–18 Fr (ID)	55
Excluder aortic cuffs (Gore)	23.0–28.5	33.0	18 Fr (ID)	61

Abbreviations: Fr, French; ID, inner diameter; OD, outer diameter.

times limit its use in the tightly angulated aorta. Features of the various devices are summarized in Table 1.

PATTERNS OF GRAFT FAILURE

As described in AAST 2, the advantages and lowered mortality and paraplegia rates were offset by an approximately 20% device-related complication rate [3]. The endoleak rate was 14.4%, half of which underwent open exploration for resolution [3]. Several patterns of graft failure have been observed over the combined experience with endograft repair for blunt aortic injury. One pitfall leading to graft failure has been in the appropriate sizing of devices. One particular issue was with the over sizing of the Gore TAG device. The smallest available TAG device is 26 mm in diameter and attempts were made to place it in aortas as small as 19 mm. This practice has been associated with reported collapse of the device [21]. An additional issue with the TAG device is that even when properly sized, if a portion of the device encroaches into the horizontal portion of the aortic arch, a bird-beak effect could occur (Fig. 3). Device collapse has also been reported in this setting [22].

However, even when devices are properly sized and care is taken to minimize the bird-beak effect, device failure and endoleaks do occur. In evaluating patterns of graft failure in the authors' own experience, they identified that distance from the left subclavian artery to the area of injury and the acuity of the aortic arch angle were both significantly associated with device failure (Fig. 4). The mean distance from the origin of the left subclavian artery to the site of injury was 2.2 cm in repairs without graft failure and 1.2 cm ($P = .04$)

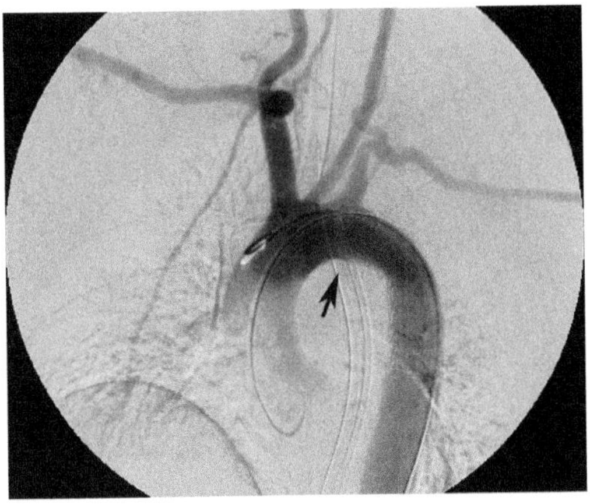

Fig. 3. Completion aortogram demonstrating incomplete apposition of the proximal portion of the endograft to the lesser curvature of the aorta creating a distinctive bird's-beak defect (*arrow*). When severe, this lack of apposition can lead to device collapse.

in repairs that experienced graft failure, such as endoleak or device collapse [5]. Further evaluation of prerepair angiograms revealed anatomic patterns associated with graft failure (Fig. 5). All device failures in the authors' experience occurred in the Type IV injury, in which there was a bend in the aorta

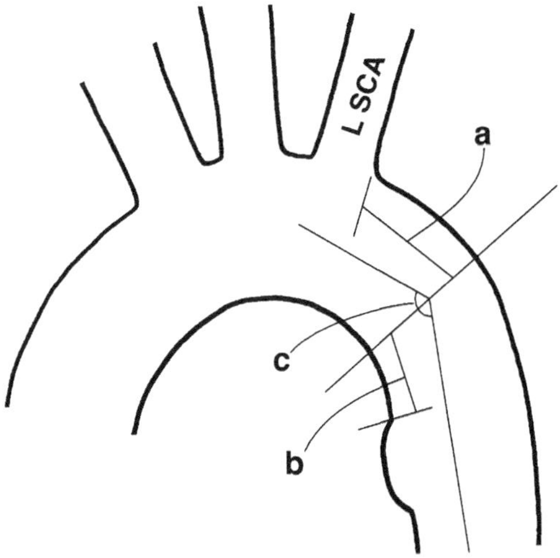

Fig. 4. Anatomic relationships of aorta in setting of blunt injury. a, distance from LSCA to the sharpest bend in the descending thoracic aorta; b, distance form bend to site of injury; c, angle made at sharpest bend in the descending thoracic aorta. *Reproduced from* Neschis DG, Moainie S, Flinn WR, et al. Endograft Repair of Traumatic Aortic Injury: A Technique in Evolution. Ann Surg 2009;250(3):377–83; with permission.

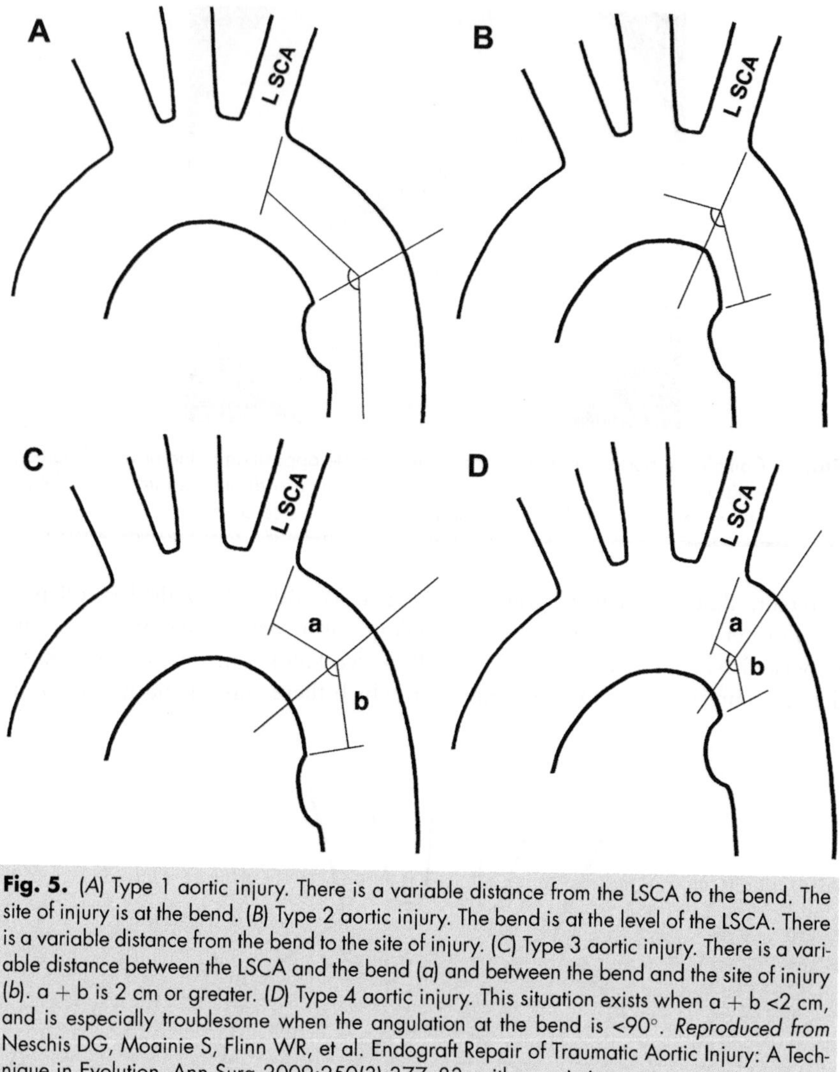

Fig. 5. (*A*) Type 1 aortic injury. There is a variable distance from the LSCA to the bend. The site of injury is at the bend. (*B*) Type 2 aortic injury. The bend is at the level of the LSCA. There is a variable distance from the bend to the site of injury. (*C*) Type 3 aortic injury. There is a variable distance between the LSCA and the bend (*a*) and between the bend and the site of injury (*b*). a + b is 2 cm or greater. (*D*) Type 4 aortic injury. This situation exists when a + b <2 cm, and is especially troublesome when the angulation at the bend is <90°. *Reproduced from* Neschis DG, Moainie S, Flinn WR, et al. Endograft Repair of Traumatic Aortic Injury: A Technique in Evolution. Ann Surg 2009;250(3):377–83; with permission.

within the planned proximal coverage zone *and* the total length of that coverage zone was less than 2 cm in length [5].

SUMMARY

Endograft repair has clearly revolutionized the treatment of traumatic aortic injury. Numerous studies, both retrospective and prospective, have documented the advantages with respect to lower mortality and lower paraplegia rates as compared with traditional open repair [3,23–27]. Additionally, 2 recent meta-analyses of the published literature both reported significantly lower mortality and paraplegia rates with endovascular repair [28,29]. These clear improvements, however, come at an increased rate of device-related complications [3].

Currently, newer devices designed to adapt to more acute bends in the proximal thoracic aorta are in the multicenter trial phase. These devices are also expected to be available in a wider range of diameters and lengths, including smaller diameter devices required to treat younger patients. A conformable Gore TAG design is undergoing trials in the United States. Trials of the Talent thoracic device for the treatment of blunt aortic injury are also ongoing. We await the results of the ongoing multicenter trials and expect that with improvements in technology, the vast majority of patients with traumatic aortic injury can be treated without open thoracic aortic surgery.

The long-term durability and natural history of thoracic endograft devices, however, are unknown. Continued regular follow-up is recommended, although this can be difficult in this young population of patients. Because follow-up may be ongoing for decades, the need to identify a potential problem has to be weighed against the oncologic risks of repeated radiation exposure.

References

[1] Semba CP, Kato N, Kee ST, et al. Acute rupture of the descending thoracic aorta: repair with use of endovascular stent-grafts. J Vasc Interv Radiol 1997;8(3):337–42.

[2] Fabian TC, Richardson JD, Croce MA, et al. Prospective study of blunt aortic injury: multicenter trial of the American Association for the Surgery of Trauma. J Trauma 1997;42(3): 374–80 [discussion: 380–3].

[3] Demetriades D, Velmahos GC, Scalea TM, et al. Operative repair or endovascular stent graft in blunt traumatic thoracic aortic injuries: results of an American Association for the Surgery of Trauma Multicenter Study. J Trauma 2008;64(3):561–70 [discussion: 570–1].

[4] Demetriades D, Velmahos GC, Scalea TM, et al. Diagnosis and treatment of blunt thoracic aortic injuries: changing perspectives. J Trauma 2008;64(6):1415–8 [discussion: 1418–9].

[5] Neschis DG, Moainie S, Flinn WR, et al. Endograft repair of traumatic aortic injury-a technique in evolution: a single institution's experience. Ann Surg 2009;250(3):377–82.

[6] Parmley LF, Mattingly TW, Manion WC, et al. Nonpenetrating traumatic injury of the aorta. Circulation 1958;17(6):1086–101.

[7] Fabian TC, Davis KA, Gavant ML, et al. Prospective study of blunt aortic injury: helical CT is diagnostic and antihypertensive therapy reduces rupture. Ann Surg 1998;227(5):666–76 [discussion: 676–7].

[8] Kipfer B, Leupi F, Schuepbach P, et al. Acute traumatic rupture of the thoracic aorta: immediate or delayed surgical repair? Eur J Cardiothorac Surg 1994;8(1):30–3.

[9] Pate JW, Fabian TC, Walker W. Traumatic rupture of the aortic isthmus: an emergency? World J Surg 1995;19(1):119–25 [discussion: 125–6].

[10] Symbas PN, Sherman AJ, Silver JM, et al. Traumatic rupture of the aorta: immediate or delayed repair? Ann Surg 2002;235(6):796–802.

[11] Malhotra AK, Fabian TC, Croce MA, et al. Minimal aortic injury: a lesion associated with advancing diagnostic techniques. J Trauma 2001;51(6):1042–8.

[12] van Prehn J, van Herwaarden JA, Muhs BE, et al. Difficulties with endograft sizing in a patient with traumatic rupture of the thoracic aorta: the possible influence of hypovolemic shock. J Vasc Surg 2008;47(6):1333–6.

[13] Patel NH, Hahn D, Comess KA. Blunt chest trauma victims: role of intravascular ultrasound and transesophageal echocardiography in cases of abnormal thoracic aortogram. J Trauma 2003;55(2):330–7.

[14] Neschis DG, Moaine S, Gutta R, et al. Twenty consecutive cases of endograft repair of traumatic aortic disruption: lessons learned. J Vasc Surg 2007;45(3):487–92.
[15] Hoornweg LL, Dinkelman MK, Goslings JC, et al. Endovascular management of traumatic ruptures of the thoracic aorta: a retrospective multicenter analysis of 28 cases in The Netherlands. J Vasc Surg 2006;43(6):1096–102 [discussion: 1102].
[16] Dorros G, Cohn JM. Adenosine-induced transient cardiac asystole enhances precise deployment of stent-grafts in the thoracic or abdominal aorta. J Endovasc Surg 1996;3(3):270–2.
[17] Pornratanarangsi S, Webster MW, Alison P, et al. Rapid ventricular pacing to lower blood pressure during endograft deployment in the thoracic aorta. Ann Thorac Surg 2006;81(5): e21–3.
[18] Brenner DJ, Hall EJ. Computed tomography–an increasing source of radiation exposure. N Engl J Med 2007;357(22):2277–84.
[19] Rosenthal D, Wellons ED, Burkett AB, et al. Endovascular repair of traumatic thoracic aortic disruptions with "stacked" abdominal endograft extension cuffs. J Vasc Surg 2008;48(4): 841–4.
[20] Panos A. Late retrograde aortic perforation by the uncovered part of an endograft: an increasing complication. Hellenic J Cardiol 2007;48(2):115–6.
[21] Idu MM, Reekers JA, Balm R, et al. Collapse of a stent-graft following treatment of a traumatic thoracic aortic rupture. J Endovasc Ther 2005;12(4):503–7.
[22] Steinbauer MG, Stehr A, Pfister K, et al. Endovascular repair of proximal endograft collapse after treatment for thoracic aortic disease. J Vasc Surg 2006;43(3):609–12.
[23] Kasirajan K, Heffernan D, Langsfeld M. Acute thoracic aortic trauma: a comparison of endoluminal stent grafts with open repair and nonoperative management. Ann Vasc Surg 2003;17(6):589–95.
[24] Rousseau H, Dambrin C, Marcheix B, et al. Acute traumatic aortic rupture: a comparison of surgical and stent-graft repair. J Thorac Cardiovasc Surg 2005;129(5):1050–5.
[25] Ott MC, Stewart TC, Lawlor DK, et al. Management of blunt thoracic aortic injuries: endovascular stents versus open repair. J Trauma 2004;56(3):565–70.
[26] Midgley PI, Mackenzie KS, Corriveau MM, et al. Blunt thoracic aortic injury: a single institution comparison of open and endovascular management. J Vasc Surg 2007;46(4): 662–8.
[27] Moainie SL, Neschis DG, Gammie JS, et al. Endovascular stenting for traumatic aortic injury: an emerging new standard of care. Ann Thorac Surg 2008;85(5):1625–9 [discussion: 1629–30].
[28] Tang GL, Tehrani HY, Usman A, et al. Reduced mortality, paraplegia, and stroke with stent graft repair of blunt aortic transections: a modern meta-analysis. J Vasc Surg 2008;47(3): 671–5.
[29] Xenos ES, Abedi NN, Davenport DL, et al. Meta-analysis of endovascular vs open repair for traumatic descending thoracic aortic rupture. J Vasc Surg 2008;48(5):1343–51.

Advances in Surgery 44 (2010) 293–311
ADVANCES IN SURGERY

Update on Familial Pancreatic Cancer

Ralph H. Hruban, MD[a,b,*], Marcia I. Canto, MD, MHS[b,c], Michael Goggins, MD[a,b,c], Richard Schulick, MD, PhD[b,d], Alison P. Klein, PhD[a,b,e]

[a]Department of Pathology, The Sol Goldman Pancreatic Cancer Research Center, The Johns Hopkins University School of Medicine, 401 North Broadway, Weinberg 2242, Baltimore, MD 21231, USA
[b]Department of Oncology, The Sol Goldman Pancreatic Cancer Research Center, The Johns Hopkins University School of Medicine, 401 North Broadway, Weinberg 2242, Baltimore, MD 21231, USA
[c]Department of Gastroenterology, The Sol Goldman Pancreatic Cancer Research Center, The Johns Hopkins University School of Medicine, 1830 East Monument Street, Room 427, Baltimore, MD 21205, USA
[d]Department of Surgery, The Sol Goldman Pancreatic Cancer Research Center, The Johns Hopkins University School of Medicine, 600 North Wolfe Street, Blalock 685, Baltimore, MD 21287, USA
[e]Department of Epidemiology, Bloomberg School of Public Health, The Johns Hopkins University, 615 North Wolfe Street, Baltimore, MD 21205, USA

Approximately 10% of pancreatic cancers may have a familial basis [1,2]. Individuals with a family history of pancreatic cancer have an increased risk of developing pancreatic and extrapancreatic malignancies, and an individual's risk of developing pancreatic cancer can be quantified based on their family cancer history [1,3,4].

Although some of the aggregation of pancreatic cancer in families is due to chance, and some to shared environmental exposures such as cigarette smoking, much of this aggregation has a genetic basis [5]. Several of the genes responsible for the familial clustering of pancreatic cancer have been discovered. For example, germline mutations in the *BRCA2* gene cause familial breast cancer, and individuals with germline *BRCA2* gene mutations have an approximately 3.5-fold increased risk of pancreatic cancer [6–12]. Germline mutations in the *p16/CDKN2A* gene cause the familial atypical multiple mole melanoma (FAMMM) syndrome, and these individuals have a 13- to 37-fold increased risk of pancreatic cancer [10,13–23]. Inherited mutations in the *STK11* gene cause the Peutz-Jeghers syndrome, and individuals with Peutz-Jeghers have a 130-fold increased risk of pancreatic cancer [24–30]. The discovery of these

*Corresponding author. Department of Pathology, The Johns Hopkins Hospital, The Sol Goldman Pancreatic Cancer Research Center, Weinberg 2242, 401 North Broadway, Baltimore, MD 21231. *E-mail address:* rhruban@jhmi.edu.

0065-3411/10/$ – see front matter
doi:10.1016/j.yasu.2010.05.011

familial pancreatic cancer genes has helped identify cellular pathways important for the development of pancreatic cancer, it has provided a basis for genetic counseling of individuals with a family history of pancreatic cancer, and it has established a foundation for prioritizing patients for screening for early preinvasive disease [21,29,31–33]. In addition, the discovery of familial pancreatic cancer genes has also led to the development of gene-specific therapies, as shown by the remarkable sensitivity of pancreatic cancers harboring mutations in the *BRCA2* gene to poly[ADP-ribose] polymerase (PARP) inhibitors and to mitomycin C [34–41].

Familial pancreatic cancer and whole genome sequencing are timely topics. For example, this year the *PALB2* gene was discovered to be a familial pancreatic cancer susceptibility gene through complete, unbiased, sequencing of all of the protein-coding genes in a single patient's cancer [42,43]. As the speed of next-generation sequencing technologies increases and the costs decrease, the discovery of several new familial pancreatic cancer genes can be foreseen in the coming years.

The known genetic syndromes account for less than 20% of the observed familial aggregation of pancreatic cancer, and the discovery of additional familial pancreatic cancer genes remains one of the most exciting opportunities in pancreatic cancer research [1,2]. As these genes are discovered, the challenge will be to use these scientific breakthroughs to improve clinical care.

USING FAMILY HISTORY TO ASSESS CANCER RISK

As recognition that pancreatic cancer aggregates in families grows, more and more surgeons are being asked by their patients: "*I have a family history of pancreatic cancer, what is my risk of developing cancer?*" A body of evidence-based medicine has been developed to answer this question, and it is clear that individuals with a family history of pancreatic cancer have an increased risk of pancreatic and of extrapancreatic malignancies [4,44,45].

Family history and pancreatic cancer

Several large epidemiologic studies have established that a family history of pancreatic cancer increases one's risk of developing the disease [4,44,46–52]. For example, Amundadottir and colleagues [44] correlated the risk of a variety of cancers with family cancer history by linking the Iceland Cancer Registry with the deCODE genealogic database. A first-degree relationship is a parent-child or sibling-sibling relationship, and Icelanders with a first-degree family relative with pancreatic cancer had a 2.33-fold increased risk of developing pancreatic cancer themselves [44]. Similar observations have been made in a large number of case-control and cohort studies, and it is now clear that having a single close relative with pancreatic cancer doubles one's risk of developing the disease [4,44,46–52].

Klein and colleagues [4] extended these analyses by prospectively following thousands of patients with a family history of pancreatic cancer. Individuals with 2 first-degree relatives with pancreatic cancer had a 6-fold increased risk of developing pancreatic cancer, and individuals with 3 or more first-degree relatives with pancreatic cancer had a 14- to 32-fold increased risk [4]. Using these and other data, Wang and colleagues [3] have developed a risk prediction tool, called PancPRO, that can be used to quantify an individual's risk of developing pancreatic cancer based on their family history of pancreatic cancer. PancPRO is available free online (http://astor.som.jhmi.edu/BayesMendel/pancpro.html, accessed September 1, 2009) and can be used to answer the question posed earlier by our hypothetical patient. Fig. 1 shows 3 pedigrees of similar structure but differing family histories of pancreatic cancer. The counselee shown with an arrow in Fig. 1A is predicted to have a 3.3% chance of developing pancreatic cancer by the age of 70 years. This risk increases to ~7% if this patient's mother rather than his/her maternal aunt had a history pancreatic cancer (Fig. 1B) or if his/her brother also has a history of pancreatic cancer (Fig. 1C) [3]. Without knowing the gene responsible for the aggregation of pancreatic cancer in a family, clinicians can still provide their patients with quantitative estimates of their absolute lifetime pancreatic cancer risks.

It is important to put this risk in perspective, because the average patient may be unduly alarmed by relative risks. Pancreatic cancer is a rare disease, averaging 9 per 100,000 per year in the United States [53]. A relative risk (RR) of 2 increases an individual's risk to ~18 per 100,000 per year, less than a fiftieth of 1 percent per year. This incidence increases with age, particularly after the age of 50 years, culminating in a lifetime risk of developing pancreatic cancer of 1%. Contrast this with the risk of a woman developing breast cancer. The National Cancer Institute estimates that 12.7% of women born in the United States today will develop breast cancer at some time in their lives. Even having a 2-fold increased risk of developing pancreatic cancer, most patients with a family history of pancreatic cancer will not develop the disease themselves. For this reason it is important to explain relative and absolute risks to patients.

Family history and extrapancreatic malignancies

The risk of cancer is not confined to one organ in most familial cancer syndromes [45,54,55]. For example, patients with hereditary nonpolyposis colorectal cancer (HNPCC) syndrome have an increased risk of developing cancer of the colorectum, endometrium, ovary, stomach, ureter, renal pelvis, and pancreas [56]. Epidemiologic studies have recently shown that the same is true for familial pancreatic cancer; patients with a family history of pancreatic cancer have an increased risk of extrapancreatic malignancies [45,54,55]. Wang and colleagues [45] followed families enrolled in the National Familial Pancreas Tumor Registry (http://pathology.jhu.edu/pancreas/nfptr) and found that overall cancer mortality is increased in the members of sporadic pancreatic cancer kindreds (defined as at least a single pancreatic cancer in the kindred, but not an affected pair of first-degree relatives; RR 1.55, 95% confidence interval [CI] 1.39–1.73) and in familial pancreatic cancer kindreds (defined as a family with at least a pair of first-degree relatives with pancreatic cancer; RR 1.41, 95% CI

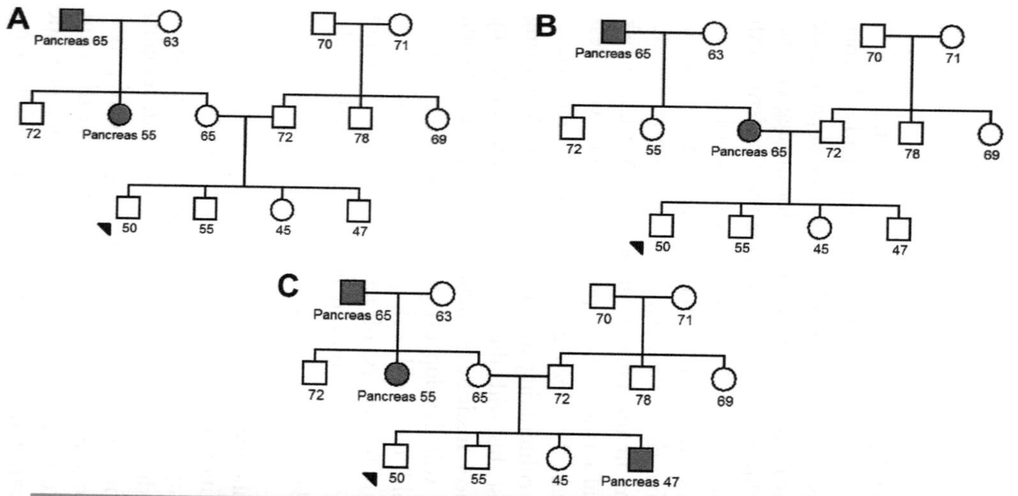

Pedigree	Carrier Probability	Proband's Estimated Risk of Pancreatic Cancer by age 60	70	80
A	22%	1.2%	3.3%	5.3%
B	44%	2.4%	6.6%	10.1%
C	49%	2.6%	7.3%	11.1%
General Population*	0.7%	0.14%	0.46%	0.93%

*Devcan Version 6.4.0, April 2009, National Cancer Institute (http://srab.cancer.gov/devcan/).
Source: SEER 17 areas (San Francisco, Connecticut, Detroit, Hawaii, Iowa, New Mexico, Seattle, Utah, Atlanta, San Jose-Monterey, Los Angeles, Alaska Native Registry, Rural Georgia, California excluding SF/SJM/LA, Kentucky, Louisiana and New Jersey).

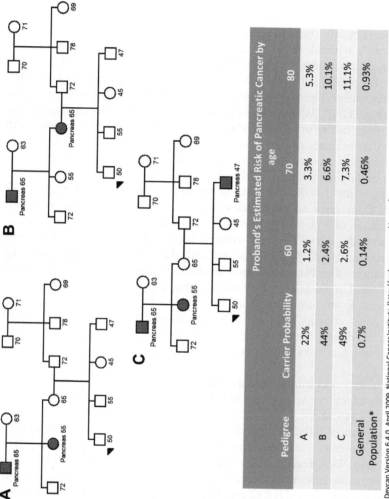

Fig. 1. Three pedigrees with different risks of pancreatic cancer: one of the counselees (*A, arrow*) is predicted to have a 3.3% chance of developing pancreatic cancer by the age of 70 years. This risk increases to ~7% if the patient's mother, rather than his/her maternal aunt had a history of pancreatic cancer (*B*) or if his/her brother also has a history of pancreatic cancer (*C*).

1.26–1.58). Relatives of patients with familial pancreatic cancer had an increased risk of dying from breast cancer (RR 1.66, 95% CI 1.15–2.34), ovarian (RR 2.05, 95% CI 1.10–3.49), and bile duct cancers (RR 2.89, 95% CI 1.04–6.39) [45].

In addition to the associations identified without knowledge of the gene involved, as noted earlier, several known genetic syndromes increase the risk of pancreatic and extrapancreatic malignancies (Table 1). For example, individuals with Peutz-Jeghers syndrome have an increased risk of developing cancers of esophagus, stomach, small intestine, colon, pancreas, breast, lung, ovary, and uterus [27,28]. Similarly, a personal history of young-onset breast cancer with or without a family history of pancreatic cancer (particularly in patients with Ashkenazi Jewish ancestry) could suggest the presence of a familial breast-ovarian cancer syndrome involving one of the breast cancer–related genes (*BRCA1* or *BRCA2*). These genes, particularly *BRCA2*, are associated with a high risk of breast, ovarian, and prostate cancer and moderate risk for pancreatic cancer [6–12]. Surgeons should be aware that patients with a strong family history of pancreatic cancer are at higher risk for developing extrapancreatic malignancies.

Intraductal papillary mucinous neoplasms and extrapancreatic neoplasms

Intraductal papillary mucinous neoplasms (IPMNs) are precursors to invasive pancreatic cancer, and patients with an IPMN have an increased risk of developing invasive pancreatic cancer [53]. Patients with a personal history of IPMN also have an increased risk of developing an extrapancreatic neoplasm. Excess rates of gastric and colonic epithelial neoplasms have been reported in patients with IPMNs [57–60]. This finding suggests the possibility of a common predisposing genetic susceptibility, but no specific hereditary syndrome linking IPMNs with gastric and colonic neoplasms has been established.

Individuals with a family history of pancreatic cancer, as well as those with a personal history of an IPMN, have an increased risk of developing pancreatic and selected extrapancreatic malignancies. These findings have two immediate implications for surgeons. First, a good family cancer history should be obtained from all patients. Do not simply document whether a patient has a family history of cancer; carefully document which family members have had cancer, which types of cancer they have had, and how each affected individual is related to the patient. Second, as discussed in detail later in this review, knowledge of these increased risks can help guide clinical management.

FAMILIAL PANCREATIC CANCER GENES

We have handled the question of risk assessment using family cancer history, but in most instances an individual's family cancer history is, at best, just a surrogate for gene status, and determining the specific gene responsible for a given patient's cancer can have significant clinical implications. A patient

Table 1
Syndromes associated with pancreatic cancer

Genetic syndrome	Gene(s)	Increased risk of pancreatic cancer	Risk of pancreatic cancer by age 70 y (%)	Other malignancies
No family history	None	RR = 1	0.5	None
Two first-degree relatives with pancreatic cancer	Unknown in most cases	6-fold	3	Breast, ovarian, and bile duct
Hereditary breast and ovarian cancer	*BRCA2, FANC-C, FANC-G, PALB2*	3.5-fold to 10-fold	2–5	Breast, ovarian, prostate
FAMMM	*p16/CDKN2A*	9-fold to 47-fold	5–24	Melanoma
Three or more first-degree relatives with pancreatic cancer	Unknown in most cases	14- to 32-fold	7–16	Breast, ovarian, and bile duct
Familial pancreatitis	*PRSS1, SPINK1*	50- to 80-fold	25–40	None
Peutz-Jeghers	*STK11*	132-fold	60	Small intestine, lung, esophagus, stomach, breast, lung, uterus, ovary

Abbreviation: FAMMM, familial atypical multiple mole melanoma.

might come to the office and ask "*I have a family history of pancreatic cancer; can I undergo genetic testing, and, if so, for which genes?*"

Although we believe that this question is often best answered by a trained cancer genetic counselor (see www.nsgc.org to find a local genetic counselor), it is important for surgeons to know the major genes responsible for the familial aggregation of pancreatic cancer (see Table 1).

BRCA2 and other fanconi anemia pathway genes

BRCA2 is probably the best characterized of all of the familial pancreatic cancer genes. Germline (inherited) mutations in the *BRCA2* gene increase the risk of breast, ovarian and prostate cancer, and increase the risk of pancreatic cancer 3.5- to 10-fold [6–12]. Although breast cancer develops in most families with a *BRCA2* gene mutation, the absence of breast cancer in a family should not be used to exclude germline *BRCA2* mutations, because Goggins and colleagues [8] reported that pancreatic cancer can run in *BRCA2* gene mutation–carrying families without an apparent association with breast cancer. Germline *BRCA2* mutations are particularly common in individuals of Ashkenazi Jewish heritage [61–65]. It has been calculated that 1% of the Ashkenazi Jewish population carries a germline *BRCA2* gene mutation, the 6174delT mutation, and these individuals, in addition to an increased risk of breast, ovarian and prostate cancer, have a 10-fold increased risk of developing pancreatic cancer [61–65]. Individuals without a Jewish heritage can also carry a germline *BRCA2* gene mutation, but these mutations are more widely distributed throughout the gene and, overall, it is estimated that only 1 in every 400 to 800 individuals carries a mutation in *BRCA2* [66].

Clinical genetic testing for germline *BRCA2* gene mutations is commercially available through Myriad Genetics (http://www.myriad.com/products/bracanalysis.php). Testing should be considered in patients with a strong family history of pancreatic cancer, especially if the patient or other family members have been diagnosed with bilateral or young age of onset breast or ovarian cancer, and if the individual is of Ashkenazi Jewish heritage. A clinical tool is available to help clinicians identify who would best benefit from genetic testing for *BRCA2* gene mutations (http://astor.som.jhmi.edu/BayesMendel/brcapro.html), but this model does not include pancreatic or prostate cancers as a risk criterion.

The protein product of the *BRCA2* gene functions in the same DNA repair pathway as the Fanconi anemia proteins to repair DNA cross-linking damage [67]. Germline mutations in genes coding for other members of the pathway, including *FANC-C* and *FANC-G*, have also been linked to the familial clustering of pancreatic cancer [67,68]. Germline *BRCA1* gene mutations have been reported in only a few patients with familial pancreatic cancer [69–72].

Most recently, the *PALB2* gene has been discovered to be a familial pancreatic cancer gene [42]. The *PALB2* gene codes for a protein that binds to the Brca2 protein and helps to localize Brca2, and possibly also Brca1, to the nucleus [73]. Indeed, PALB2 stands for partner and localizer of BRCA2. Jones and colleagues [42] discovered that *PALB2* is a familial pancreatic cancer gene by sequencing all of the genes in a pancreatic cancer from a single patient with familial pancreatic cancer. This achievement highlights the potential of whole genome sequencing to discover the causes of inherited diseases. The *PALB2* gene finding has been confirmed, and *PALB2* seems to account for 1% to 3% of familial pancreatic cancer [42,43].

The *BRCA2* gene story provides several important lessons. First, as noted earlier, many familial cancer genes do not increase the risk of just 1 cancer type. Germline *BRCA2* gene mutations increase the risk of breast, ovarian, prostate, and pancreatic cancer [6,66,74–77]. Once the gene is found in a family, lives can be saved by screening gene carriers for these extrapancreatic neoplasms and, in selected cases, by prophylactic surgery [6,66,74–77]. Second, *BRCA2* shows that, once a gene is found and its function determined, then genes coding for other members of the same pathway can be screened to see whether they also contribute to familial pancreatic cancer. Germline mutations in 4 members of the Fanconi anemia pathway, *BRCA2*, *FANC-C*, *FANC-G*, and *PALB2*, can cause familial pancreatic cancer [42,43,67,68]. As is discussed in greater detail later, *BRCA2* gene mutations are also an example of the potential power of gene-specific therapies [34–41].

p16/CDKN2A and FAMMM

Germline mutations in the *p16/CDKN2A* gene cause about 30% to 40% of FAMMM syndrome, a syndrome characterized my multiple nevi, multiple atypical nevi, and an increased risk of melanoma (Fig. 2). Patients with FAMMM caused by *p16/CDKN2A* gene mutations also have a 9-fold to 47-fold increased risk of developing pancreatic cancer [10,13–23,78]. For example, de Snoo and colleagues [17] studied 22 families with the *p16*-Leiden founder mutation who had attended a surveillance clinic, and found that

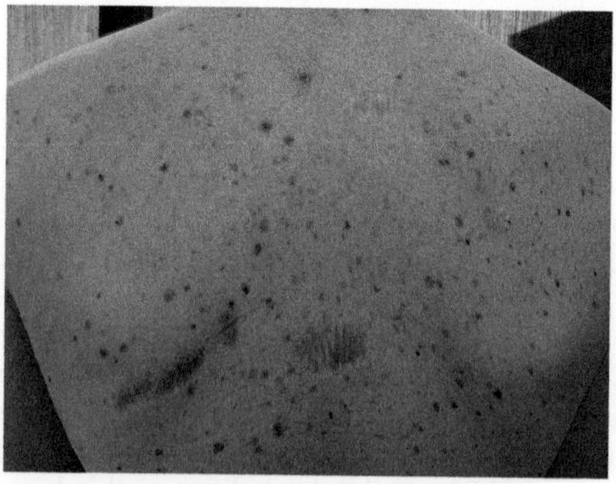

Fig. 2. Familial atypical multiple mole melanoma syndrome: this patient has multiple melanocytic nevi, some of which were atypical. Note the surgical scars. (*Courtesy of* Dr Rhoda M. Alani.)

carriers of the mutation have a 47-fold increased risk of developing pancreatic cancer (RR 46.6, 95% CI 24.7–76.4). Similarly, Lynch and colleagues [21] followed 8 families with the FAMMM and pancreatic carcinoma in concert with a germline *p16/CDKN2A* mutation and reported 4 incidences of melanoma and pancreatic carcinoma as double primaries in the same individuals. It is important to recognize the FAMMM syndrome because lives can be saved by screening at-risk individuals for extrapancreatic neoplasms, in this case atypical nevi and early curable melanomas [79].

STK11 and the Peutz-Jeghers syndrome

The Peutz-Jeghers syndrome is an autosomal dominant syndrome characterized by melanocytic macules on the lips and buccal mucosa, and hamartomatous polyps of the gastrointestinal tract (Fig. 3) [24–30]. In addition to gastrointestinal and breast cancer, patients with the Peutz-Jeghers syndrome have a high risk of developing pancreatic cancer [24–30]. An obligate carrier of the gene developed pancreatic cancer in the kindred first described by Jeghers and colleagues [80]. Hearle and colleagues [28] reported that 80% of *STK11* mutation carriers develop cancer by the age of 60 years, and Giardiello and colleagues [26,27] reported that patients with the syndrome have a 132-fold increased risk of developing pancreatic cancer (CI 44, 261). The extremely high risk of pancreatic cancer in patients with the Peutz-Jeghers syndrome highlights the clinical need to develop effective screening tests for early curable pancreatic neoplasia in at-risk patients [24–30].

A first step in screening patients with the Peutz-Jeghers syndrome for curable disease will be to characterize the lesions that precede the development of invasive cancer in these patients. Preliminary analyses correlating histopathology with genetics have shown that some patients with Peutz-Jeghers develop IPMNs as the result of their genetic defect [30,81]. Because IPMNs typically grow to several centimeters in size before they invade, these data suggest that some curable pancreatic precursor lesions should be detectable and treatable in patients with Peutz-Jeghers.

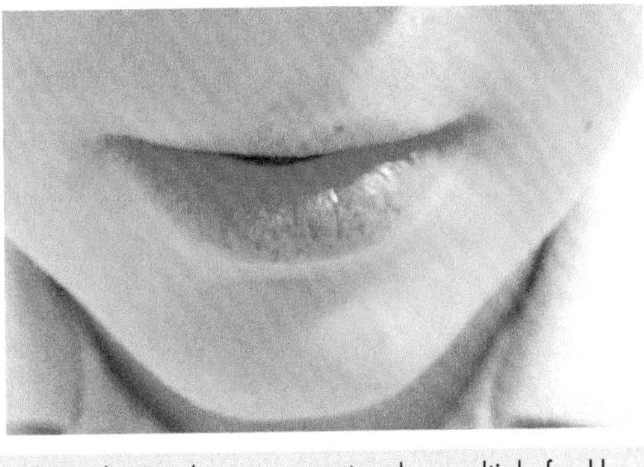

Fig. 3. Peutz-Jeghers syndrome: this young patient has multiple freckles on his lips. These may fade with age. (*Courtesy of* Dr Francis Giardiello.)

PRSS1, *SPINK1*, and familial pancreatitis

Familial pancreatitis, also known as hereditary pancreatitis, is characterized by recurrent episodes of severe acute pancreatitis starting at a young age [82]. Most patients ultimately develop chronic pancreatitis. Germline mutations in the *PRSS1* and *SPINK1* genes have been shown to cause familial pancreatitis [83–85]. Germline mutations in *PRSS1* lead to an autosomal dominant form of inheritance [85]. Germline mutations in *SPINK1* increase the risk of developing pancreatitis, but the RR is small (2- to 5-fold) and most patients with *SPINK1* mutations never develop pancreatitis [86]. Patients with familial pancreatitis have as high as a 40% lifetime risk of developing pancreatic cancer [87,88]. As is discussed in greater detail later, some of these patients elect to have prophylactic pancreatectomy.

Other genes

Linkage analyses have suggested that chromosome 4q may harbor a pancreatic cancer susceptibility gene, and Pogue-Geile and colleagues [89] suggested that this gene is palladin (*PALLD*). However, follow-up studies on *PALLD* have failed to confirm that it is a significant familial pancreatic cancer gene [90–94].

The familial adenomatous polyposis (FAP) syndrome is characterized by the development of more than 100 adenomatous polyps of the colon [95]. The small bowel can also be affected. It has been suggested that patients with FAP have an increased risk of pancreatic cancer, but some of the apparent increased risk may simply be the result of misclassification of duodenal adenocarcinomas as pancreatic primaries [95].

HNPCC syndrome is characterized by early-onset colon cancer and an increased risk of carcinomas of the endometrium, ovary, bile duct, kidney, bladder, ureter, and skin [96]. HNPCC is caused by inherited mutations in one of the DNA mismatch repair genes, including *hMSH2*, *hMLH1*, *hPMS1*, *hPMS2*, and *hMSH6*/*GTBP* [1]. There have been several case reports of patients with HNPCC developing pancreatic cancer, but the exact contribution of HNPCC to the familial clustering of pancreatic cancer is poorly defined [1,97,98].

Although genetic testing may be of benefit to many families, the genetic basis of more than 80% of the clustering of pancreatic cancer in families remains unknown. Many families with an aggregation of pancreatic cancer may harbor mutations in yet-to-be-identified genes and they will not be found to carry mutations in the genes mentioned earlier. Mutations in the *BRCA2* gene account for 6% to 12% of families with at least 2 pancreatic cancers, *PALB2* 1% to 3%, and the remaining genes account for less than 1% of familial pancreatic cancer.

THERAPEUTIC IMPLICATIONS

So far, this review has quantified the risk of pancreatic cancer and identified some of the genes responsible for familial pancreatic cancer. However, there is a third question from our hypothetical patient: "*I have a germline mutation in a cancer predisposition gene; can this knowledge be used to guide my treatment?*" The answer depends on the patient's specific gene mutation.

Targeting *BRCA2* gene mutations

BRCA2-targeted therapies show that the discovery of a familial pancreatic cancer gene can lead to the development of gene-specific therapies. In the laboratory, pancreatic cancer cell lines harboring biallelic mutations in the *BRCA2* gene are extremely sensitive to mitomycin C and to PARP inhibitors [34–41]. These drugs target the pathway controlling repair of DNA cross-linking damage, which is inactivated in *BRCA2* mutant cells [34–41]. Normal cells, with a functional copy of the *BRCA2* gene, can repair the DNA injury caused by these agents, whereas cancer cells with biallelic inactivating mutations in the *BRCA2* gene do not produce functional Brca2 protein and cannot repair the damage from these agents [34–41]. The cancer cells are killed, whereas the normal cells survive. These results in the laboratory are now being translated to the clinic, and there are several reports of significant clinical responses in patients with *BRCA2* mutant cancers [34–41]. These findings suggest a scenario in which a patient's genotype can be used to identify the most effective therapy for that patient.

Prophylactic surgery in patients with familial pancreatitis

The increased risk of cancer in patients with familial pancreatitis is confined to the pancreas, and many patients with familial pancreatitis have severe exocrine and endocrine pancreatic insufficiency [87,88]. Some of these patients therefore consider prophylactic total pancreatectomy [99–101]. Although this surgery will eliminate the patient's significant risk of developing pancreatic cancer, the benefit of prophylactic surgery has to be weighed against the significant risks of total pancreatectomy [101]. The main complication of total pancreatectomy is brittle diabetes and, although there is now increasing experience in managing diabetes after total pancreatectomy, there is an increased risk of morbidity and mortality associated with this surgery [99,100,102–104]. Some have considered the option of islet autotransplantation, but the cell of origin for pancreatic cancer is not known, and the risk of autotransplanting a potential neoplastic cell remains a theoretical concern [99,100,102–104].

As more familial pancreatic cancer genes are discovered, genetic testing might eventually be used routinely to determine an individual's risk and to guide therapy should they develop disease.

SCREENING FOR EARLY NEOPLASIA

Our hypothetical patient, recognizing the value of prevention, next asks: "*I have seen several of my family members die of pancreatic cancer, and I do not want to suffer the same fate. Are any screening tests available?*" There are no clinically proven effective screening tests available for the early detection of pancreatic cancer at this time. Serum CA19–9 levels have been suggested as a possible test, but the assay lacks the sensitivity and specificity needed to screen for pancreatic cancer [105].

However, several screening tests are being evaluated in clinical trials, and several approaches hold promise.

Canto and colleagues [31,106] studied endoscopic ultrasound (EUS) as a screening test for asymptomatic members of at-risk families. This trial, called Cancer of the Pancreas Screening (CAPS), screened asymptomatic patients with a strong family history of pancreatic cancer, as well as asymptomatic patients with the Peutz-Jeghers syndrome. Almost 10% of the asymptomatic individuals screened were found to have a lesion in their pancreas that resulted in surgery [31,106]. Most of these lesions were IPMNs, and one-fourth of the precursors discovered on screening had significant dysplasia (carcinoma in situ), showing that curable precancerous lesions can be detected and treated in asymptomatic at-risk individuals [31,106–108]. Other groups using EUS-based or abdominal magnetic resonance imaging (MRI) to screen individuals with multiple affected family members or germline mutation carriers have also detected and treated IPMNs, pancreatic intraepithelial neoplasia (PanIN), and invasive pancreatic ductal adenocarcinomas [109,110]. A group in The Netherlands recently reported a low diagnostic yield for screening for pancreatic neoplasia, but the study included subjects in a lower-risk population with only 2 affected relatives [111]. Clearly, identifying the correct group to screen is a critical first step in developing an effective screening test.

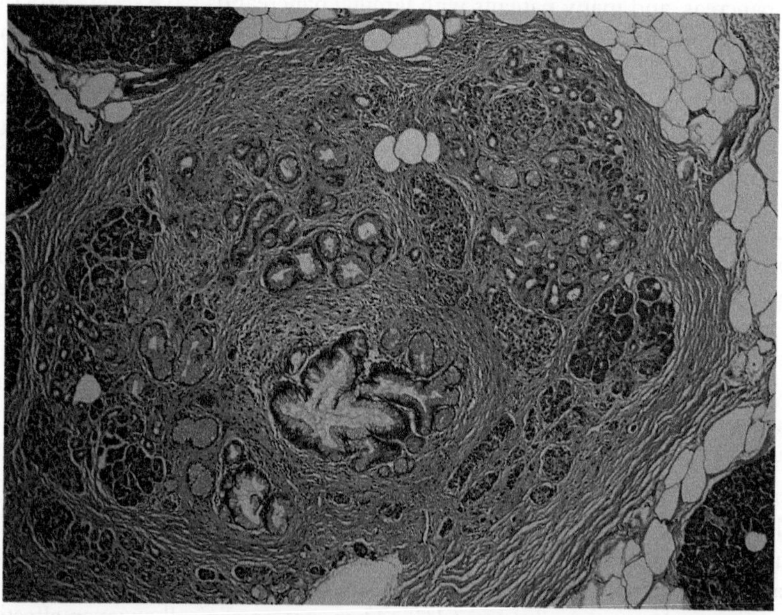

Fig. 4. Lobulocentric atrophy associated with PanIN lesion. The lobule of pancreatic parenchyma surrounding this small PanIN lesion is remarkable for fibrosis and acinar dropout.

The screening and surgical resection of early curable neoplasms in at-risk individuals in the CAPS and other similar trials has also provided a unique opportunity for pathologists to study the morphology of unadulterated precursor lesions in individuals with a strong family history of pancreatic cancer [108,112]. Three observations can be drawn from these morphologic studies. First, PanINs are often associated with lobulocentric atrophy (Fig. 4) [111]. Although PanIN lesions are small, most are associated with larger areas of lobulocentric atrophy and fibrosis [112]. Second, PanINs in patients with a strong family history of pancreatic cancer are often multifocal [112]. As many as 20% of the smaller ducts in some patients contain PanIN lesions [112]. Third, the combination of lobulocentric atrophy and multifocality of PanIN often produces grossly appreciable changes in the pancreas, and these changes can be detected by EUS [112–114]. Although single PanIN lesions are almost always too small to be appreciated grossly, larger PanINs (2–5 mm) can be seen by EUS as anechoic nonseptated lesions, often indistinguishable from saccular dilatations of branch ducts along the main duct or small branch duct IPMNs. Multifocal PanINs, together with their multiple foci of associated lobulocentric atrophy, produce a mosaic of fibrosis, atrophy, and uninvolved parenchyma, changes that are similar to chronic pancreatitis [112]. These changes are often detectable by EUS using standard criteria for the diagnosis of chronic pancreatitis, such as heterogeneous parenchyma, multifocal lobularity, and dilated main and branch pancreatic ducts [112,114].

Thus, although there are no clinically proven effective methods to screen at-risk individuals for early pancreatic neoplasia, several EUS-based studies have established that it is possible, in principle, to detect curable pancreatic neoplasms in asymptomatic at-risk patients. As the resolution of imaging improves and as our knowledge of precursor lesions grows, we believe that multifocal PanIN lesions will be detectable in clinical practice.

THE FUTURE

The coming year will see an expansion of our understanding of familial pancreatic cancer. Next-generation sequencing will allow researchers to sequence candidate familial pancreatic cancer genes on a scale unimaginable just a few years ago. Investigators at Johns Hopkins University are planning to sequence the coding genomes of a series of patients with familial pancreatic cancer. The resultant information will offer unparalleled opportunities to improve patient care. Investigators at Johns Hopkins have also formed an international screening and surveillance consortium involving 25 countries from North America, Europe, Australia, and Asia. It is hoped that this consortium will define the best methods to assess pancreatic cancer risk, increase our understanding of the natural history of apparently benign precancerous neoplasms, and define the survival benefit, if any, of treating premalignant neoplasms in high-risk individuals.

Surgeons will be at the forefront of this progress, translating these advances to patient care. Surgical management will not simply be operating to resect a well-defined, but incurable, invasive carcinoma. An integration of clinical history, family cancer history, gene status, imaging, and surgical skill will be needed to identify and treat early curable pancreatic neoplasia.

References

[1] Shi C, Hruban RH, Klein AP. Familial pancreatic cancer. Arch Pathol Lab Med 2009;133(3):365–74.
[2] Permuth-Wey J, Egan KM. Family history is a significant risk factor for pancreatic cancer: results from a systematic review and meta-analysis. Fam Cancer 2009;8(2):109–17.
[3] Wang W, Chen S, Brune KA, et al. PancPRO: risk assessment in individuals with a family history of pancreatic cancer. J Clin Oncol 2007;25(11):1417–22.
[4] Klein AP, Brune KA, Petersen GM, et al. Prospective risk of pancreatic cancer in familial pancreatic cancer kindreds. Cancer Res 2004;64(7):2634–8.
[5] Klein AP, Beaty TH, Bailey-Wilson JE, et al. Evidence for a major gene influencing risk of pancreatic cancer. Genet Epidemiol 2002;23(2):133–49.
[6] Cancer risks in BRCA2 mutation carriers. The Breast Cancer Linkage Consortium. J Natl Cancer Inst 1999;91(15):1310–6.
[7] Couch FJ, Johnson MR, Rabe KG, et al. The prevalence of BRCA2 mutations in familial pancreatic cancer. Cancer Epidemiol Biomarkers Prev 2007;16(2):342–6.
[8] Goggins M, Schutte M, Lu J, et al. Germline BRCA2 gene mutations in patients with apparently sporadic pancreatic carcinomas. Cancer Res 1996;56:5360–4.
[9] Hahn SA, Greenhalf B, Ellis I, et al. BRCA2 germline mutations in familial pancreatic carcinoma. J Natl Cancer Inst 2003;95(3):214–21.
[10] Lal G, Liu G, Schmocker B, et al. Inherited predisposition to pancreatic adenocarcinoma: role of family history and germ-line p16, BRCA1, and BRCA2 mutations. Cancer Res 2000;60:409–16.
[11] Murphy KM, Brune KA, Griffin CA, et al. Evaluation of candidate genes MAP2K4, MADH4, ACVR1B, and BRCA2 in familial pancreatic cancer: deleterious BRCA2 mutations in 17%. Cancer Res 2002;62(13):3789–93.
[12] van Asperen CJ, Brohet RM, Meijers-Heijboer EJ, et al. Cancer risks in BRCA2 families: estimates for sites other than breast and ovary. J Med Genet 2005;42(9):711–9.
[13] Gruis NA, Sandkuiji LA, van der Velden PA, et al. CDKN2 explains part of the clinical phenotype in Dutch familial atypical multiple-mole melanoma (FAMMM) syndrome families. Melanoma Res 1995;5:169–77.
[14] Lynch HT, Fusaro RM. Pancreatic cancer and the familial atypical multiple mole melanoma (FAMMM) syndrome. Pancreas 1991;6:127–31.
[15] Bartsch DK, Sina-Frey M, Lang S, et al. CDKN2A germline mutations in familial pancreatic cancer. Ann Surg 2002;236(6):730–7.
[16] Borg A, Sandberg T, Nilsson K, et al. High frequency of multiple melanomas and breast and pancreas carcinomas in CDKN2A mutation-positive melanoma families. J Natl Cancer Inst 2000;92(15):1260–6.
[17] de Snoo FA, Bishop DT, Bergman W, et al. Increased risk of cancer other than melanoma in CDKN2A founder mutation (p16-Leiden)-positive melanoma families. Clin Cancer Res 2008;14(21):7151–7.
[18] de vos tot Nederveen Cappel WH, Offerhaus GJ, van Puijenbroek M, et al. Pancreatic carcinoma in carriers of a specific 19 base pair deletion of CDKN2A/p16 (p16-leiden). Clin Cancer Res 2003;9(10 Pt 1):3598–605.
[19] Goldstein AM, Fraser MC, Struewing JP, et al. Increased risk of pancreatic cancer in melanoma-prone kindreds with p16INK4 mutations. N Engl J Med 1995;333(15):970–4.
[20] Lynch HT, Brand RE, Lynch JF, et al. Genetic counseling and testing for germline p16 mutations in two pancreatic cancer-prone families. Gastroenterology 2000;119(6):1756–60.

[21] Lynch HT, Brand RE, Hogg D, et al. Phenotypic variation in eight extended CDKN2A germline mutation familial atypical multiple mole melanoma-pancreatic carcinoma-prone families: the familial atypical mole melanoma-pancreatic carcinoma syndrome. Cancer 2002;94(1):84–96.
[22] Moskaluk CA, Hruban RH, Lietman AS, et al. Novel germline p16$^{(INK4)}$ allele (Asp145Cys) in a family with multiple pancreatic carcinomas. Mutations in brief no. 148. Online. Hum Mutat 1998;12(1):70–3.
[23] Vasen HF, Gruis NA, Frants RR, et al. Risk of developing pancreatic cancer in families with familial atypical multiple mole melanoma associated with a specific 19 deletion of p16 (p16-Leiden). Int J Cancer 2000;87(6):809–11.
[24] Boardman LA, Thibodeau SN, Schaid DJ, et al. Increased risk for cancer in patients with the Peutz-Jeghers syndrome. Ann Intern Med 1998;128:896–9.
[25] Bowlby LS. Pancreatic adenocarcinoma in an adolescent male with Peutz-Jeghers syndrome. Hum Pathol 1986;17:97–9.
[26] Giardiello FM, Welsh SB, Hamilton SR, et al. Increased risk of cancer in the Peutz-Jeghers syndrome. N Engl J Med 1987;316(24):1511–4.
[27] Giardiello FM, Brensinger JD, Tersmette AC, et al. Very high risk of cancer in familial Peutz-Jeghers syndrome. Gastroenterology 2000;119:1447–53.
[28] Hearle N, Schumacher V, Menko FH, et al. Frequency and spectrum of cancers in the Peutz-Jeghers syndrome. Clin Cancer Res 2006;12(10):3209–15.
[29] Latchford A, Greenhalf W, Vitone LJ, et al. Peutz-Jeghers syndrome and screening for pancreatic cancer. Br J Surg 2006;93(12):1446–55.
[30] Su GH, Hruban RH, Bova GS, et al. Germline and somatic mutations of the STK11/LKB1 Peutz-Jeghers gene in pancreatic and biliary cancers. Am J Pathol 1999;154(6): 1835–40.
[31] Canto MI, Goggins M, Hruban RH, et al. Screening for early pancreatic neoplasia in high-risk individuals: a prospective controlled study. Clin Gastroenterol Hepatol 2006;4(6): 766–81.
[32] Axilbund JE, Brune KA, Canto MI, et al. Patient perspective on the values of genetic counseling for familial pancreatic cancer. Hered Cancer Clin Pract 2005;3(3):115–22.
[33] Kluijt I, Cats A, Fockens P, et al. Atypical familial presentation of FAMMM syndrome with a high incidence of pancreatic cancer: case finding of asymptomatic individuals by EUS surveillance. J Clin Gastroenterol 2009;43(9):853–7.
[34] van der Heijden MS, Brody JR, Dezentje DA, et al. In vivo therapeutic responses contingent on Fanconi anemia/BRCA2 status of the tumor. Clin Cancer Res 2005;11(20):7508–15.
[35] Helleday T, Bryant HE, Schultz N. Poly(ADP-ribose) polymerase (PARP-1) in homologous recombination and as a target for cancer therapy. Cell Cycle 2005;4(9):1176–8.
[36] Bryant HE, Schultz N, Thomas HD, et al. Specific killing of BRCA2-deficient tumours with inhibitors of poly(ADP-ribose) polymerase. Nature 2005;434(7035):913–7.
[37] Donawho CK, Luo Y, Luo Y, et al. ABT-888, an orally active poly(ADP-ribose) polymerase inhibitor that potentiates DNA-damaging agents in preclinical tumor models. Clin Cancer Res 2007;13(9):2728–37.
[38] Abbott DW, Freeman ML, Holt JT. Double-strand break repair deficiency and radiation sensitivity in *BRCA2* mutant cancer cells. J Natl Cancer Inst 1998;90(13):978–85.
[39] Hay T, Jenkins H, Sansom OJ, et al. Efficient deletion of normal Brca2-deficient intestinal epithelium by poly(ADP-ribose) polymerase inhibition models potential prophylactic therapy. Cancer Res 2005;65(22):10145–8.
[40] James E, Waldron-Lynch MG, Saif MW. Prolonged survival in a patient with BRCA2 associated metastatic pancreatic cancer after exposure to camptothecin: a case report and review of literature. Anticancer Drugs 2009;20(7):634–8.
[41] McCabe N, Lord CJ, Tutt AN, et al. BRCA2-deficient CAPAN-1 cells are extremely sensitive to the inhibition of poly(ADP-ribose) polymerase: an issue of potency. Cancer Biol Ther 2005;4(9):934–6.

[42] Jones S, Hruban RH, Kamiyama M, et al. Exomic sequencing identifies PALB2 as a pancreatic cancer susceptibility gene. Science 2009;324(5924):217.
[43] Tischkowitz M, Sabbaghian N, Hamel N, et al. Analysis of the gene coding for the BRCA2-interacting protein PALB2 in familial and sporadic pancreatic cancer. Gastroenterology 2009;137(3):1183–6.
[44] Amundadottir LT, Thorvaldsson S, Gudbjartsson DF, et al. Cancer as a complex phenotype: pattern of cancer distribution within and beyond the nuclear family. PLoS Med 2004;1(3):e65.
[45] Wang L, Brune KA, Visvanathan K, et al. Elevated cancer mortality in the relatives of pancreatic cancer patients. Clin Cancer Res 2009;18(11):2829–34.
[46] Coughlin SS, Calle EE, Patel AV, et al. Predictors of pancreatic cancer mortality among a large cohort of United States adults. Cancer Causes Control 2000;11(10):915–23.
[47] Falk RT, Pickle LW, Fontham ET, et al. Life-style risk factors for pancreatic cancer in Louisana: a case-control study. Am J Epidemiol 1988;128(2):324–36.
[48] Fernandez E, La Vecchia C, D'Avanzo B, et al. Family history and the risk of liver, gallbladder, and pancreatic cancer. Cancer Epidemiol Biomarkers Prev 1994;3:209–12.
[49] Ghadirian P, Boyle P, Simard A, et al. Reported family aggregation of pancreatic cancer within a population-based case-control study in the Francophone community in Montreal, Canada. Int J Pancreatol 1991;10:183–96.
[50] Hassan MM, Bondy ML, Wolff RA, et al. Risk factors for pancreatic cancer: case-control study. Am J Gastroenterol 2007;102(12):2696–707.
[51] Hemminki K, Li X. Familial and second primary pancreatic cancers: a nationwide epidemiologic study from Sweden. Int J Cancer 2003;103(4):525–30.
[52] Silverman DT, Schiffman M, Everhart J, et al. Diabetes mellitus, other medical conditions and familial history of cancer as risk factors for pancreatic cancer. Br J Cancer 1999;80(11):1830–7.
[53] Hruban RH, Pitman MB, Klimstra DS. Tumors of the pancreas. Atlas of tumor pathology. Fourth Series, Fascicle. 6th edition. Washington, DC: American Registry of Pathology and Armed Forces Institute of Pathology; 2007.
[54] Lumadue JA, Griffin CA, Osman M, et al. Familial pancreatic cancer and the genetics of pancreatic cancer. Surg Clin North Am 1995;75:845–55.
[55] McWilliams RR, Rabe KG, Olswold C, et al. Risk of malignancy in first-degree relatives of patients with pancreatic carcinoma. Cancer 2005;104(2):388–94.
[56] Lynch HT, Lanspa SJ, Smyrk T, et al. Hereditary nonpolyposis colorectal cancer (Lynch syndromes I & II). Genetics, pathology, natural history, and cancer control, part 1. Cancer Genet Cytogenet 1991;53:143–60.
[57] Baumgaertner I, Corcos O, Couvelard A, et al. Prevalence of extrapancreatic cancers in patients with histologically proven intraductal papillary mucinous neoplasms of the pancreas: a case-control study. Am J Gastroenterol 2008;103(11):2878–82.
[58] Sugiyama M, Atomi Y. Extrapancreatic neoplasms occur with unusual frequency in patients with intraductal papillary mucinous tumors of the pancreas. Am J Gastroenterol 1999;94(2):470–3.
[59] Kamisawa T, Tu Y, Egawa N, et al. Malignancies associated with intraductal papillary mucinous neoplasm of the pancreas. World J Gastroenterol 2005;11(36):5688–90.
[60] Eguchi H, Ishikawa O, Ohigashi H, et al. Patients with pancreatic intraductal papillary mucinous neoplasms are at high risk of colorectal cancer development. Surgery 2006;139(6):749–54.
[61] Figer A, Irmin L, Geva R, et al. The rate of the 6174delT founder Jewish mutation in BRCA2 in patients with non-colonic gastrointestinal tract tumours in Israel. Br J Cancer 2001;84(4):478–81.
[62] McClain MR, Nathanson KL, Palomaki GE, et al. An evaluation of BRCA1 and BRCA2 founder mutations penetrance estimates for breast cancer among Ashkenazi Jewish women. Genet Med 2005;7(1):34–9.

[63] Neuhausen S, Gilewski T, Norton L, et al. Recurrent *BRCA2* 6174delT mutations in Ashkenazi Jewish women affected by breast cancer. Nat Genet 1996;13:126–8.
[64] Oddoux C, Struewing JP, Clayton MC, et al. The carrier frequency of the BRCA2 6174delT mutation among Ashkenazi Jewish individuals is approximately 1%. Nat Genet 1996;14:188–90.
[65] Ozcelik H, Schmocker B, DiNicola N, et al. Germline BRCA2 6174delT mutations in Ashkenazi Jewish pancreatic cancer patients. Nat Genet 1997;16:17–8.
[66] Liede A, Karlan BY, Narod SA. Cancer risks for male carriers of germline mutations in BRCA1 or BRCA2: a review of the literature. J Clin Oncol 2004;22(4):735–42.
[67] van der Heijden MS, Yeo CJ, Hruban RH, et al. Fanconi anemia gene mutations in young-onset pancreatic cancer. Cancer Res 2003;63(10):2585–8.
[68] Couch FJ, Johnson MR, Rabe K, et al. Germ line Fanconi anemia complementation group C mutations and pancreatic cancer. Cancer Res 2005;65(2):383–6.
[69] Thompson D, Easton DF. Cancer incidence in BRCA1 mutation carriers. J Natl Cancer Inst 2002;94(18):1358–65.
[70] Al Sukhni W, Rothenmund H, Eppel BA, et al. Germline BRCA1 mutations predispose to pancreatic adenocarcinoma. Hum Genet 2008;124(3):271–8.
[71] Axilbund JE, Argani P, Kamiyama M, et al. Absence of germline BRCA1 mutations in familial pancreatic cancer patients. Cancer Biol Ther 2009;8(2):131–5.
[72] Ford D, Easton DF, Bishop DT, et al. Risks of cancer in BRCA1-mutation carriers. Breast Cancer Linkage Consortium. Lancet 1994;343(8899):692–5.
[73] Zhang F, Ma J, Wu J, et al. PALB2 Links BRCA1 and BRCA2 in the DNA-damage response. Curr Biol 2009;19(6):524–9.
[74] Antoniou AC, Pharoah PD, Narod S, et al. Breast and ovarian cancer risks to carriers of the BRCA1 5382insC and 185delAG and BRCA2 6174delT mutations: a combined analysis of 22 population based studies. J Med Genet 2005;42(7):602–3.
[75] Satagopan JM, Offit K, Foulkes W, et al. The lifetime risks of breast cancer in Ashkenazi Jewish carriers of BRCA1 and BRCA2 mutations. Cancer Epidemiol Biomarkers Prev 2001;10(5):467–73.
[76] Struewing JP, Hartge P, Wacholder S, et al. The risk of cancer associated with specific mutations of BRCA1 and BRCA2 among Ashkenazi Jews. N Engl J Med 1997;336:1401–8.
[77] Tulinius H, Olafsdottir GH, Sigvaldason H, et al. The effect of a single BRCA2 mutation on cancer in Iceland. J Med Genet 2002;39(7):457–62.
[78] Goldstein AM, Chan M, Harland M, et al. High-risk melanoma susceptibility genes and pancreatic cancer, neural system tumors, and uveal melanoma across GenoMEL. Cancer Res 2006;66(20):9818–28.
[79] Mesters I, Jonkman L, Vasen H, et al. Skin self-examination of persons from families with familial atypical multiple mole melanoma (FAMMM). Patient Educ Couns 2009;75(2):251–5.
[80] Jeghers H, McKusick VA, Katz KH. Generalized intestinal polyposis and melanin spots of the oral mucosa, lips and digits. N Engl J Med 1949;241(25):992–1005.
[81] Sato N, Rosty C, Jansen M, et al. STK11/LKB1 Peutz-Jeghers gene inactivation in intraductal papillary-mucinous neoplasms of the pancreas. Am J Pathol 2001;159(6):2017–22.
[82] Gorry MC, Gabbaizedeh D, Furey W, et al. Mutations in the cationic trypsinogen gene are associated with recurrent acute and chronic pancreatitis. Gastroenterology 1997;113(4):1063–8.
[83] Witt H, Luck W, Hennies HC, et al. Mutations in the gene encoding the serine protease inhibitor, Kazal type 1 are associated with chronic pancreatitis. Nat Genet 2000;25(2):213–6.
[84] las Heras-Castano G, Castro-Senosiain B, Fontalba A, et al. Hereditary pancreatitis: clinical features and inheritance characteristics of the R122C mutation in the cationic trypsinogen gene (PRSS1) in six Spanish families. JOP 2009;10(3):249–55.

[85] Whitcomb DC, Gorry MC, Preston RA, et al. Hereditary pancreatitis is caused by a mutation in the cationic trypsinogen gene. Nat Genet 1996;14:141–5.
[86] Schneider A, Suman A, Rossi L, et al. SPINK1/PSTI mutations are associated with tropical pancreatitis and type II diabetes mellitus in Bangladesh. Gastroenterology 2002;123(4): 1026–30.
[87] Lowenfels AB, Maisonneuve P, Cavallini G, et al. Pancreatitis and the risk of pancreatic cancer. International Hereditary Pancreatitis Study Group. N Engl J Med 1993;328: 1433–7.
[88] Lowenfels AB, Maisonneuve EP, Dimagno YE, et al. Hereditary pancreatitis and the risk of pancreatic cancer. International Hereditary Pancreatitis Study Group. J Natl Cancer Inst 1997;89(6):442–6.
[89] Pogue-Geile KL, Chen R, Bronner MP, et al. Palladin mutation causes familial pancreatic cancer and suggests a new cancer mechanism. PLoS Med 2006;3(12):e516.
[90] Earl J, Yan L, Vitone LJ, et al. Evaluation of the 4q32-34 locus in European familial pancreatic cancer. Cancer Epidemiol Biomarkers Prev 2006;15(10):1948–55.
[91] Klein AP, Borges M, Griffith M, et al. Absence of deleterious palladin mutations in patients with familial pancreatic cancer. Cancer Epidemiol Biomarkers Prev 2009;18(4): 1328–30.
[92] Salaria SN, Illei PB, Walter KM, et al. Palladin is overexpressed in the non-neoplastic stroma of infiltrating ductal adenocarcinomas of the pancreas, but is only rarely overexpressed. Cancer Biol Ther 2007;6(3):324–8.
[93] Slater E, Amrillaeva V, Fendrich V, et al. Palladin mutation causes familial pancreatic cancer: absence in European families. PLoS Med 2007;4(4):e164.
[94] Zogopoulous G, Rothenmund H, Eppel A, et al. The P239S palladin variant does not account for a significant fraction of hereditary or early onset pancreas cancer. Hum Genet 2007;121(5):635–7.
[95] Giardiello FM, Offerhaus GJ, Lee DH, et al. Increased risk of thyroid and pancreatic carcinoma in familial adenomatous polyposis. Gut 1993;34:1394–6.
[96] Lynch HT, Smyrk TC, Watson P, et al. Genetics, natural history, tumor spectrum, and pathology of hereditary nonpolyposis colorectal cancer: an updated review. Gastroenterology 1993;104:1535–49.
[97] Lynch HT, Voorhees GJ, Lanspa SJ, et al. Pancreatic carcinoma and hereditary nonpolyposis colorectal cancer: a family study. Br J Cancer 1985;52:271–3.
[98] Kastrinos F, Mukherjee B, Tayob N, et al. Risk of pancreatic cancer in families with Lynch syndrome. JAMA 2009;302(16):1790–5.
[99] Keim V. Identification of patients with genetic risk factors of pancreatitis: impact on treatment and cancer prevention. Dig Dis 2003;21(4):346–50.
[100] Davis B, Lowy AM. Surgical management of hereditary pancreatic cancer. Med Clin North Am 2000;84(3):749–59.
[101] Charpentier KP, Brentnall TA, Bronner MP, et al. A new indication for pancreas transplantation: high grade pancreatic dysplasia. Clin Transplant 2004;18(1):105–7.
[102] Blondet JJ, Carlson AM, Kobayashi T, et al. The role of total pancreatectomy and islet autotransplantation for chronic pancreatitis. Surg Clin North Am 2007;87(6):1477–501, x.
[103] Jethwa P, Sodergren M, Lala A, et al. Diabetic control after total pancreatectomy. Dig Liver Dis 2006;38(6):415–9.
[104] Billings BJ, Christein JD, Harmsen WS, et al. Quality-of-life after total pancreatectomy: is it really that bad on long-term follow-up? J Gastrointest Surg 2005;9(8):1059–66.
[105] Homma T, Tsuchiya R. The study of the mass screening of persons without symptoms and of the screening of outpatients with gastrointestinal complaints or icterus for pancreatic cancer in Japan, using CA19-9 and elastase-1 or ultrasonography. Int J Pancreatol 1991;9:119–24.
[106] Canto MI, Goggins M, Yeo CJ, et al. Screening for pancreatic neoplasia in high-risk individuals: an EUS-based approach. Clin Gastroenterol Hepatol 2004;2(7):606–21.

[107] Rulyak SJ, Kimmey MB, Veenstra DL, et al. Cost-effectiveness of pancreatic cancer screening in familial pancreatic cancer kindreds. Gastrointest Endosc 2003;57(1):23–9.
[108] Brentnall TA, Bronner MP, Byrd DR, et al. Early diagnosis and treatment of pancreatic dysplasia in patients with a family history of pancreatic cancer. Ann Intern Med 1999;131(4):247–55.
[109] Kurtz RC, Simon J, Ludwig E, et al. A pancreatic cancer screening program for familial high-risk individuals [abstract]. Gastroenterology 2007;132(Suppl 2):199.
[110] Poley JW, Kluijt I, Gouma DJ, et al. The yield of first-time endoscopic ultrasonography in screening individuals at a high risk of developing pancreatic cancer. Am J Gastroenterol 2009;104(9):2175–81.
[111] Langer P, Kann PH, Fendrich V, et al. 5 years of prospective screening of high risk individuals from familial pancreatic cancer - families. Gut 2009;58(10):1410–8.
[112] Brune KA, Abe T, Canto MI, et al. Multifocal neoplastic precusor lesions associated with lobular atrophy of the pancreas in patients having a strong family history of pancreatic cancer. Am J Surg Pathol 2006;30(9):1067–76.
[113] Takaori K, Matsusue S, Fujikawa T, et al. Carcinoma in situ of the pancreas associated with localized fibrosis: a clue to early detection of neoplastic lesions arising from pancreatic ducts. Pancreas 1998;17(1):102–5.
[114] Aimoto T, Uchida E, Nakamura Y, et al. Multicentric pancreatic intraepithelial neoplasias (PanINs) presenting with the clinical features of chronic pancreatitis. J Hepatobiliary Pancreat Surg 2008;15(5):549–53.

Advances in Surgery 44 (2010) 313–325

ADVANCES IN SURGERY

ELSEVIER
MOSBY

The Role of PET Scanning in Pancreatic Cancer

Oscar K. Serrano, MD[a], Muhammad A. Chaudhry, MD[b], Steven D. Leach, MD[a,*]

[a]Department of Surgery, The Sol Goldman Pancreatic Cancer Research Center, The Sidney Kimmel Comprehensive Cancer Center, The Johns Hopkins Hospital, 733 North Broadway, Baltimore, MD 21205, USA
[b]Department of Nuclear Medicine, The Sol Goldman Pancreatic Cancer Research Center, The Sidney Kimmel Comprehensive Cancer Center, The Johns Hopkins Hospital, 733 North Broadway, Baltimore, MD, USA

Pancreatic ductal adenocarcinoma ranks as the fourth leading cause of cancer-related death in the United States [1]. Despite improvements in surgery, chemotherapy, and radiation treatment in the last few decades, long-term survival rate of patients with pancreatic cancer remains dismal, with a median survival of 8 to 12 months in patients with localized disease, and 3 to 6 months in patients with metastatic disease [2]. With a 1-year survival rate of 19% and a 5-year survival rate of 4% for all stages [3], superior techniques for early diagnosis and innovative methods for treatment are urgently needed.

Historically, the only means to achieve long-term survival has been through surgical resection. Unfortunately, the diagnosis is often made late in the course of the disease, when the tumor has spread to lymph nodes or nearby structures such as blood vessels or nerve roots, making surgical resection impossible. At present, less than 25% of patients present with resectable tumors. Even after surgery, median disease-free survival is 13.4 months for patients treated with adjuvant gemcitabine and 6.9 months for untreated patients [2], suggesting that pancreatic cancer evolves into a systemic disease early in the disease process before detection is possible with current imaging modalities.

The symptoms of pancreatic cancer are somewhat nonspecific, and initially tend to be ignored or inadequately treated by patient and caretaker. Consequently, patients tend to seek medical treatment at a later stage of the disease. Tumors located in the head and body of the pancreas exhibit symptoms that are brought on by compression of surrounding structures: the biliary ductal system, mesenteric and celiac nerves, the pancreatic duct, and the duodenum [4]. Frequently, painless jaundice is the initial clinical sign that prompts a medical workup. However, many patients experience precursory periods of

*Corresponding author. *E-mail address:* stleach@jhmi.edu.

0065-3411/10/$ – see front matter
doi:10.1016/j.yasu.2010.05.007

abdominal or back pain, followed by obstructive jaundice. Other signs include the development of diabetes mellitus, malabsorption, or even bouts of acute pancreatitis [4]. For pancreatic tail lesions, symptoms are characteristically related to tumor size, with pain in the left upper quadrant or pain radiations toward the back. Most of these patients present with metastatic disease because of the size of their tumor.

At present, techniques to detect early disease are not available. However, accurate diagnosis and staging is of utmost importance to determine the most appropriate and successful treatment plan. Initially, a patient who presents with symptoms suggestive of biliary obstruction undergoes ultrasonography (US) after ruling out other sources of pathology through clinical acumen and biochemical tests. US often provides reliable information about the size and site of a tumor, diameter of the biliary tree, and the specific site of obstruction. Although US has been reported to be as accurate as computed tomography (CT) in detecting liver metastases [5] and provides some indication of local resectability [6], it is a modality that is uniformly operator-dependent. Its accuracy of identifying pancreatic tumors varies widely, between 57% and 81% [7].

The current gold standard for the diagnosis and staging of pancreatic cancer is thin-slice (1–3 mm), contrast-enhanced, dual-phased multidetector helical CT. By obtaining thin-slice images, multifaceted reconstructions can be made that provide greater anatomic detail and demonstrate the relationship between a suspected pancreatic mass and adjacent structures crucial to a potential surgical resection [8]. At present, the criteria for unresectability of a pancreatic tumor includes presence of distant metastases, malignant ascites or pleural effusion, vascular encasement, and abutment of the tumor to major blood vessels extending more than 50% of the vessel circumference [8]. At present, CT can reliably demonstrate unresectability in almost 100% of cases [9]. However, a recent meta-analysis of 1823 patients reported an overestimate of resectability by helical CT in as many as 20% of patients who were found to be inoperable at surgery [10].

Once a pancreatic mass has been ascertained with CT, typically an endoscopic ultrasound (EUS) is performed in an effort to obtain a needle biopsy for a pathologic diagnosis. EUS enables visualization of the entire pancreas and allows biopsies of suspicious areas to be performed. It also accurately determines local vascular invasion and lymph node involvement with similar results to CT. EUS has been demonstrated to have superior sensitivity and specificity compared with CT in evaluating tumors less than 3 cm in diameter [11].

In cases where biliary decompression becomes necessary before surgery, or as a means of obtaining symptomatic control in advanced disease, endoscopic retrograde cholangiopancreatography (ERCP) provides a therapeutic and diagnostic modality. ERCP allows visualization of the ductal structures, and also provides a method to obtain biopsy samples or brushings [12]. In addition, with ERCP biliary stents can be inserted without the need to pierce the liver parenchyma. However, a 4% to 8% incidence of postprocedure pancreatitis is noted in most prospective randomized trials, and although 90% of these cases are considered mild, the potential for severe cases still exists and must be weighed [13].

The aforementioned modalities, albeit critical in establishing a diagnosis of pancreatic cancer, have limitations, especially when dealing with small lesions. Furthermore, neither of these imaging methods can confidently discern between inflammatory or benign lesions versus cancer. The emergence of positron emission tomography (PET) technology has given rise to the use of functional imaging as an adjunct to provide a more accurate means of delineating between benign and malignant pancreatic processes. Because PET relies on the detection of functional activity rather than lesion size alone, it provides the advantage of being able to differentiate benign from malignant disease. Consequently, when added as an adjunct to current imaging modalities, PET has the potential to reduce overall false-positive, false-negative, and indeterminate rates. The reduction of false positives diminishes unnecessary laparoscopy, while reduction of false negatives leads to earlier detection of small, localized tumors that may be more amenable to surgery [14].

^{18}FLUORODEOXYGLUCOSE-PET

Fluorodeoxyglucose labeled with radioactive fluorine (^{18}F) coupled with PET (^{18}FDG-PET) is a noninvasive functional imaging technique that exploits the difference in biochemistry of normal and abnormal tissue. ^{18}FDG is actively transported into living cells just like any other glucose molecule via native glucose transporters. Typically, physiologic radiotracer uptake is noted in highly metabolically-active tissue such as myocardium, liver and bowel, and the urinary bladder because of renal excretion of the radiotracer (Fig. 1). Because tumors have enhanced glucose uptake and normal pancreas has low glucose utilization rate, ^{18}FDG readily accumulates in malignant cells and can be detected by a PET camera [15]. Once the molecule is transported into the cytosol, ^{18}FDG is phosphorylated by the enzyme hexokinase during the initial reaction of the glycolytic pathway. Therefore, ^{18}FDG-PET measures cellular glycolysis, which indirectly reflects cellular metabolism and growth. Moreover, pancreatic adenocarcinoma cells generally lack the enzyme that breaks down ^{18}FDG, essentially trapping ^{18}FDG in the cytosol and thereby generating large repositories within the tumor, amplifying the signal intensity in comparison with the surrounding tissue [14].

^{18}FDG-PET has been established as an important diagnostic tool in clinical oncology. At present, ^{18}FDG is the most widely used biochemical tracer to measure abnormal cellular metabolism. However, the role of ^{18}FDG-PET in the evaluation of primary pancreatic adenocarcinoma has not been conclusively established. Furthermore, its utility in evaluating tumor response to neoadjuvant or adjuvant chemoradiotherapy or in the evaluation of recurrent disease after surgical resection is still unclear. In this review, the authors assess the evolving application and relevance of ^{18}FDG-PET in the preoperative diagnosis, staging, and postoperative surveillance of pancreatic cancer.

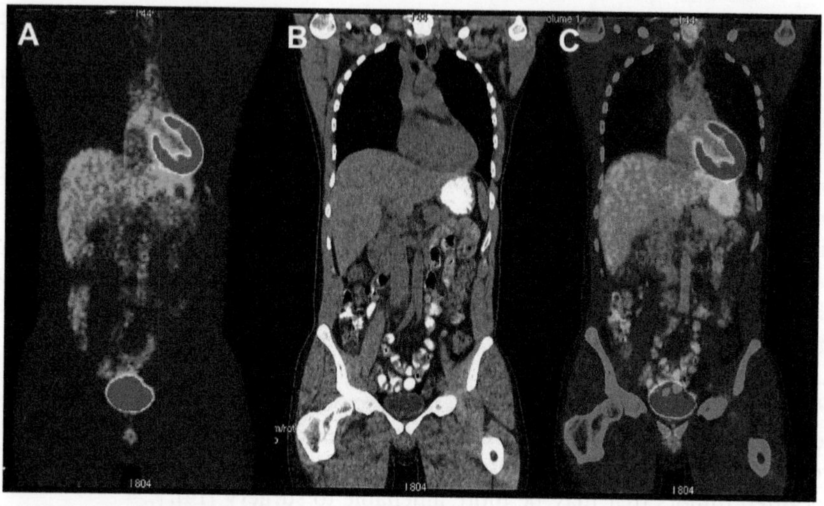

Fig. 1. Coronal ^{18}FDG-PET (*A*), CT (*B*), and fused PET/CT (*C*) images in a normal human subject. Physiologic radiotracer uptake is noted in myocardium, hepatic parenchyma, bowel, and urinary bladder.

PREOPERATIVE DIAGNOSIS OF PANCREATIC CARCINOMA

EUS and CT imaging both provide precise anatomic delineation of tumor position and extension with respect to surrounding structures, but they are not always able to reliably differentiate between malignant and benign diseases [16]. For instance, the distinction of pancreatic cancer from focal pancreatitis remains a diagnostic conundrum because the latter may have a CT appearance that is indistinguishable from that of malignancy (Fig. 2). Because of selective uptake of ^{18}FDG by neoplastic cells, ^{18}FDG-PET allows the segregation of malignant lesions in the pancreas (Fig. 3). The pancreas is not normally visualized on PET, and therefore a "hot spot" within the peripancreatic tissue would usually be considered abnormal [17].

Several studies have demonstrated ^{18}FDG-PET to be more accurate than conventional imagining modalities in the preoperative workup for a suspected pancreatic cancer (Table 1). Recently a meta-analysis was published, which looked at 17 studies in order to assess the diagnostic accuracy of ^{18}FDG-PET as an adjunct to CT versus CT alone [14]. The study included only articles that reported primary data on at least 12 patients. In addition, all studies reported biopsy-confirmed pancreatic adenocarcinoma or long-term follow-up of patients as a reference standard for detection of pancreatic malignancy [14].

In their meta-analysis, Orlando and colleagues [14] reported that among 290 individuals with pancreatic adenocarcinoma, there were 50 and 27 false negatives by CT and ^{18}FDG-PET, respectively. Of the malignancies that were missed by CT, ^{18}FDG-PET detected 42 (84%) and of those missed by ^{18}FDG-PET, CT detected 19 (70%). Among 120 individuals with benign

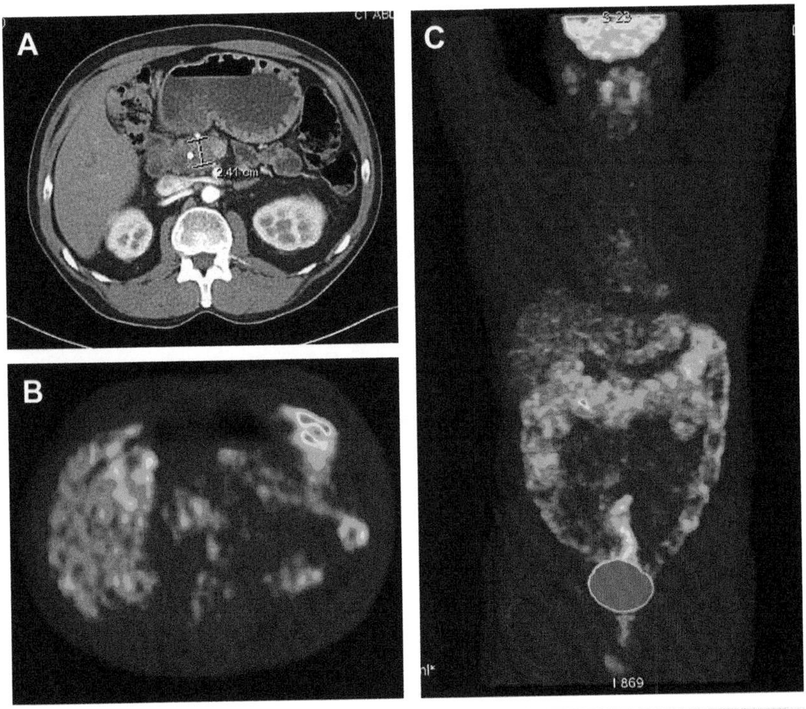

Fig. 2. Contrast-enhanced transaxial CT image showing a 2.4-cm mass at the head of the pancreas in the setting of chronic pancreatitis (*A*). Transaxial ^{18}FDG-PET does not reveal discernible ^{18}FDG uptake in the region of the pancreatic head. Normal physiologic activity is noted in liver parenchyma and bowel (*B*). Maximum-intensity projection (MIP) images reveal physiologic radiotracer distribution within brain, nasopharynx, liver, bowel, and bladder (*C*). No abnormal ^{18}FDG accumulation is noted in the region of pancreatic head.

disease, there were 39 false positives by CT and 19 by ^{18}FDG-PET. ^{18}FDG-PET detected 26 (67%) of those missed by CT, and CT detected 8 (42%) of those missed by ^{18}FDG-PET. The investigators concluded that overall, 89 individuals were misdiagnosed by CT, and that addition of ^{18}FDG-PET reduced that number to 21 (84% detection rate). The pooled sensitivities and specificities from this meta-analysis is summarized in Table 2 . Together, these results suggest that the addition of ^{18}FDG-PET as an adjunct in the workup of a pancreatic mass improves the ability to discriminate between patients with and without pancreatic cancer.

One of the most notable strengths of adding ^{18}FDG-PET in conjunction with CT in the diagnostic workup of a suspected pancreatic cancer is its ability to detect small lesions (Fig. 4). In one study, ^{18}FDG-PET was found to have a sensitivity of 100% in detecting pancreatic lesions less than 2 cm in size, compared with 18% for CT alone [35]. This analysis highlights the importance

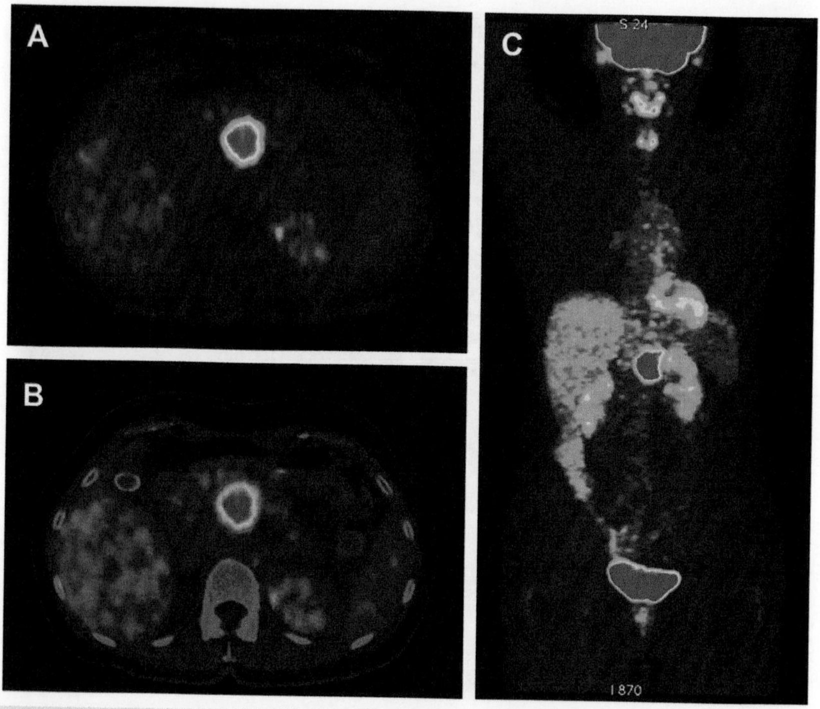

Fig. 3. ^{18}FDG-PET images in a patient presenting with a pancreatic mass. Transaxial PET images reveal intensely ^{18}FDG-avid disease in the pancreatic head region (*A*). Fused PET/CT transaxial images reveal ^{18}FDG-avid disease involving the pancreatic head (*B*). MIP images reveal ^{18}FDG-avid pancreatic adenocarcinoma (*C*). Physiologic radiotracer accumulation is noted in the brain, nasopharynx, liver, kidneys, bowel, and bladder.

of the semiquantitative nature of ^{18}FDG-PET for a disease that is commonly discovered at such a late stage in its course. Furthermore, the diagnostic accuracy of ^{18}FDG-PET is enhanced by the ability to quantify injected tracer using the established standard uptake values (SUVs), which is a calculation of the activity concentration divided by the injected dose per body weight.

STAGING PANCREATIC CARCINOMA

Because PET scans the whole body concurrently, it can accurately stage patients with a new diagnosis of pancreatic cancer. Pancreatic staging is performed using the American Joint Committee on Cancer TNM staging system [36]. Stage I refers to tumors that are confined to the pancreas; stage II is characterized by extrapancreatic extension; stage III by lymph node involvement; and stage IV by distant metastases. T staging should be evaluated with imaging modalities that demonstrate the tumor with its relationship to adjacent organs and vascular structures, such as US, EUS, or CT. With poor spatial resolution,

Table 1
Description of studies evaluating the sensitivity and specificity of PET and CT

Study	Year	PET (No. of patients)	CT (No. of patients)	Country	PET sensitivity	PET specificity	CT sensitivity	CT specificity
Bares et al [18]	1993	15	15	Germany	92%	100%	95%	50%
Bares et al [19]	1994	40	40	Germany	89%	85%	100%	23%
Inokuma et al [20]	1995	46	46	Japan	94%	82%	89%	73%
Kato et al [21]	1995	24		Japan	93%	78%		
Ho et al [22]	1996	14	14	USA	100%	67%	25%	100%
Zimny et al [23]	1997	106		Germany	89%	53%		
Keogan et al [24]	1998	37	37	USA	88%	83%	75%	83%
Rajput et al [25]	1998	13	13	USA	82%	100%	73%	0%
Imdahl et al [26]	1999	48	48	Germany	96%	100%	50%	44%
Delbeke et al [27]	1999	65	65	USA	92%	58%	65%	62%
Diederichs et al [28]	2000	122	101	Germany	88%	87%	95%	91%
Sendler et al [29]	2000	43	43	Germany	71%	64%	74%	73%
Nakamoto et al [30]	2000	47		Japan	100%	80%		
Koyama et al [31]	2001	86	86	Japan	82%	81%	91%	38%
Kasperk et al [32]	2001	103	103	Germany	92%	58%	85%	89%
Papós et al [33]	2002	22	22	Hungary	100%	88%	100%	56%
Kalady et al [15–17,34]	2002	54	54	USA	88%	92%	65%	87%

Table 2
Pooled sensitivity and specificity for CT alone and PET in the setting of a positive and negative CT

	Sensitivity	Specificity
CT alone	81%	66%
PET (in setting of positive CT)	92%	68%
PET (in setting of negative CT)	73%	86%

Data from Orlando LA, Kulasingam SL, Matchar DB. Meta-analysis: the detection of pancreatic malignancy with positron emission tomography. Aliment Pharmacol Ther 2004;20(10):1063–70.

^{18}FDG-PET limits the ability to visualize these relationships, and EUS is the best modality for T staging.

N staging is difficult to estimate with current imaging modalities, a phenomenon that has been attributed to the proximity of regional peripancreatic lymph nodes to the primary tumor [37]. However, ^{18}FDG-PET appears to be the most useful in M staging, where distant disease is readily apparent as a focus of ^{18}FDG uptake (Fig. 5). The 3 most common organs involved by metastatic pancreatic adenocarcinoma are the liver, the lungs, and the bone marrow, in that order. In a study of 89 patients, the sensitivity and specificity of ^{18}FDG-PET for detecting hepatic metastases were reported to be 70% and 95%, respectively [28]. Similarly, another study of 168 preoperative patients found ^{18}FDG-PET to have a sensitivity of 68% and a specificity of 95% [38].

A tabulated review of the ^{18}FDG-PET literature on staging for pancreatic carcinoma, which included 461 patients, reports weighted averages for sensitivity and specificity of 83% and 82%, respectively, compared with 65% and 61% for CT [39].

POSTOPERATIVE SURVEILLANCE OF PANCREATIC CARCINOMA

Unfortunately, the dismal survival rates even for resected pancreatic cancer limit studies on postoperative surveillance. An increase in tumor markers,

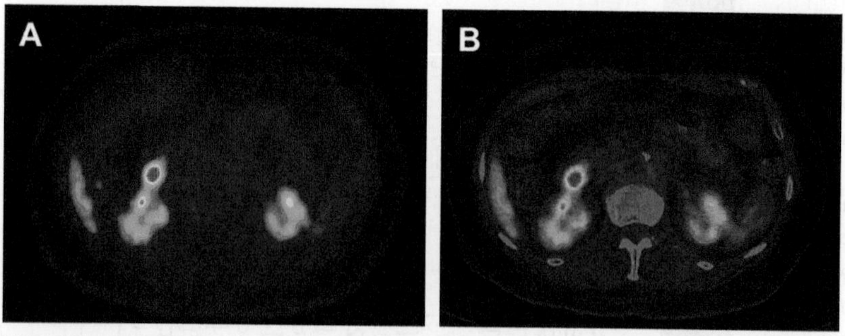

Fig. 4. ^{18}FDG-PET and fused PET/CT in a patient with pancreatic adenocarcinoma. Transaxial PET images reveal focal ^{18}FDG accumulation in the region of the pancreatic head (*A*). Also noted is physiologic uptake in kidneys. Transaxial Fused PET/CT images reveal a 1.9-cm pancreatic adenocarcinoma in ampullary region (*B*).

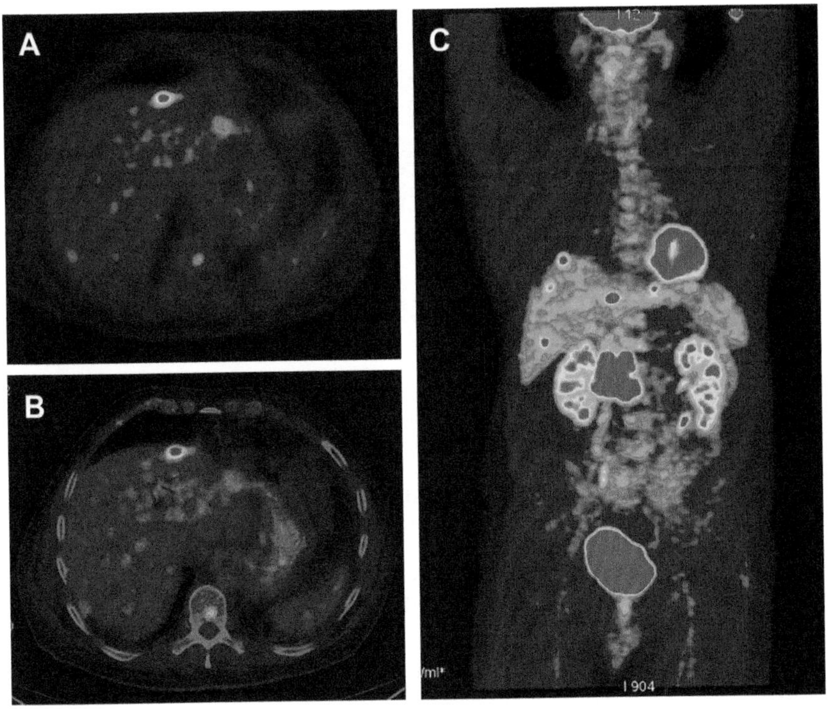

Fig. 5. ^{18}FDG-PET images from a patient with pancreatic adenocarcinoma and liver metastases. Transaxial PET images reveal ^{18}FDG-avid metastatic involvement of anterior left hepatic lobe region (*A*). Transaxial fused PET/CT images reveal ^{18}FDG-avid metastatic disease in the left hepatic lobe (*B*). MIP images reveal ^{18}FDG-avid metastatic disease involving the hepatic parenchyma (*C*). Physiologic uptake is noted in brain, myocardium, kidneys, bowel, and bladder.

such as carbohydrate antigen 19-9, in the postoperative setting makes differentiating between disease recurrence and postsurgical or radiotherapy changes with conventional CT or magnetic resonance imaging difficult. Few studies have been performed on the use of ^{18}FDG-PET to follow tumor response to neoadjuvant and adjuvant chemoradiotherapy.

In one particular study [35], 9 patients were scanned before and after neoadjuvant chemoradiation. ^{18}FDG-PET successfully demonstrated histologic evidence of chemoradiation-induced tumor necrosis in all 4 patients who appeared to have had at least a 50% reduction in tumor SUV (Fig. 6). Of note, none of these patients demonstrated size reduction by CT. These 4 patients went on to resection, which demonstrated 20% to 80% tumor necrosis in the surgical specimen. In this study, 2 patients demonstrated an increase in SUV, which was corroborated by an increase in tumor size by CT [35].

In the same study, 8 patients were evaluated for recurrence after surgical resection based on indeterminate CT findings or after an increase in tumor

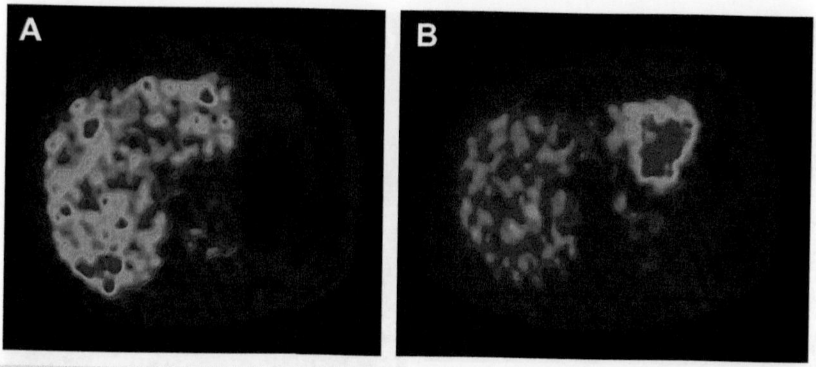

Fig. 6. ^{18}FDG-PET images from a patient with pancreatic adenocarcinoma and multiple liver metastases. Prechemotherapy transaxial evaluation reveals diffuse metastatic involvement of hepatic parenchyma (*A*). Postchemotherapy transaxial PET images reveal interval resolution of intense focal ^{18}FDG uptake (*B*). Mild ^{18}FDG uptake is seen physiologically. Of note, the large area in the left upper quadrant is myocardium.

markers was discovered. All patients were noted to have regions of increased ^{18}FDG uptake, 4 in the surgical bed and 4 in new hepatic metastases [35].

A more recent study of 31 patients suspected of having recurrent disease showed that 96% of local recurrences were detected with ^{18}FDG-PET, whereas only 23% were detected with conventional CT [40].

Therefore, ^{18}FDG-PET has been suggested to be useful in the postoperative setting when CT is unable to differentiate postoperative or postradiation fibrosis at the surgical bed, when evaluating new hepatic lesions too small to perform biopsy, or in patients with rising tumor markers and a negative conventional workup [37].

EMERGING MODALITIES: ^{18}FDG-PET/CT

Combined ^{18}FDG-PET and CT has had a significant impact on cancer imaging. The ability of CT to map out tissue attenuation for correction of PET images and the ability to register the functional information provided by ^{18}FDG-PET with the anatomic data have resulted in remarkable improvements in diagnostic accuracy (see Figs. 2 and 3).

The role of ^{18}FDG-PET/CT image fusion in pancreatic cancer was examined by 2 studies. One study retrospectively fused CT and ^{18}FDG-PET images, resulting in an improved sensitivity. Sensitivity for ^{18}FDG-PET/CT fusion was 89.1%, versus 76% for CT alone and 84.4% for ^{18}FDG-PET alone [41]. Image fusion also resulted in improved sensitivity for detecting lymph node metastasis (^{18}FDG-PET, 25.8%; CT, 25.8%; ^{18}FDG-PET/CT 32.3%) [41].

In a second study, ^{18}FDG-PET/CT was found to have similar accuracy for detecting pancreatic cancer when compared with ^{18}FDG-PET alone [42]. However, 16% of patients were spared unnecessary surgery because of the detection of CT-occult metastases by ^{18}FDG-PET/CT, thereby leading to overall cost-effectiveness [42]. The investigators concluded that despite requiring multiple additional studies, ^{18}FDG-PET/CT resulted in significant cost saving, thereby justifying the studies.

SUMMARY

The strength of functional imaging lies in its ability to detect malignant disease irrespective of lesion morphology. In this setting, ^{18}FDG-PET can complement management by providing a more accurate diagnosis. When combined as an adjunct to CT, ^{18}FDG-PET can increase the sensitivity, specificity, and accuracy for detecting a pancreatic malignancy, especially in patients in whom CT alone fails to identify a discrete mass or in whom biopsy results are indeterminate. This capability is accentuated with small lesions of the pancreas.

^{18}FDG-PET is significantly more sensitive in detecting metastatic disease than conventional CT imaging. Moreover, ^{18}FDG-PET is able to differentiate tumor response to therapy in the postoperative setting, and could potentially serve to monitor recurrence patterns in the setting of neoadjuvant or adjuvant chemoradiotherapy.

Finally, as ^{18}FDG-PET/CT fusion modalities become more widespread and technical advances in image acquisition progress, ^{18}FDG-PET will continue to have an increasing role in the diagnosis, staging, and surveillance of pancreatic cancer, integrating anatomic information with functional imaging.

References

[1] Greenlee RT, Murray T, Bolden S, et al. Cancer statistics, 2000. CA Cancer J Clin 2000;50:7.
[2] Nieto J, Grossbard ML, Kozuch P. Metastatic pancreatic cancer 2008: is the glass less empty? Oncologist 2008;13(5):562–76.
[3] Ries LAG, Kosary CL, Hankey BF, editors. SEER Cancer statistics review 1973–1997, Table XXI-4. Bethesda (MD): National Cancer Institute; 1999.
[4] Li D, Xie K, Wolff R, et al. Pancreatic cancer. Lancet 2004;363(9414):1049–57.
[5] Minniti S, Bruno C, Biasiutti C, et al. Sonography versus helical CT in identification and staging of pancreatic ductal adenocarcinoma. J Clin Ultrasound 2003;31(4):175–82.
[6] Clarke DL, Thomson SR, Madiba TE, et al. Preoperative imaging of pancreatic cancer: a management-oriented approach. J Am Coll Surg 2003;196(1):119–29.
[7] Haycox A, Lombard M, Neoptolemos J, et al. Review article: current practice and future perspectives in detection and diagnosis of pancreatic cancer. Aliment Pharmacol Ther 1998;12(10):937–48.
[8] Smith SL, Rajan PS. Imaging of pancreatic adenocarcinoma with emphasis on multidetector CT. Clin Radiol 2004;59(1):26–38.
[9] Fuhrman GM, Charnsangavej C, Abbruzzese JL, et al. Thin-section contrast-enhanced computed tomography accurately predicts the resectability of malignant pancreatic neoplasms. Am J Surg 1994;167(1):104–11 [discussion: 111–3].
[10] Bipat S, Phoa SS, van Delden OM, et al. Ultrasonography, computed tomography and magnetic resonance imaging for diagnosis and determining resectability of pancreatic adenocarcinoma: a meta-analysis. J Comput Assist Tomogr 2005;29(4):438–45.
[11] Mertz HR, Sechopoulos P, Delbeke D, et al. EUS, PET, and CT scanning for evaluation of pancreatic adenocarcinoma. Gastrointest Endosc 2000;52(3):367–71.
[12] Graham RA, Bankoff M, Hediger R, et al. Fine-needle aspiration biopsy of pancreatic ductal adenocarcinoma: loss of diagnostic accuracy with small tumors. J Surg Oncol 1994;55(2): 92–4.

[13] Abdel Aziz AM, Lehman GA. Pancreatitis after endoscopic retrograde cholangio-pancreatography. World J Gastroenterol 2007;13(19):2655–68.
[14] Orlando LA, Kulasingam SL, Matchar DB. Meta-analysis: the detection of pancreatic malignancy with positron emission tomography. Aliment Pharmacol Ther 2004;20(10):1063–70.
[15] Berberat P, Friess H, Kashiwagi M, et al. Diagnosis and staging of pancreatic cancer by positron emission tomography. World J Surg 1999;23(9):882–7.
[16] Gangi S, Fletcher JG, Nathan MA, et al. Time interval between abnormalities seen on CT and the clinical diagnosis of pancreatic cancer: retrospective review of CT scans obtained before diagnosis. AJR Am J Roentgenol 2004;182(4):897–903.
[17] Kostakoglu L, Agress H Jr, Goldsmith SJ. Clinical role of FDG PET in evaluation of cancer patients. Radiographics 2003;23(2):315–40.
[18] Bares R, Klever P, Hellwig D, et al. Pancreatic cancer detected by positron emission tomography with ^{18}F-labelled deoxyglucose: method and first results. Nucl Med Commun 1993;14(7):596–601.
[19] Bares R, Klever P, Hauptmann S, et al. ^{18}F- fluorodeoxyglucose PET in vivo evaluation of pancreatic glucose metabolism for detection of pancreatic cancer. Radiology 1994;192(1):79–86.
[20] Inokuma T, Tamaki N, Torizuka T, et al. Evaluation of pancreatic tumors with positron emission tomography and ^{18}F-fluorodeoxyglucose: comparison with CT and US. Radiology 1995;195(2):345–52.
[21] Kato T, Fukatsu H, Ito K, et al. Fluorodeoxyglucose positron emission tomography in pancreatic cancer: an unsolved problem. Eur J Nucl Med 1995;22(1):32–9.
[22] Ho CL, Dehdashti F, Griffeth LK, et al. FDG-PET evaluation of indeterminate pancreatic masses. J Comput Assist Tomogr 1996;20(3):363–9.
[23] Zimny M, Bares R, Fass J, et al. ^{18}Fluorine-fluorodeoxyglucose positron emission tomography in the differential diagnosis of pancreatic carcinoma: a report of 106 cases. Eur J Nucl Med 1997;24(6):678–82.
[24] Keogan MT, Tyler D, Clark L, et al. Diagnosis of pancreatic carcinoma: role of FDG PET. AJR Am J Roentgenol 1998;171(6):1565–70.
[25] Rajput A, Stellato TA, Faulhaber PF, et al. The role of fluorodeoxyglucose and positron emission tomography in the evaluation of pancreatic disease. Surgery 1998;124(4):793–7.
[26] Imdahl A, Nitzsche E, Krautmann F, et al. Evaluation of positron emission tomography with 2-[^{18}F]fluoro-2-deoxy-D-glucose for the differentiation of chronic pancreatitis and pancreatic cancer. Br J Surg 1999;86(2):194–9.
[27] Delbeke D, Rose DM, Chapman WC, et al. Optimal interpretation of FDG PET in the diagnosis, staging and management of pancreatic carcinoma. J Nucl Med 1999;40(11):1784–91.
[28] Diederichs CG, Staib L, Vogel J, et al. Values and limitations of ^{18}F-fluorodeoxyglucose-positron-emission tomography with preoperative evaluation of patients with pancreatic masses. Pancreas 2000;20(2):109–16.
[29] Sendler A, Avril N, Helmberger H, et al. Preoperative evaluation of pancreatic masses with positron emission tomography using ^{18}F-fluorodeoxyglucose: diagnostic limitations. World J Surg 2000;24(9):1121–9.
[30] Nakamoto Y, Higashi T, Sakahara H, et al. Delayed ^{18}F-fluoro-2-deoxy-D-glucose positron emission tomography scan for differentiation between malignant and benign lesions in the pancreas. Cancer 2000;89(12):2547–54.
[31] Koyama K, Okamura T, Kawabe J, et al. Diagnostic usefulness of FDG PET for pancreatic mass lesions. Ann Nucl Med 2001;15(3):217–24.
[32] Kasperk RK, Riesener KP, Wilms K, et al. Limited value of positron emission tomography in treatment of pancreatic cancer: surgeon's view. World J Surg 2001;25(9):1134–9.

[33] Papós M, Takács T, Trón L, et al. The possible role of ^{18}F-FDG positron emission tomography in the differential diagnosis of focal pancreatic lesions. Clin Nucl Med 2002;27(3): 197–201.
[34] Kalady MF, Clary BM, Clark LA, et al. Clinical utility of positron emission tomography in the diagnosis and management of periampullary neoplasms. Ann Surg Oncol 2002;9(8): 799–806.
[35] Rose DM, Delbeke D, Beauchamp RD, et al. ^{18}Fluorodeoxyglucose-positron emission tomography in the management of patients with suspected pancreatic cancer. Ann Surg 1999;229(5):729–37.
[36] Greene FL. TNM staging for malignancies of the digestive tract: 2003 changes and beyond. Semin Surg Oncol 2003;21(1):23–9.
[37] Delbeke D, Pinson CW. Pancreatic tumors: role of imaging in the diagnosis, staging, and treatment. J Hepatobiliary Pancreat Surg 2004;11(1):4–10.
[38] Fröhlich A, Diederichs CG, Staib L, et al. Detection of liver metastases from pancreatic cancer using FDG PET. J Nucl Med 1999;40(2):250–5.
[39] Gambhir SS, Czernin J, Schwimmer J, et al. A tabulated summary of the FDG PET literature. J Nucl Med 2001;42(Suppl 5):1S–93S.
[40] Ruf J, Lopez Hänninen E, Oettle H, et al. Detection of recurrent pancreatic cancer: comparison of FDG-PET with CT/MRI. Pancreatology 2005;5(2–3):266–72.
[41] Lemke AJ, Niehues SM, Hosten N, et al. Retrospective digital image fusion of multidetector CT and ^{18}F-FDG PET: clinical value in pancreatic lesions—a prospective study with 104 patients. J Nucl Med 2004;45(8):1279–86.
[42] Heinrich S, Goerres GW, Schäfer M, et al. Positron emission tomography/computed tomography influences on the management of resectable pancreatic cancer and its cost-effectiveness. Ann Surg 2005;242(2):235–43.

Advances in Surgery 44 (2010) 327–346

ELSEVIER
MOSBY

ADVANCES IN SURGERY

Reoperative Surgery for the Zollinger-Ellison Syndrome

Stephen R. Grobmyer, MD*, Steven N. Hochwald, MD
Division of Surgical Oncology, Department of Surgery, University of Florida, 1600 SW Archer Road, Room 6165, PO Box 100109, Gainesville, FL 32610, USA

The Zollinger-Ellison syndrome (ZES) is a syndrome of gastric acid hypersecretion and severe peptic ulcer disease caused by a gastrin-producing neruoendocrine tumor [1]. ZES is a rare syndrome with an incidence of 1 to 3 cases per 1×10^6 people per year in the United States [2]. ZES occurs as either a component of multiple endocrine neoplasia type 1 (MEN-1) (20% of cases) or more commonly as sporadic disease (80% of cases) [3–6]. Approaches to treatment of patients with ZES have evolved from surgical management of the stomach [7–9] and medical management of acid hypersecretion [10,11]. The modern approach is based on an improved understanding of the disease pathobiology of ZES and is focused on surgical removal of the site(s) of gastrinoma [12–15]. This approach most effectively addresses the 2 clinical problems that arise in patients with ZES: gastric acid hypersecretion and removal of tumor with metastatic potential [13]. Primary surgery in ZES is appropriately considered and performed in many patients with ZES: with curative intent; [13,16] to reduce the likelihood of developing metastatic disease; [13] to prolong survival; [17] and/or to palliate symptoms associated with hypergastrinemia and its sequelae [17,18]. Gastrinomas in sporadic disease and those arising in the setting of MEN-1 have different patterns of presentation and natural histories leading to recommendations for distinct therapeutic approaches to ZES in these 2 settings.

Although primary surgery for sporadic ZES using modern approaches is associated with an initial biochemical cure in many cases, most patients do eventually suffer from persistent or recurrent disease following initial surgery [13]. Reoperation can play a role in the optimal management of patients with persistent or recurrent ZES [17,19,20]. The indications for reoperation in sporadic gastrinoma include (1) failed initial surgery with persistence of hypergastrinemia or image-detectable persistent disease, (2) image-detectable recurrence of disease following initial curative surgery, and (3) control of

*Corresponding author. *E-mail address*: stephen.grobmyer@surgery.ufl.edu.

0065-3411/10/$ – see front matter
doi:10.1016/j.yasu.2010.05.006

symptoms related to hypergastrinemia and reduced dependence on acid suppression therapy.

Decisions about when and if to reoperate on patients with ZES requires a detailed knowledge of: current approaches for optimizing primary operative results in sporadic ZES and ZES associated with MEN-1 [16]; tumor biology and natural history of ZES [21]; imaging and biochemical strategies for detecting recurrent gastrinoma [17]; and the role of medical therapy for gastrinoma [22]. In this review, consideration is given to these factors in the context of clinical decision making regarding reoperation for patients with ZES.

MODERN APPROACH TO PRIMARY SPORADIC ZES

The management of ZES has evolved significantly in the last 30 years from operations designed to manage the sequelae of gastric acid hypersecretion to operations aimed at removal of the primary gastrinoma to improve overall survival and provide long-term relief of hypergastrinemia [16]. An understanding of the current concepts in management of primary gastrinoma is essential as these concepts may need to be applied when considering reoperation in ZES. This is particularly true for the subset of patients in whom complete initial operative exploration is not performed.

Diagnosis of ZES

ZES must be differentiated from other conditions associated with hypergastrinemia [23]. Patients should be off acid suppression therapy for accurate diagnosis of ZES including proton pump inhibitors for 1 week and histamine antagonists for 2 days. All patients with ZES have a fasting serum gastrin level greater than 100 pg/mL with gastric pH less than 2 [24]. Most patients with ZES have fasting gastrin level greater than 1000 pg/mL [24]. High basal acid output (>15 mEq/h) is diagnostic of ZES [25] (or >5 mEq/h in patients with previous acid-reducing surgery [18]).

Secretin stimulation testing is useful for confirming ZES in patients with otherwise equivocal test results [25]. An increase in serum gastrin greater than 200 pg/mL following intravenous administration of a 2 U/kg bolus of secretin is consistent with ZES. The secretin stimulation test can be useful in diagnosing ZES in patients in whom proton pump inhibitors cannot be held [26].

Imaging of tumors in ZES

Once a biochemical diagnosis is made, imaging studies to localize and determine the extent of disease are useful and should be performed [18,25]. Preoperative imaging studies most commonly used presently are: somatostatin receptor scintigraphy (SRS), computed tomography (CT) scan, magnetic resonance imaging (MRI), and endoscopic ultrasound [23]. SRS is the most sensitive test for detecting primary and metastatic gastrinoma [27]. The preoperative use of SRS has been reported to often prompt a change in management plans [2]. Tumor size is an important determinant of imaging sensitivity of gastrinoma [28]. Small tumors including small duodenal primary tumors are difficult to image using any of these techniques [28]. For detection and evaluation of liver metastases, SRS is the most sensitive followed by MRI and CT [25]. Information on the anatomic location of liver tumors is essential for surgical planning and is best obtained from CT or MRI. At present, more invasive imaging studies including selective angiography and venous sampling are being used on a more limited basis for identifying otherwise occult sites of disease [18,25,29].

Location of primary tumors in sporadic ZES

Eighty percent of gastrinomas are found in the gastrinoma triangle defined by the junction of the cystic duct and common bile duct, the second and third portions of the duodenum, and the junction of the head and neck of the pancreas [30]. In sporadic ZES, most (~80%) gastrinomas are found in the duodenum or pancreas (Fig. 1) with a minority occurring in regions outside the pancreaticoduodenal area including the small bowel, stomach, lung, and heart [31]. Duodenal tumors are more common than pancreatic tumors in sporadic disease in a ratio of 3:1 [23]. Duodenal gastrinomas are small (1 cm); 25% are less than 0.5 cm thus making them not detectable with standard imaging studies (SRS, CT, MRI, and endoscopy) in some cases.

Primary operative management for sporadic ZES

All patients with sporadic ZES and without a medical contraindication to surgery or widespread metastatic disease should undergo initial operative management with intent to resect the primary tumor and identifiable sites of metastatic disease, even when initial imaging examinations do not identify the site of the primary lesion [13,25]. Standard tests that should be performed before operative exploration include CT scan or MRI, SRS, and endoscopic evaluation of the entire duodenum including endoscopic ultrasound evaluation of the entire pancreas.

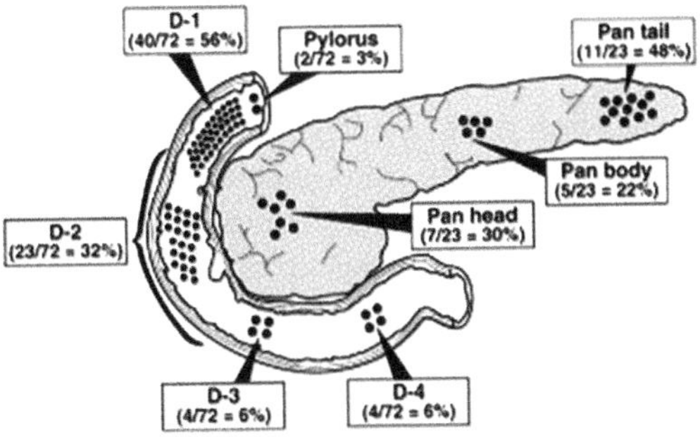

Fig. 1. Location of sporadic gastrinomas from reported series of patients. Each dot represents a gastrinoma from a single patient. *Reproduced from* Norton JA, Jensen RT. Current surgical management of Zollinger-Ellison syndrome (ZES) in patients without multiple endocrine neoplasia-type1 (MEN1). Surg Oncol Aug 2003;12(2):145–51; with permission.

Operative maneuvers in the management of primary sporadic ZES should include Kocher maneuver; transillumination of the duodenum; [32] palpation of the duodenum, pancreas, and nodes in the gastrinoma triangle; inspection and palpation of the liver, intraoperative ultrasound of the pancreatic head and liver, and routine duodenotomy [15,17,33,34]. Among these maneuvers, routine duodenotomy is associated with the highest rate of identification of duodenal primary tumors [28,34].

Duodenal primary gastrinomas in sporadic ZES should be completely excised and this can typically be accomplished through excision and primary closure [13,35]. Pancreatic head gastrinomas can commonly be enucleated although in some patients large size or position will rarely mandate pancreaticoduodenectomy [17]. Routine pancreaticoduodenectomy is not indicated in patients with sporadic ZES [17]. Distal pancreatic lesions can be managed with enucleation or distal pancreatectomy (preferably splenic preserving).

Fifty to 60% of duodenal primary gastrinomas are associated with lymph node metastases. Enlarged and/or suspicious regional lymph nodes should be removed at the time of primary surgery. Although its effect on survival is unknown, regional lymphadenectomy should be strongly considered at the time of initial exploration as this may increase biochemical cure rates [14,17,34,36]. In addition, lymph node primary gastrinomas have been described [36]. Nodal basins most commonly involved vary with the site of the primary lesion in the duodenum or pancreas [28].

Intraoperative serum gastrin determination following secretin administration has been suggested by some to be useful in the operative management of patients with primary gastrinoma to confirm cure before operative closure [37–39]. However, with modern surgical approaches including duodenotomy and high initial biochemical cure rates in patients with sporadic disease based on advances in the understanding of the pathobiology of ZES, the value of the routine use of this assay in the management of primary sporadic disease remains controversial [23,35]. This assay may best be used in reoperation for ZES.

Clinical outcomes following primary surgery for sporadic ZES

Biochemical cure following surgical management of ZES is defined as: normalization of fasting serum gastrin, normalization of stimulation testing, and absence of recurrent or persistent disease on imaging studies [13,25]. Persistent disease is defined as failure to normalize gastrin and stimulated gastrin levels in the postoperative period [28].

Initial biochemical cure rates using modern approaches including routine duodenotomy are approximately 60% initially, 50% at 5 years, and 35% long-term (Fig. 2) [12,13,35]. Hence, in long-term follow-up, even with modern imaging and surgical approaches, most patients will develop and require management of persistent or recurrent gastrinoma. This is likely because of unrecognized occult metastatic disease at the time of initial surgery.

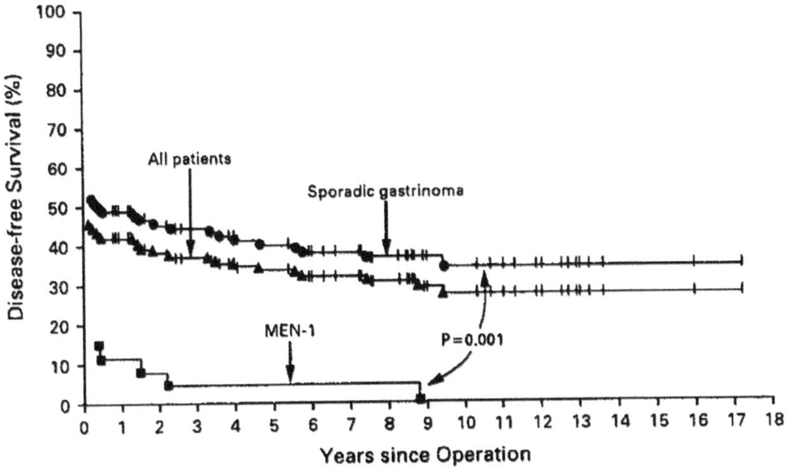

Fig. 2. Disease-free survival following 180 operations for ZES. *Reproduced from* Norton JA, Fraker DL, Alexander HR, et al. Surgery to cure the Zollinger-Ellison syndrome. N Engl J Med 1999;341(9):635–44; with permission.

In those patients presenting with disease limited to the primary site ± regional lymph nodes, long-term overall survival rates are excellent following a properly performed initial operation in modern series [16]. Disease-specific survival rates have been reported to be 100% at 5 years and 95% at 10 years [16].

Clinical follow-up following initial surgery for sporadic ZES

Recommendations for clinical follow-up of patients following initial surgery varies according to the findings and results of the initial operation. Before discharge, fasting serum gastrin determinations and secretin stimulation testing is helpful in identifying the patients in whom biochemical cure has been achieved [20,40–42]. Normalization of postoperative testing has also been shown to correlate with durable biochemical cure at 5 years [41]. When biochemical cure has been achieved, patients may be followed annually with clinical examination with particular attention to the development of symptoms such as heartburn or reflux that may be associated with recurrence as well as fasting gastrin and secretin stimulation testing [25]. Both tests are necessary because neither is completely sensitive to detect recurrence [43]. Routine imaging is not used in the follow-up of these patients as it has not been shown to detect recurrences earlier than blood tests [25]. Imaging studies including SRS and CT scanning are performed for patients who develop new symptoms that may be consistent with recurrent disease or who demonstrate changes in gastrin or stimulated gastrin levels [25]. In patients with persistent or recurrent disease, fasting serum gastrin and stimulated gastrin levels are monitored and imaged on a more frequent basis (CT and SRS) to detect disease progression [25]. Progressive symptoms or increasing requirement for medical acid suppression should prompt more frequent or invasive imaging examinations in attempt to localize sites of disease amenable to surgery or other intervention.

Molecular/biochemical markers of disease progression in ZES

The identification of molecular and biochemical markers of progression for patients with ZES is potentially useful for making decisions about risk of recurrence and in making therapeutic choices in patients with recurrent or metastatic disease (reviewed in [31]). Serum gastrin levels at presentation do correlate with the extent of disease in patients with sporadic ZES but do not predict disease progression, and the test has not been shown to be reliable in deciding which patients benefit from therapeutic interventions [44]. Similarly, chromogranin A levels are increased in patients with ZES but are not predictive of disease progression [45,46]. Molecular markers, including human epidermal growth factor receptor (HER-2) [47] and insulinlike growth factor 1 receptor [48], have been investigated but have not affected clinical approaches to date.

REOPERATION FOR SPORADIC ZES

Reoperation in patients with sporadic ZES should be considered in 4 subsets of patients: (1) those with persistent disease following incomplete initial surgery (eg, no duodenotomy), (2) those with persistent disease and new or progressive findings on imaging studies in whom total or near total resection is anticipated, and (3) those with recurrent disease after initial biochemical cure in whom total or near total resection is anticipated, and (4) for control of hypergastrinemia and its sequelae.

Routine initial surgery in patients diagnosed with ZES has been shown to be associated with the possibility of long-term cure [13] and improved survival [16]. Long-term survival after reoperation for ZES has also been demonstrated [20]. However, the true effect of reoperation for persistent or recurrent disease on overall survival in patients with ZES is unclear and, as a result, the decision for reoperation requires significant clinical judgment [49]. Although achieving eugastrinemia with reoperation is possible, long-term survival rates seem to be independent of achieving biochemical cure [20,49].

Sites of persistent or recurrent disease include the duodenum, small bowel, peripancreatic or portal lymph nodes, and liver in addition to numerous other less common sites [19,20]. Liver is a common site of metastatic disease and a common cause of disease-specific mortality in patients with ZES. Specific issues related to management of patients with liver metastases from gastrinoma are discussed separately later.

The group of patients with sporadic ZES most likely to benefit from reoperation are those in whom an incomplete initial operation (without duodenotomy) was performed [16]. In these patients, reoperation is indicated with increased serum tests (fasting gastrin or secretin stimulation test) even with negative imaging studies; gastrinomas can most commonly be found in the duodenum using techniques of palpation and transillumination as discussed earlier. Zogakis and colleagues [28] reported on 8 patients with sporadic ZES who had persistent disease following an initial operation in which no duodenetomy was performed. In all 8 cases, a duodenal primary tumor was identified at reoperation with the performance of a duodentomy. Norton and colleagues [35] reported finding a duodenal gastrinoma at reoperation in 6 of 10 patients in whom duodenotomy had not been initially performed for either sporadic or familial ZES. Removal of a primary gastrinoma in this setting can result in long-term cure and likely affects overall survival to the same extent as a properly performed initial operation using modern techniques.

Following the initial operation, with modern techniques for preoperative evaluation and surgical exploration including duodenotomy, 50% to 60% of patients with sporadic ZES will have an initial biochemical cure and 40% to 50% will have persistent biochemical evidence of disease. Among those with initial biochemical cure, approximately half will develop evidence of recurrent disease in long-term follow-up [13]. For these patients with persistent or recurrent disease following an initial operation, clinical, serologic, and radiographic follow-up is indicated as discussed earlier. Reoperation should be limited to and considered in patients who develop new findings on tumor localization studies during the follow-up period.

Gastrinoma identification has been reported at the time of reoperation to range between 65% and 100% and biochemical cure rates have been reported in 35% [19] to 44% [50] of patients. These rates are slightly lower than the biochemical cure rates reported for primary surgery for sporadic disease in modern series [16]. Reoperation resulting in biochemical cure has been reported in the following clinical scenarios: no tumor identified at primary operation, following initial resection of a duodenal gastrinoma, following initial enucleation of a pancreatic tumor, and following multiple reoperations for recurrent or persistent disease [19,20]. Long-term biochemical cure in the reoperative setting is not uncommon and durable biochemical cure of up to 12 years has been reported following reoperation for ZES [20] (Fig. 3). However, decisions for reoperation must be made in the context of the overall condition (comorbidities, age, medical condition, and previous surgical history) of a patient particularly in light of the reported mortality rates of up to 6% associated with reoperation for ZES [19] and the lack of clear association between reoperation and improved overall survival for most cases.

Radioguided surgery using radiolabeled octreotide has been reported by some investigators to facilitate gastrinoma localization [51,52]. However, the effect of radioguidance on surgical cure rates either at the time of primary operation or reoperation has not been well defined and the use of intraoperative radioguidance for improving outcomes remains investigational at present. Serum gastrin assay determinations may also have a role in the reoperative setting but the role of this intraoperatively has likewise not been well defined [37–39].

Reoperation for palliation with debulking of disease may be indicated in selected patients with metastatic gastrinoma [53]. In terms of overall survival, Ellison and colleagues [49] found no effect on overall survival in patients undergoing a R2 resection for metastatic gastrinoma and have advocated

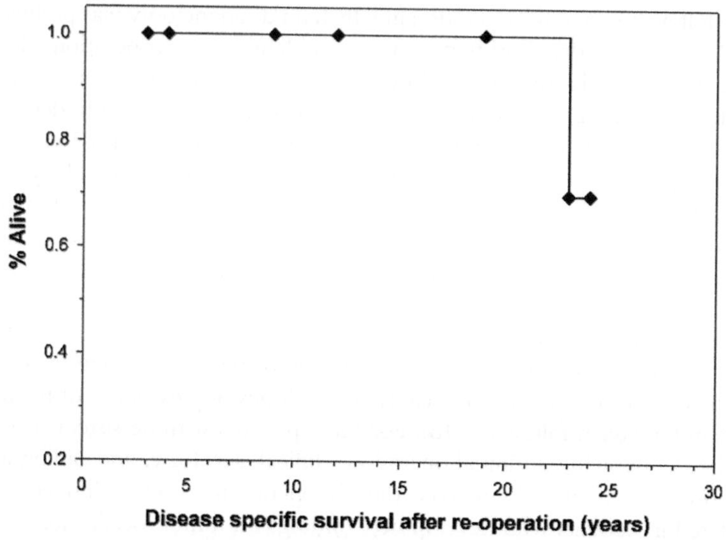

Fig. 3. Disease-specific survival for 9 patients undergoing reoperation for sporadic ZES. Median patient follow-up was 14 years. *Reproduced from* Grobmyer SR, Vogel SB, McGuigan JE, et al. Reoperative surgery in sporadic Zollinger-Ellison syndrome: long term results. J Am Coll Surg 2009;208(5):718–22; with permission.

attempted resection in those in whom either R0 or R1 is believed to be possible. On the other hand, Norton and colleagues [53] have shown that extended resection including multiorganectomy can be safely performed in selected patients with advanced metastatic neuroendocrine tumors and that debulking can be associated with long-term survival, although recurrence rates are high.

MODERN APPROACHES TO ZES IN THE SETTING OF MEN-1

Disagreement concerning the lethality of pancreatic endocrine neoplasms associated with MEN-1 still exists and many consider the pancreatic neoplasms to be fairly indolent. Doherty and colleagues [54] analyzed 34 distinct kindreds for cause and age of death and found that 46% died of causes related to their endocrine neoplasms at a median age of 47 years and that pancreatic islet cell neoplasms were the most common cause of death. However, the variability in inactivating mutations of the MEN-1 tumor suppressor gene results in varied prevalence and behavior of pancreatic endocrine neoplasms in different kindreds [55].

Because the clinical phenotype varies widely, the management of patients with MEN-1 and ZES remains challenging and controversial. Patients with MEN-1 undergoing operation for ZES are rarely, if ever, cured [56]. Norton and colleagues [57] have reported on 81 patients with ZES and MEN-1; these patients were managed prospectively with observation (all patients with tumors <2.5 cm in size or those with diffuse liver metastases) or surgery all patients with a single tumor 2.5–6 cm in size or 2 or more lesions 2.5 cm in diameter or larger or 1 lesion larger than 6 cm. Pancreatic endocrine tumors were found in all patients at surgery. Most patients undergoing surgery had multiple tumors. Of the patients undergoing resection, 46% had a distal pancreatectomy, 8% had a hepatic resection, 4% had a Whipple procedure, and 62% had a duodenal resection. No patient was cured at 5 years follow-up. Mean follow-up from surgery was 6.9 years, and during follow-up liver metastases developed in 6% of the patients. The survival rate was similar for patients with 1 or more tumors greater than 2.5 cm in size. However, the survival rate was significantly worse for those patients presenting with liver metastases [13,57].

The goal of surgery in patients with MEN-1 and ZES is not biochemical cure but to remove the primary tumor before the development of liver metastases. The risk of liver metastases is associated with the size of the primary pancreatic gastrinoma. Patients with small (<1 cm) primary pancreatic gastrinomas have a 4% rate of liver metastases compared with 28% with gastrinomas that are 1 to 3 cm in size and 61% for tumors greater than 3 cm. Therefore, some recommend resection of the primary tumor when it is 2 cm or greater [58]. Whether resection of the primary tumor really decreases the rate of liver metastases or if liver metastases are related to more aggressive biology in a subset of gastrinomas in MEN-1 is not known.

The operation of choice for ZES in MEN-1 is still under debate but enucleation of the primary tumor and avoidance of radical resection (unless enucleation is not possible) is preferred [23,56]. This recommendation is based on the difficulty of achieving biochemical cure in MEN-1 and ZES despite radical resection, such as pancreaticoduodenectomy. In addition, following a pancreaticoduodenectomy, anatomy is altered and additional surgery to remove recurrent tumor may be exceedingly difficult. It may also be challenging to treat liver metastases because of poor tolerance of embolization following pancreaticoduodenectomy with increased chance of liver abscess. In addition to therapy directed at a known pancreatic tumor in a patient with MEN-1, duodenal primary gastrinomas are frequently found in MEN-1 patients with ZES. It is not known if duodenotomy and palpation and subsequent removal of small tumors from the duodenum provide much benefit. However, if the goal is to prevent metastatic disease, then duodenotomy with palpation should be incorporated into a planned resection for a larger dominant pancreatic tumor.

On the other hand, Thompson and colleagues [5] have long advocated an aggressive surgical approach for pancreatic endocrine neoplasms in patients with MEN-1 and ZES because their interpretation is that the incidence of malignancy is similar to that in patients with sporadic islet cell neoplasms. Their preferred surgical approach is a distal pancreatectomy to the level of the superior mesenteric vein, enucleation of any significant neoplasms in the pancreatic head or uncinate process, duodenotomy and excision of any neoplasms in the first to fourth portion of the duodenum as indicated by increased basal or stimulated gastrin levels, a peripancreatic lymph node dissection including nodes in the porta hepatis and along the hepatic artery, and a prophylactic cholecystectomy [59]. The incidence of eugastrinemia on long-term follow-up has been impressive by others who have used this approach [60]. This approach must be recognized as having higher morbidity rates compared with more conservative resections/therapy and still results in a relatively high biochemical or clinical recurrence rate of ZES despite radical resection.

REOPERATION FOR ZES IN MEN-1

Long-term studies show that most patients with ZES and MEN-1 are not biochemically cured. At present the indications for reoperation and the type of operation are largely undefined and controversial. Studies on reoperation for ZES and MEN-1 are limited. Jensen and colleagues [19] reported their results for reoperation in 2 patients with ZES and MEN-1. The indication for reoperation was identification of disease on imaging during follow-up. One of the patients had his entire duodenum carpeted with small tumors and lymph node involvement around the pancreatic head. The other patient had 2 duodenal tumors and lymph node involvement near the first portion of the duodenum. In another series, 3 patients with ZES and MEN-1 underwent reoperation for biochemical recurrent disease and a lesion seen on imaging. Two of 3 patients are free of disease 3 and 5 years after pancreaticoduodenectomy. The third patient has biochemical evidence of recurrent disease [60]. It is clear that with limited data, indications and rationale for reoperation in patients with ZES and MEN-1 have to be made on a case by case basis.

Reoperation following limited initial operation for ZES in MEN-1

Following a limited initial operation for ZES in MEN-1, such as enucleation, patients should be followed with serum gastrin and secretin stimulation tests. If these are abnormal, SRS and CT scan are recommended. The indications for reoperation are similar to those before the first operation. If recurrent disease is detected, reoperation should be performed to prevent the development of liver metastases and is generally reserved for tumors greater than 2 cm in size [61]. Reoperation should be performed with care taken to examine the pancreas fully and consideration should be given to duodenotomy and excision of palpable tumors. A lymphadenectomy should be completed to encompass the portal and hepatic artery lymph nodes as well as nodes in the peripancreatic location around the pancreatic head.

Reoperation following aggressive initial operation for ZES in MEN-1

Thompson and colleagues [62] have recently described their results for completion pancreatectomy and duodenectomy for recurrent MEN-1 pancreaticoduodenal endocrine neoplasms. All patients (n = 49) underwent an initial aggressive resection as described earlier. Of these patients, 8 of 49 (16%) required completion pancreatectomy and duodenectomy. Seven of these 8 patients required an additional pancreatic or duodenal operation in the interim such that the median number of operations for either resection of recurrent pancreatic neoplasms or duodenal gastrinomas was 2 before completion pancreatectomy. Postoperative complications were frequent including 1 bilioenteric anastomotic leak, 1 pulmonary embolism, a bowel obstruction requiring reoperation and a late enterocutaneous fistula. Severe diabetes mellitus managed with an insulin pump occurred in 3 patients and standard insulin therapy in the remaining 5 patients. The investigators concluded from their report that completion pancreatectomy and duodenectomy is difficult but outcomes are acceptable. They also concluded that initial alternative pancreatic resections that preserve pancreatic mass and allow future pancreas-preserving operations should be considered.

REOPERATION FOR MANAGEMENT OF LIVER METASTASES IN ZES

Two distinct patterns of tumor dissemination to the liver have been observed in patients with gastrinoma. Most patients with metastatic gastrinoma to the liver present with these lesions; a minority of patients develop liver metastases years after the initial diagnosis [63]. Also, the development of hepatic metastases in large series of patients with gastrinoma followed for many years is infrequent [64]. In a series of 185 patients followed prospectively, liver metastases were present in 24% of patients and correlated with the size of the primary tumor. Liver metastases occurred more often ($P<.00001$) with pancreatic than duodenal primary tumors. In those with liver metastases, the duodenal primary tumors were smaller than pancreatic tumors [65]. It seems that there is a benign and malignant form of ZES distinguished in part by the presence or subsequent development of liver metastases. In addition, it has been described that the growth rate of metastatic gastrinoma varies markedly in different patients. Sutliff and colleagues [66] followed 19 patients with metastatic gastrinoma to the liver. Imaging was performed at 4- to 6-month intervals and the metastases growth rate was calculated. Twenty-six percent of patients had no growth for a mean follow-up time of 29 months, 32% had slow growth (1%–50% increase in volume per month) in a 19-month period, and 42% had rapid growth (>50% volume increase per month) in an 11-month period. In patients with rapid growth, 62% died; none of the patients in the other 2 groups died. The growth rate needs to be considered in determining the timing and type of antitumor therapy.

Patients with multiple liver metastases from ZES can generally feel well and remain functional while being maintained on medical acid suppressive therapy. However, in most patients, the tumor(s) progress over time. Some investigators have indicated that only patients found to have gastrinoma in the liver at initial examination are at risk for death from progressive tumor growth. Such growth has been reported to result in inanition or hepatic failure [63]. In 27 patients with gastrinoma followed by diffuse liver metastases, the 10-year survival was only 15% compared with a 95% 20-year survival in those without liver metastases. Patients with a solitary liver metastasis or fewer than 5 metastases in both liver lobes had an intermediate survival of 60% at 15 years [35]. The extent of liver metastases is therefore an important prognostic determinant of outcome. As such, an aggressive approach to the treatment of liver metastases is indicated.

Despite the absence of randomized or nonrandomized controlled studies (where the controls were similar in characteristics to the liver resection group), there is consensus that the resection of metastatic disease to the liver improves survival in ZES. Given the prolonged survival following the resection of liver metastases caused by neuroendocrine tumors, liver resection should be used as the benchmark against which all other treatments for resectable neuroendocrine disease are assessed [67]. Unfortunately, for gastrinomas as well as for other metastatic neuroendocrine tumors to the liver, less than 25% of patients have metastases that are fully resectable [68,69]. Therefore, surgery for potential cure is only possible in a small cohort of patients with metastatic disease. Several studies have reported infrequent cures for resection of metastatic gastrinoma to the liver [70,71].

Although the reported outcomes of resection for metastatic gastrinoma to the liver are limited to a few patients, extrapolation from results for gastrinomas and other gastrointestinal neuroendocrine tumors is possible. Liver resection for metastatic neuroendocrine tumor has been reported to result in early symptom control in most patients with a 5-year survival of 60%–70% (Table 1). In selected patients, a 5-year survival rate of 95% has been reported for resection of unilobar metastases [82]. In a study from the Mayo Clinic, 96% of patients achieved either a partial or complete response of their hormonal symptoms following aggressive surgical resection of neuroendocrine metastases in the liver. Symptom recurrence rate was 59% at 5 years with a median time to recurrence of 45.5 months. In addition, although survival rates were reasonable, in part because of the slow growth of well-differentiated neuroendocrine tumors, recurrence rates approached 85% at 5 years [78]. When the analysis was done between patients with complete versus those with incomplete resection, there was a significant difference in

Table 1
Selected series of resection for hepatic metastases of neuroendocrine tumors

First author	No. of patients	Symptom control (%)	Survival
Que et al [72]	74	90	73% at 4 years
Dousset et al [73]	17	88	46% at 4 years
Chen et al [74]	15	nr	73% at 5 years
Chamberlain et al [75]	34		76% at 5 years
Grazi et al [76]	19	nr	92% at 4 years
Nave et al [77]	31	nr	46% at 5 years
Sarmiento et al [78]	170	96	61% at 5 years
Gomez et al [79]	18	100	86% at 5 years
Scigliano et al [80]	41	nr	79% at 5 years
Hibi et al [81]	21	92	73% at 5 years

Abbreviation: nr, not reported.

Adapted from Sarmiento JM, Heywood G, Rubin J, et al. Surgical treatment of neuroendocrine metastases to the liver: a plea for resection to increase survival. J Am Coll Surg 2003;197(1):29–7.

survival (76% vs 91% at 5 years; median 30 vs 16 months, respectively, $P = .0004$). The liver was involved as the site of recurrence in 123 of 150 patients (82%).

Although surgery is the first consideration in patients with liver metastases of gastrinoma, many patients are not candidates for a curative resection. Radiofrequency ablation (RFA) is a locally destructive method that has been used for the treatment of these patients. Mazzaglia and colleagues [83] have reported their results using laparoscopic RFA in 63 patients with 384 neuroendocrine liver metastases. Unfortunately, gastrinoma was present in only 1 patient. Forty-nine patients underwent 1 ablation session, and 14 had repeat sessions. Significant or complete relief of symptoms was found in 70% of patients. Duration of symptom control was 11 ± 2.3 months. Local recurrence of tumor was found in 6.3% after a median follow-up of 2.8 years. RFA associated morbidity was identified in only 5%. The investigators concluded that in patients with neuroendocrine hepatic metastases and limited treatment options, RFA provides effective local control and symptom improvement. In a study of percutaneous RFA for metastatic neuroendocrine liver metastases in 19 patients followed for a median of 21 months, relief of hormone-related symptoms was achieved in 9 of 14 patients (69%). The median survival period from the diagnosis of liver metastases was 53 months [84].

Chemoembolization has been used in patients with nonresectable disease in an attempt to achieve tumor shrinkage and symptom response. Published response rates vary but symptom improvement has been reported to occur in up to 93% of patients [85,86]. Unfortunately, duration of responses are typically less than 12 months and median survival is approximately 2 years [87]. The optimal agents for embolization of metastatic disease to the liver remain controversial. Some investigators have reported prolonged overall survival for patients treated with hepatic artery chemoembolization (31.5 and 44 months) compared with those treated with hepatic artery embolization (18.2 and 39 months), however, statistical significance was not reached in either study [86,88]. In a recent review of the experience from 3 university hospitals, survival and symptom control were retrospectively compared for hepatic artery chemoembolization (HACE) and bland embolization (HAE) for hepatic neuroendocrine metastases. Pancreatic islet cell tumors were present in 40% of patients in this study. Of 100 patients managed by HACE ($n = 49$) or HAE ($n = 51$), morbidity, 30-day mortality, and symptom improvement were similar between the 2 groups (HACE vs HAE: 2.4% vs 6.6%; 0.8% vs 1.8%; and 88% vs 83%, respectively). No differences in the median survival were observed between HACE and HAE from the time of the first embolization procedure (25.5 vs 25.7 months, $P = .79$) [89]. One can conclude that the addition of intraarterial chemotherapy to embolization is not likely to provide a significant survival benefit over bland HAE.

Liver transplantation has also been used to treat metastatic liver disease in neuroendocrine tumors. In a multicenter report from France of 31 patients undergoing liver transplantation between 1989 and 1994, there were 15 cases of metastatic carcinoid and 16 cases of islet cell carcinomas. Actuarial survival rate was 59% at 1 year, 47% at 3 years and 36% at 5 years. Survival rates were significantly higher for metastatic carcinoid tumors (69% at 5 years) than for islet cell tumors (8% at 4 years) because of higher tumor-related and nontumor-related mortality rates. Based on this report, liver transplantation was not recommended for islet cell tumors [90]. In another collective review of 103 patients undergoing liver transplantation for metastatic neuroendocrine carcinoma, recurrence-free survival did not exceed 24% at 5 years. Multivariate analysis identified age greater than 50 years and transplantation combined with abdominal exenteration or pancreatic resection as adverse prognostic factors on survival [91]. The role of liver transplantation remains limited for metastatic gastrinoma. It is perhaps best reserved for young patients (<50 years old) with unresectable liver disease, who have no extrahepatic disease and have failed other local and systemic therapies.

REOPERATION IN ZES FOR MANAGEMENT OF GASTRIC-RELATED COMPLICATIONS

Presently, total gastrectomy is indicated for management of intractable peptic ulcer disease that is resistant to medical management and those who cannot or will not take oral antisecretory medications [92]. The use of total gastrectomy has become much less common in the era of proton pump inhibitors.

Parietal cell vagotomy (PCV) may have a role at the time of reoperation for ZES and has been endorsed by some [15,17,93]. PCV can reduce the acid secretory rate and may allow for a reduction of the dosage proton pump inhibitors in patients who have refractory or recurrent ZES [94]. The performance of parietal cell vagotomy may reduce the incidence of malignant carcinoids that can occur in patients with MEN-1 and ZES on long-standing proton pump inhibitors [23]. PCV should only be necessary on an infrequent basis and considered on an individual basis.

Gastric carcinoids are uncommonly found in patients with sporadic ZES. Gastric carcinoids are more common in patients with ZES and MEN-1 occurring in approximately 25% of patients [17]. In most of these cases, gastric carcinoids are small and can be managed nonsurgically. More aggressive/larger carcinoids may require gastric resection [17].

MEDICAL MANAGEMENT OF PATIENTS WITH PERSISTENT OR RECURRENT ZES

For patients with widely metastatic disease who refuse surgery or who are not medically fit for surgery, medical management with acid suppression therapy has a primary role in symptom management for patients with ZES. Acid suppression with proton pump inhibitors or antihistamines has no effect on tumor progression and metastatic spread [92,95].

Long-acting octreotide (LAR) may be of benefit in patients with metastatic gastrinoma [22]. LAR can also effectively control symptoms in patients with ZES by lowering or stabilizing serum gastrin levels although the durability of response is variable [96–98]. Octreotide is an effective, generally well-tolerated treatment in patients with metastatic gastrinoma. It is associated with stabilization of disease in approximately 50% of patients and with tumor shrinkage in approximately 5% of patients [99,100]. Reported median time to progression for patients with metastatic disease has ranged from 14 to 24 months [99,101]. Despite its effect on tumor progression, LAR has not been shown to conclusively improve overall survival in patients with metastatic gastrinoma [31,101]. Some have advocated the use of interferon alfa in combination with LAR for patients with metastatic gastrinoma [102]. The addition of interferon alfa does increase treatment-related side effects although the benefit of this combination is controversial [25,103,104]. Radiolabeled octreotide analogues are also under development for treatment of metastatic gastrinoma but their exact role in management remains incompletely defined [31].

Cytotoxic chemotherapeutics including streptozocin and doxorubicin can be considered for patients with rapidly progressive or extensive metastatic disease [22,105]. Reported response rates with this type of therapy have varied between 5% and 50 % [106]. The effect of these cytotoxic agents on overall survival is controversial [25].

SUMMARY

It is clear that a properly performed initial operation is the key to success in the management of a patient with ZES. However, reoperation is frequently a consideration in the management of patients with ZES because high rates of persistent and recurrent disease are manifest even with modern imaging and surgical approaches. In carefully selected patients, reoperation can result in durable biochemical cure and improved survival and should be considered. A thorough knowledge of the natural history of the sporadic form of ZES and ZES in the context of MEN-1, patterns of presentation, and sites of metastases are necessary to achieve the best outcome in patients with this unusual disease.

References

[1] Zollinger RM, Ellison EH. Primary peptic ulcerations of the jejunum associated with islet cell tumors of the pancreas. Ann Surg 1955;142(4):709–23 [discussion: 724–8].

[2] Gibril F, Jensen RT. Zollinger-Ellison syndrome revisited: diagnosis, biologic markers, associated inherited disorders, and acid hypersecretion. Curr Gastroenterol Rep 2004;6(6): 454–63.

[3] Underdahl LO, Woolner LB, Black BM. Multiple endocrine adenomas; report of 8 cases in which the parathyroids, pituitary and pancreatic islets were involved. J Clin Endocrinol Metab 1953;13(1):20–47.

[4] Wermer P. Genetic aspects of adenomatosis of endocrine glands. Am J Med 1954;16(3): 363–71.

[5] Thompson NW, Bondeson AG, Bondeson L, et al. The surgical treatment of gastrinoma in MEN I syndrome patients. Surgery 1989;106(6):1081–5 [discussion: 1085–6].

[6] Ellison EC. Zollinger-Ellison syndrome: a personal perspective. Am Surg 2008;74(7): 563–71.

[7] Wilson SD, Ellison EH. Survival in patients with the Zollinger-Ellison syndrome treated by total gastrectomy. Am J Surg 1966;111(6):787–91.

[8] Fox PS, Hofmann JW, Decosse JJ, et al. The influence of total gastrectomy on survival in malignant Zollinger-Ellison tumors. Ann Surg 1974;180(4):558–66.
[9] Thompson JC, Lewis BG, Wiener I, et al. The role of surgery in the Zollinger-Ellison syndrome. Ann Surg 1983;197(5):594–607.
[10] McCarthy DM. Report on the United States experience with cimetidine in Zollinger-Ellision syndrome and other hypersecretory states. Gastroenterology 1978;74(2 Pt 2): 453–8.
[11] Metz DC, Pisegna JR, Fishbeyn VA, et al. Control of gastric acid hypersecretion in the management of patients with Zollinger-Ellison syndrome. World J Surg 1993;17(4): 468–80.
[12] Howard TJ, Zinner MJ, Stabile BE, et al. Gastrinoma excision for cure. A prospective analysis. Ann Surg 1990;211(1):9–14.
[13] Norton JA, Fraker DL, Alexander HR, et al. Surgery to cure the Zollinger-Ellison syndrome. N Engl J Med 1999;341(9):635–44.
[14] Norton JA, Jensen RT. Role of surgery in Zollinger-Ellison syndrome. J Am Coll Surg 2007;205(Suppl 4):S34–7.
[15] Lorenz K, Dralle H. Surgical treatment of sporadic gastrinoma. Wien Klin Wochenschr 2007;119(19–20):597–601.
[16] Norton JA, Fraker DL, Alexander HR, et al. Surgery increases survival in patients with gastrinoma. Ann Surg 2006;244(3):410–9.
[17] Norton JA, Jensen RT. Resolved and unresolved controversies in the surgical management of patients with Zollinger-Ellison syndrome. Ann Surg 2004;240(5):757–73.
[18] Libutti SK, Alexander HR Jr. Gastrinoma: sporadic and familial disease. Surg Oncol Clin N Am 2006;15(3):479–96.
[19] Jaskowiak NT, Fraker DL, Alexander HR, et al. Is reoperation for gastrinoma excision indicated in Zollinger-Ellison syndrome? Surgery 1996;120(6):1055–62 [discussion: 1062–3].
[20] Grobmyer SR, Vogel SB, McGuigan JE, et al. Reoperative surgery in sporadic Zollinger-Ellison syndrome: longterm results. J Am Coll Surg 2009;208(5):718–22 [discussion: 722–4].
[21] Zollinger RM, Martin EW Jr, Carey LC, et al. Observations on the postoperative tumor growth behavior of certain islet cell tumors. Ann Surg 1976;184(4):525–30.
[22] Auernhammer CJ, Goke B. Medical treatment of gastrinomas. Wien Klin Wochenschr 2007;119(19–20):609–15.
[23] Morrow EH, Norton JA. Surgical management of Zollinger-Ellison syndrome; state of the art. Surg Clin North Am 2009;89(5):1091–103.
[24] Jensen RT. Gastrinomas: advances in diagnosis and management. Neuroendocrinology 2004;80(Suppl 1):23–7.
[25] Jensen RT, Niederle B, Mitry E, et al. Gastrinoma (duodenal and pancreatic). Neuroendocrinology 2006;84(3):173–82.
[26] Ellison EC, Johnson JA. The Zollinger-Ellison syndrome: a comprehensive review of historical, scientific, and clinical considerations. Curr Probl Surg 2009;46(1):13–106.
[27] Gibril F, Reynolds JC, Doppman JL, et al. Somatostatin receptor scintigraphy: its sensitivity compared with that of other imaging methods in detecting primary and metastatic gastrinomas. A prospective study. Ann Intern Med 1996;125(1):26–34.
[28] Zogakis TG, Gibril F, Libutti SK, et al. Management and outcome of patients with sporadic gastrinoma arising in the duodenum. Ann Surg 2003;238(1):42–8.
[29] Vogel SB, Wolfe MM, McGuigan JE, et al. Localization and resection of gastrinomas in Zollinger-Ellison syndrome. Ann Surg 1987;205(5):550–6.
[30] Stabile BE, Morrow DJ, Passaro E Jr. The gastrinoma triangle: operative implications. Am J Surg 1984;147(1):25–31.
[31] Gibril F, Jensen RT. Advances in evaluation and management of gastrinoma in patients with Zollinger-Ellison syndrome. Curr Gastroenterol Rep 2005;7(2):114–21.

[32] Frucht H, Norton JA, London JF, et al. Detection of duodenal gastrinomas by operative endoscopic transillumination. A prospective study. Gastroenterology 1990;99(6): 1622–7.
[33] Thompson NW, Pasieka J, Fukuuchi A. Duodenal gastrinomas, duodenotomy, and duodenal exploration in the surgical management of Zollinger-Ellison syndrome. World J Surg 1993;17(4):455–62.
[34] Thompson NW, Vinik AI, Eckhauser FE. Microgastrinomas of the duodenum. A cause of failed operations for the Zollinger-Ellison syndrome. Ann Surg 1989;209(4): 396–404.
[35] Norton JA, Alexander HR, Fraker DL, et al. Does the use of routine duodenotomy (DUODX) affect rate of cure, development of liver metastases, or survival in patients with Zollinger-Ellison syndrome? Ann Surg 2004;239(5):617–25 [discussion: 626].
[36] Norton JA, Alexander HR, Fraker DL, et al. Possible primary lymph node gastrinoma: occurrence, natural history, and predictive factors: a prospective study. Ann Surg 2003;237(5):650–7 [discussion: 657–9].
[37] Imamura M, Takahashi K, Isobe Y, et al. Curative resection of multiple gastrinomas aided by selective arterial secretin injection test and intraoperative secretin test. Ann Surg 1989;210(6):710–8.
[38] Proye C, Pattou F, Carnaille B, et al. Intraoperative gastrin measurements during surgical management of patients with gastrinomas: experience with 20 cases. World J Surg 1998;22(7):643–9 [discussion: 649–50].
[39] Kato M, Imamura M, Hosotani R, et al. Curative resection of microgastrinomas based on the intraoperative secretin test. World J Surg 2000;24(11):1425–30.
[40] McGuigan JE, Trudeau WL. Immunochemical measurement of elevated levels of gastrin in the serum of patients with pancreatic tumors of the Zollinger-Ellison variety. N Engl J Med 1968;278(24):1308–13.
[41] Alexander HR, Bartlett DL, Venzon DJ, et al. Analysis of factors associated with long-term (five or more years) cure in patients undergoing operation for Zollinger-Ellison syndrome. Surgery 1998;124(6):1160–6.
[42] Norton JA, Jensen RT. Current surgical management of Zollinger-Ellison syndrome (ZES) in patients without multiple endocrine neoplasia-type 1 (MEN1). Surg Oncol 2003;12(2): 145–51.
[43] Fishbeyn VA, Norton JA, Benya RV, et al. Assessment and prediction of long-term cure in patients with the Zollinger-Ellison syndrome: the best approach. Ann Intern Med 1993;119(3):199–206.
[44] Berger AC, Gibril F, Venzon DJ, et al. Prognostic value of initial fasting serum gastrin levels in patients with Zollinger-Ellison syndrome. J Clin Oncol 2001;19(12):3051–7.
[45] Syversen U, Mignon M, Bonfils S, et al. Chromogranin A and pancreastatin-like immunoreactivity in serum of gastrinoma patients. Acta Oncol 1993;32(2):161–5.
[46] Goebel SU, Serrano J, Yu F, et al. Prospective study of the value of serum chromogranin A or serum gastrin levels in the assessment of the presence, extent, or growth of gastrinomas. Cancer 1999;85(7):1470–83.
[47] Goebel SU, Iwamoto M, Raffeld M, et al. Her-2/neu expression and gene amplification in gastrinomas: correlations with tumor biology, growth, and aggressiveness. Cancer Res 2002;62(13):3702–10.
[48] Furukawa M, Raffeld M, Mateo C, et al. Increased expression of insulin-like growth factor I and/or its receptor in gastrinomas is associated with low curability, increased growth, and development of metastases. Clin Cancer Res 2005;11(9):3233–42.
[49] Ellison EC, Sparks J, Verducci JS, et al. 50-year appraisal of gastrinoma: recommendations for staging and treatment. J Am Coll Surg 2006;202(6):897–905.
[50] Grobmyer SR, Pieracci FM, Allen PJ, et al. Defining morbidity after pancreaticoduodenectomy: use of a prospective complication grading system. J Am Coll Surg 2007;204(3): 356–64.

[51] Woltering EA, Barrie R, O'Dorisio TM, et al. Detection of occult gastrinomas with iodine 125-labeled lanreotide and intraoperative gamma detection. Surgery 1994;116(6): 1139–46 [discussion: 1146–7].
[52] Albertario S, Forti P, Bianchi C, et al. Radioguided surgery for gastrinoma: a case report. Tumori 2002;88(3):S41–3.
[53] Norton JA, Warren RS, Kelly MG, et al. Aggressive surgery for metastatic liver neuroendocrine tumors. Surgery 2003;134(6):1057–63 [discussion: 1063–5].
[54] Doherty GM, Olson JA, Frisella MM, et al. Lethality of multiple endocrine neoplasia type I. World J Surg 1998;22(6):581–6 [discussion: 586–7].
[55] Kouvaraki MA, Shapiro SE, Cote GJ, et al. Management of pancreatic endocrine tumors in multiple endocrine neoplasia type 1. World J Surg 2006;30(5):643–53.
[56] Mortellaro VE, Hochwald SN, McGuigan JE, et al. Long-term results of a selective surgical approach to management of Zollinger-Ellison syndrome in patients with MEN-1. Am Surg 2009;75(8):730–3.
[57] Norton JA, Alexander HR, Fraker DL, et al. Comparison of surgical results in patients with advanced and limited disease with multiple endocrine neoplasia type 1 and Zollinger-Ellison syndrome. Ann Surg 2001;234(4):495–505 [discussion: 505–6].
[58] Norton JA. Gastrinoma: advances in localization and treatment. Surg Oncol Clin N Am 1998;7(4):845–61.
[59] Thompson NW. Current concepts in the surgical management of multiple endocrine neoplasia type 1 pancreatic-duodenal disease. Results in the treatment of 40 patients with Zollinger-Ellison syndrome, hypoglycaemia or both. J Intern Med 1998;243(6): 495–500.
[60] Bartsch DK, Fendrich V, Langer P, et al. Outcome of duodenopancreatic resections in patients with multiple endocrine neoplasia type 1. Ann Surg 2005;242(6):757–64 [discussion: 764–6].
[61] Norton JA, Fang TD, Jensen RT. Surgery for gastrinoma and insulinoma in multiple endocrine neoplasia type 1. J Natl Compr Canc Netw 2006;4(2):148–53.
[62] Gauger PG, Doherty GM, Broome JT, et al. Completion pancreatectomy and duodenectomy for recurrent MEN-1 pancreaticoduodenal endocrine neoplasms. Surgery 2009;146(4):801–6 [discussion: 807–8].
[63] Stabile BE, Passaro E Jr. Benign and malignant gastrinoma. Am J Surg 1985;149(1): 144–50.
[64] Friesen SR. Treatment of the Zollinger-Ellison syndrome. A 25 year assessment. Am J Surg 1982;143(3):331–8.
[65] Weber HC, Venzon DJ, Lin JT, et al. Determinants of metastatic rate and survival in patients with Zollinger-Ellison syndrome: a prospective long-term study. Gastroenterology 1995;108(6):1637–49.
[66] Sutliff VE, Doppman JL, Gibril F, et al. Growth of newly diagnosed, untreated metastatic gastrinomas and predictors of growth patterns. J Clin Oncol 1997;15(6):2420–31.
[67] Gurusamy KS, Ramamoorthy R, Sharma D, et al. Liver resection versus other treatments for neuroendocrine tumours in patients with resectable liver metastases. Cochrane Database Syst Rev 2009;2:CD007060.
[68] Yu F, Venzon DJ, Serrano J, et al. Prospective study of the clinical course, prognostic factors, causes of death, and survival in patients with long-standing Zollinger-Ellison syndrome. J Clin Oncol 1999;17(2):615–30.
[69] McEntee GP, Nagorney DM, Kvols LK, et al. Cytoreductive hepatic surgery for neuroendocrine tumors. Surgery 1990;108(6):1091–6.
[70] Norton JA, Sugarbaker PH, Doppman JL, et al. Aggressive resection of metastatic disease in selected patients with malignant gastrinoma. Ann Surg 1986;203(4):352–9.
[71] Elias D, Lasser P, Ducreux M, et al. Liver resection (and associated extrahepatic resections) for metastatic well-differentiated endocrine tumors: a 15-year single center prospective study. Surgery 2003;133(4):375–82.

[72] Que FG, Nagorney DM, Batts KP, et al. Hepatic resection for metastatic neuroendocrine carcinomas. Am J Surg 1995;169(1):36–42 [discussion: 42–3].
[73] Dousset B, Saint-Marc O, Pitre J, et al. Metastatic endocrine tumors: medical treatment, surgical resection, or liver transplantation. World J Surg 1996;20(7):908–14 [discussion: 914–5].
[74] Chen H, Hardacre JM, Uzar A, et al. Isolated liver metastases from neuroendocrine tumors: does resection prolong survival? J Am Coll Surg 1998;187(1):88–92 [discussion: 92–3].
[75] Chamberlain RS, Canes D, Brown KT, et al. Hepatic neuroendocrine metastases: does intervention alter outcomes? J Am Coll Surg 2000;190(4):432–45.
[76] Grazi GL, Cescon M, Pierangeli F, et al. Highly aggressive policy of hepatic resections for neuroendocrine liver metastases. Hepatogastroenterology 2000;47(32):481–6.
[77] Nave H, Mossinger E, Feist H, et al. Surgery as primary treatment in patients with liver metastases from carcinoid tumors: a retrospective, unicentric study over 13 years. Surgery 2001;129(2):170–5.
[78] Sarmiento JM, Heywood G, Rubin J, et al. Surgical treatment of neuroendocrine metastases to the liver: a plea for resection to increase survival. J Am Coll Surg 2003;197(1):29–37.
[79] Gomez D, Malik HZ, Al-Mukthar A, et al. Hepatic resection for metastatic gastrointestinal and pancreatic neuroendocrine tumours: outcome and prognostic predictors. HPB (Oxford) 2007;9(5):345–51.
[80] Scigliano S, Lebtahi R, Maire F, et al. Clinical and imaging follow-up after exhaustive liver resection of endocrine metastases: a 15-year monocentric experience. Endocr Relat Cancer 2009;16(3):977–90.
[81] Hibi T, Sano T, Sakamoto Y, et al. Surgery for hepatic neuroendocrine tumors: a single institutional experience in Japan. Jpn J Clin Oncol 2007;37(2):102–7.
[82] Ahlman H, Westberg G, Wangberg B, et al. Treatment of liver metastases of carcinoid tumors. World J Surg 1996;20(2):196–202.
[83] Mazzaglia PJ, Berber E, Milas M, et al. Laparoscopic radiofrequency ablation of neuroendocrine liver metastases: a 10-year experience evaluating predictors of survival. Surgery 2007;142(1):10–9.
[84] Gillams A, Cassoni A, Conway G, et al. Radiofrequency ablation of neuroendocrine liver metastases: the Middlesex experience. Abdom Imaging 2005;30(4):435–41.
[85] Wallace S, Ajani JA, Charnsangavej C, et al. Carcinoid tumors: imaging procedures and interventional radiology. World J Surg 1996;20(2):147–56.
[86] Ruutiainen AT, Soulen MC, Tuite CM, et al. Chemoembolization and bland embolization of neuroendocrine tumor metastases to the liver. J Vasc Interv Radiol 2007;18(7):847–55.
[87] Perry LJ, Stuart K, Stokes KR, et al. Hepatic arterial chemoembolization for metastatic neuroendocrine tumors. Surgery 1994;116(6):1111–6 [discussion: 1116–7].
[88] Gupta S, Johnson MM, Murthy R, et al. Hepatic arterial embolization and chemoembolization for the treatment of patients with metastatic neuroendocrine tumors: variables affecting response rates and survival. Cancer 2005;104(8):1590–602.
[89] Pitt SC, Pitt HA, Baker MS, et al. Small pancreatic and periampullary neuroendocrine tumors: resect or enucleate? J Gastrointest Surg 2009;13(9):1692–8.
[90] Le Treut YP, Delpero JR, Dousset B, et al. Results of liver transplantation in the treatment of metastatic neuroendocrine tumors. A 31-case French multicentric report. Ann Surg 1997;225(4):355–64.
[91] Lehnert T. Liver transplantation for metastatic neuroendocrine carcinoma: an analysis of 103 patients. Transplantation 1998;66(10):1307–12.
[92] Bonfils S, Landor JH, Mignon M, et al. Results of surgical management in 92 consecutive patients with Zollinger-Ellison syndrome. Ann Surg 1981;194(6):692–7.
[93] Jensen RT. Should the 1996 citation for Zollinger-Ellison syndrome read: "Acid-reducing surgery in, aggressive resection out". Am J Gastroenterol 1996;91(6):1067–70.

[94] McArthur KE, Richardson CT, Barnett CC, et al. Laparotomy and proximal gastric vagotomy in Zollinger-Ellison syndrome: results of a 16-year prospective study. Am J Gastroenterol 1996;91(6):1104–11.
[95] Brennan MF, Jensen RT, Wesley RA, et al. The role of surgery in patients with Zollinger-Ellison syndrome (ZES) managed medically. Ann Surg 1982;196(3):239–45.
[96] Mozell E, Woltering EA, O'Dorisio TM, et al. Effect of somatostatin analog on peptide release and tumor growth in the Zollinger-Ellison syndrome. Surg Gynecol Obstet 1990;170(6):476–84.
[97] Mozell EJ, Cramer AJ, O'Dorisio TM, et al. Long-term efficacy of octreotide in the treatment of Zollinger-Ellison syndrome. Arch Surg 1992;127(9):1019–24 [discussion: 1024–6].
[98] Saijo F, Naito H, Funayama Y, et al. Octreotide in control of multiple liver metastases from gastrinoma. J Gastroenterol 2003;38(9):905–8.
[99] Shojamanesh H, Gibril F, Louie A, et al. Prospective study of the antitumor efficacy of long-term octreotide treatment in patients with progressive metastatic gastrinoma. Cancer 2002;94(2):331–43.
[100] Granberg D, Jacobsson H, Oberg K, et al. Regression of a large malignant gastrinoma on treatment with Sandostatin LAR: a case report. Digestion 2008;77(2):92–5.
[101] Rinke A, Muller HH, Schade-Brittinger C, et al. Placebo-controlled, double-blind, prospective, randomized study on the effect of octreotide LAR in the control of tumor growth in patients with metastatic neuroendocrine midgut tumors: a report from the PROMID Study Group. J Clin Oncol 2009;27(28):4656–63.
[102] Pisegna JR, Slimak GG, Doppman JL, et al. An evaluation of human recombinant alpha interferon in patients with metastatic gastrinoma. Gastroenterology 1993;105(4):1179–83.
[103] Joensuu H, Katka K, Kujari H. Dramatic response of a metastatic carcinoid tumour to a combination of interferon and octreotide. Acta Endocrinol (Copenh) 1992;126(2):184–5.
[104] Faiss S, Pape UF, Bohmig M, et al. Prospective, randomized, multicenter trial on the antiproliferative effect of lanreotide, interferon alfa, and their combination for therapy of metastatic neuroendocrine gastroenteropancreatic tumors–the International Lanreotide and Interferon Alfa Study Group. J Clin Oncol 2003;21(14):2689–96.
[105] Moertel CG, Lefkopoulo M, Lipsitz S, et al. Streptozocin-doxorubicin, streptozocin-fluorouracil or chlorozotocin in the treatment of advanced islet-cell carcinoma. N Engl J Med 1992;326(8):519–23.
[106] Arnold R, Rinke A, Schmidt C, et al. Endocrine tumours of the gastrointestinal tract: chemotherapy. Best Pract Res Clin Gastroenterol 2005;19(4):649–56.

Advances in Surgery 44 (2010) 347–360

ADVANCES IN SURGERY

Computerized Physician Order Entry System in a Surgical Practice

William M. Stone, MD

Division of Vascular Surgery, Mayo Clinic, 5777 East Mayo Boulevard, Phoenix, AZ 85525, USA

The quality of health care provided in the United States has come under increased scrutiny over the past several years. Specifically, patient safety has become a national initiative driven not only by patients but also by governmental agencies. It has been well documented that medication errors in particular are potentially avoidable and harmful [1]. The Institute of Medicine reports, *To Err is Human* and *Crossing the Quality Chasm: A New Health System for the 21st Century* [2,3], suggest that reporting systems of errors should be used for potentially preventing these errors. Most health care organizational efforts have involved some sort of information technology solution for the elimination of such errors [2]. In 2004, President Bush established by executive order the Office of National Coordinator for Health Information Technology. This office was created to assure the establishment of electronic forms of medical records throughout the United States by 2014. In addition, the Institute of Medicine has called for the use of electronic prescribing systems in all health care organizations by 2010 [3]. This combination is felt to provide the appropriate platform for reduction or potential elimination of medication errors. Recommendations from the industry-based Leapfrog Group has additionally enhanced interest in technological solutions for prescribing errors [4].

Computerized physician order entry (CPOE) systems have proved successful for the reduction of medication errors in hospital settings [5]. The obvious benefit would be derived from yielding accurate, legible, and timely orders. The interpretation of handwritten orders can be difficult. Fig. 1 represents a typical set of handwritten orders that can be confusing and lead to subjective interpretation by uneducated personnel. On the second line, the dosage of Tegretol appears to be 400 mg, when in actuality it is 100 mg. The handwritten hanging "g" causes this confusion. In addition, drug-to-drug interaction review is facilitated through these systems to minimize potentially harmful and avoidable events. Formulary adherence is facilitated by CPOE systems, which subsequently results in decreased drug expenditures [6].

Most published reviews of the impact of CPOE implementation to date describe the processes for establishment of CPOE systems, reduction of

E-mail address: stone.william@mayo.edu.

0065-3411/10/$ – see front matter
doi:10.1016/j.yasu.2010.05.010

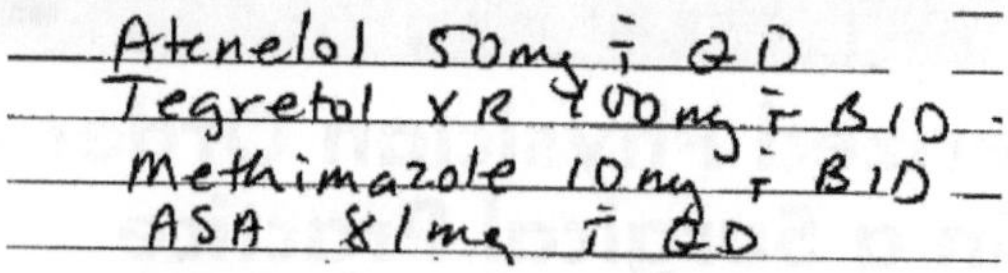

Fig. 1. Example of handwritten orders.

medication errors, physician behavioral change, and costs. Most reviews have shown beneficial effects on the turnaround time of the physician ordering process. In addition, many have shown increased time requirements for physicians and, although medication errors are reduced, mixed results have been reported when the outcome of patient safety is measured. These reviews involve inpatient medical services, including ICU settings, psychiatric wards, pediatric services, and various medical specialties. There have been no reviews of the impact of these ordering systems on multispecialty surgical practices. Accordingly, we conducted a review of the impact of implementation of a CPOE system within a multispecialty academic surgical practice.

In addition to standard CPOE systems, other electronic support systems have been devised to enhance the beneficial effect of CPOE systems. Decision support systems (DSSs) are designed to assist in clinical decision making for providers by linking specific patient characteristics to database information. These systems can be used independently but most frequently are used in conjunction with a CPOE system. The automated process can be beneficial in providing evidenced-based guidelines and access to results to providers in a timely fashion. At present, DSSs have been shown to decrease length of stay, decrease drug costs, improve preventive care, decrease medication errors, and improve drug administration [7]. These systems add to the complexity of the ordering process and are continually evolving and will play an increasingly important role in quality and safety for patient care. This article does not focus on these DSSs but primarily discusses the impact of CPOE systems.

ORDERING PROCESS TIME

Most of the evaluations of the ordering process have revealed a distinct increase in the amount of time required for clinical providers using CPOE. This includes any provider that is inputting orders to be implemented. Five published reports have evaluated the actual time required for physician ordering times comparing a paper-based system to an electronic system. Four of these showed a significant increase in the time required to input orders, but one review revealed a decrease in time required to input laboratory orders [8–12]. In addition, several studies have focused on the physician's perception of the time required. All of these studies suggested an increase in time requirement by physicians and, importantly, suggested that this detracted from the time available for patients [13,14]. It has been shown that the efficiency of inputting orders by providers does improve over time [15]. Amusan and colleagues [15] found that rounding times decreased from a mean of 18.79

minutes before CPOE implementation and decreased to 12.97 minutes 5 months after implementation ($P = .0011$).

Most of the reviews have focused on physician time, which is only a subset of the ordering process. After implementation of CPOE, physicians and nurses transform to spending more time on computers. The system provides access to all orders along the entire chain of patient care. Modifications in ordering can occur in such a manner as to expedite and accelerate clinical processes. Standard order sets, which can be modified to fit a specific providers needs, also adds to efficiency. When studies have evaluated the entire ordering process in aggregate, there have been significant time savings noted. There is a greatly diminished need for clerical work and transcription of orders. Nursing staff does not have the redundant task of trying to clarify written orders that are illegible. Pharmacy times are also reduced in the electronic ordering environment. The pharmacists require less time spent having to discuss medication-to-medication interaction and clarifying dosages and allergies; additionally, there is a greater adherence to the hospital formulary [16,17]. These reduced times provide a more efficient model of clinical care.

In our own review, we found the time savings substantial [18]. Order implementation times (defined as time from initiation of the order to order being available to nursing, radiology, or laboratory) as well as provider time was recorded for written and electronic ordering. Using a personal digital assistant (PDA), order entry time (time for provider to find patient record and write the order) was measured for written orders by hidden observation of providers in the ordering process. Data for the electronic ordering entry time (time for provider to access record and enter the order) were obtained electronically. Device log-on time was obtained through electronic measurement of time to access a patient's medical record on the electronic devices used by the providers. Four electronic devices were used for patient record access, including standard desktop computers, modified desktop computers with streamlined access software, standard laptop computers, and thin laptops (personal computers [PCs]). Order implementation times were obtained electronically and with hidden direct observation.

For written orders, the systematic process used is outlined in Fig. 2. Blinded, direct observation with PDA recording of data entry was performed on 53 order entry sessions. This included samples from 6:45 AM until 7:30 PM. Staff surgeons performed 21 (39.6%) of the recorded order entry sessions. Physician assistants performed 22 (41.5%) sessions and surgical residents and fellows performed 10 (18.9%). Average time for a provider to find a chart was 2 minutes and 3 seconds with a standard deviation of 4 minutes and 1 second (range, 1 second to 30 minutes and 1 second) (Fig. 3). Mean number of orders entered per written order session was 4.3 (range, 1 to 34 orders). Mean time for writing all of the orders during an order session was 2 minutes and 39 seconds (range, 3 seconds to 16 minutes, 2 seconds) with mean time per order of 37 seconds.

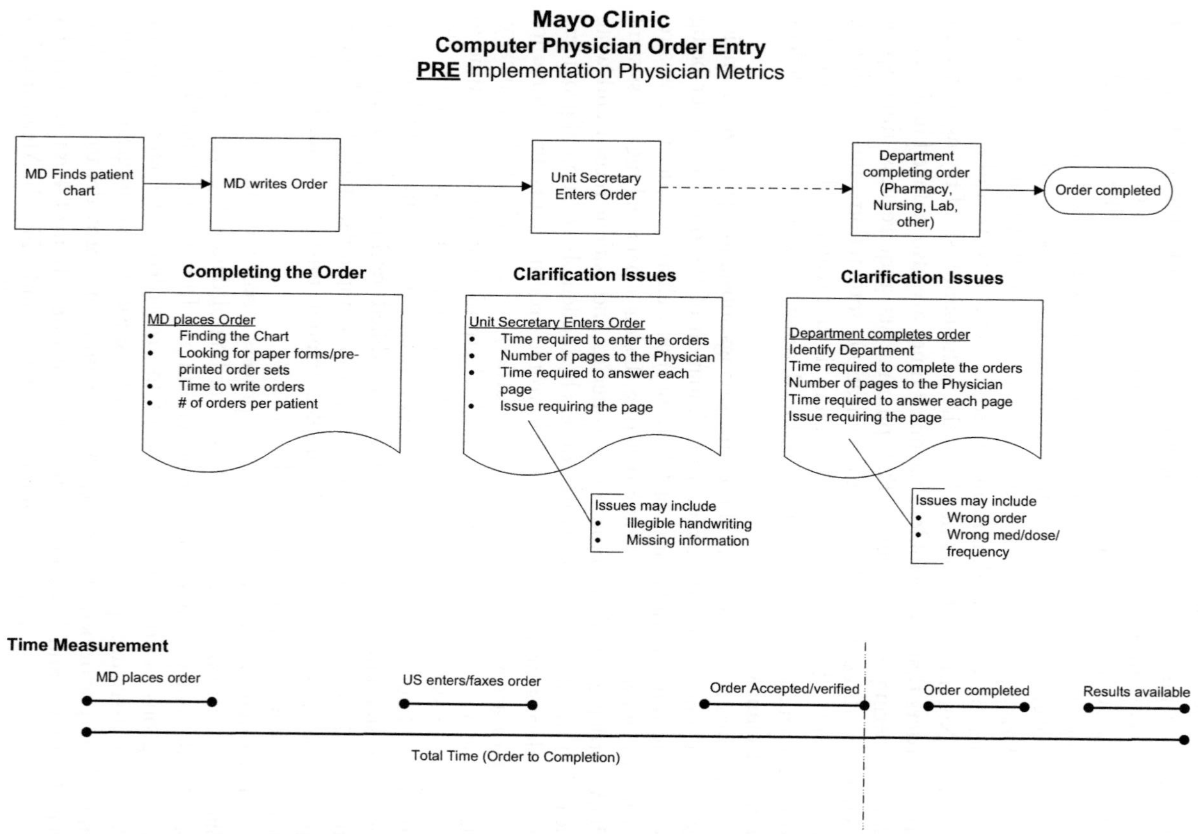

Fig. 2. Written order process. (*From* Stone WM, Smith BE, Shaft, et al. The impact of a computerized physician order entry system. J Am Coll Surg 2009;208:304–13; with permission.)

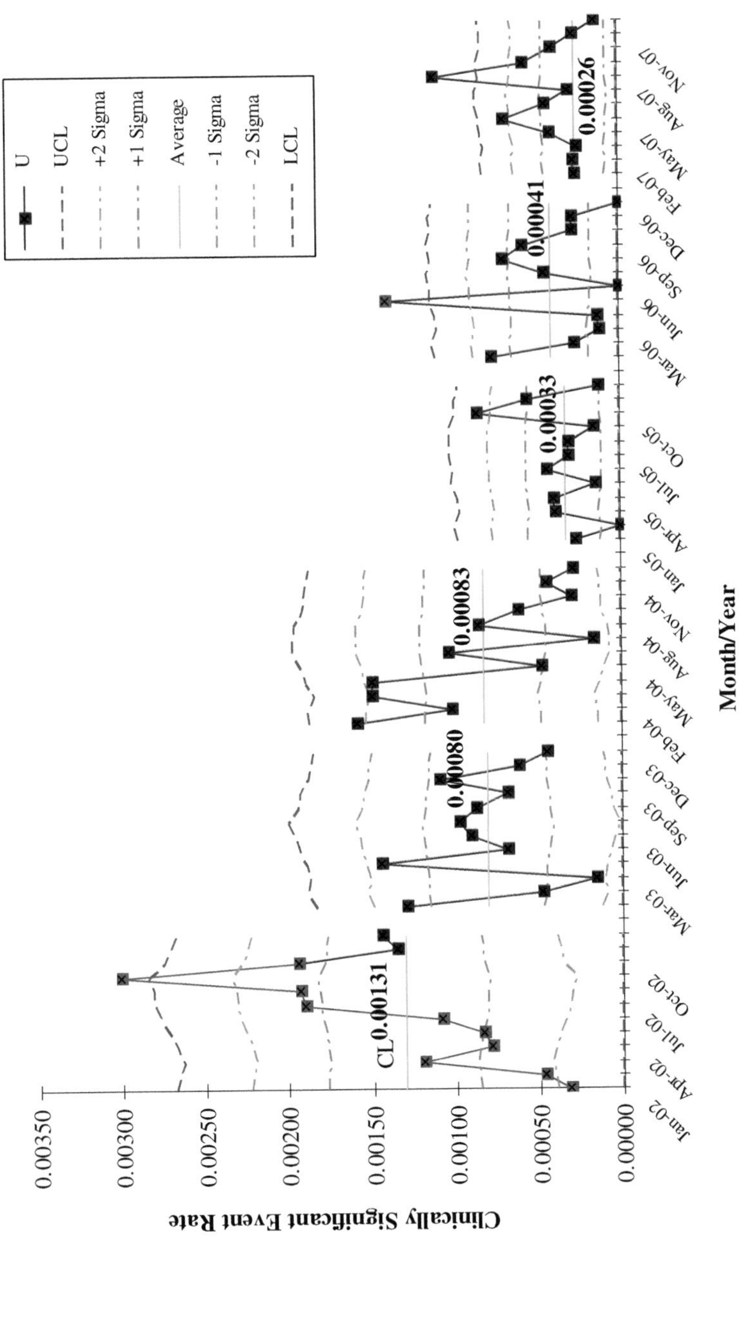

Fig. 3. Mayo Clinic Hospital patient safety score. (*From* Stone WM, Smith BE, Shaft, et al. The impact of a computerized physician order entry system. J Am Coll Surg 2009;208:304–13; with permission.)

The next step in the written ordering process involves a unit secretary, who transcribes an order and makes it available to nursing, radiology, and laboratory. The unit secretary average time for routine written orders was 51 minutes and 24 seconds (medications, 45 minutes; laboratory orders, 41 minutes; radiology orders, 56 minutes; dietary orders, 55 minutes; nursing orders, 47 minutes; and other orders, 62 minutes). If orders were given verbally (not written), average unit secretary time was 10 minutes and 30 seconds (medications, 12 minutes; laboratory orders, 10 minutes; radiology orders, 3 minutes; and nursing orders, 16 minutes). For all written orders (routine, admission, discharge, verbal, stat, and so forth), the average time from completion of writing the orders until available for nursing services was 38 minutes and 24 seconds (Fig. 4).

Electronic orders were tabulated for 100 sample order sessions on 4 random days over a 4-month period. Providers had access to four electronic devices to enter orders on patients. These included a standard laptop, standard desktop, thin PC, and a modified desktop for easier access. Device log-on and patient activation times were recorded for each electronic device. Log-on and activation time was longest using standard desktop devices (1 minute and 1 second) followed by thin PC (57 seconds), modified desktop (yellow screen) (30 seconds), and laptop (28 seconds) ($P=$ not significant) (Fig. 5). Mean number of electronic orders entered per session was 8.12 (range, 2 to 60). Time required to enter an individual order per order with the electronic ordering system had a mean of 27 seconds per order (range, 1 second to 19 minutes).

When evaluating time in aggregate, before implementation of CPOE, time from physician needing to place an order to receipt by nurse was 41.2 minutes. This included 2.05 minutes to find the chart, 0.72 minutes to write the order, and 38.4 minutes for unit secretary clarification and transcription. After CPOE, time from physician entering an order to having it accessible to the nurse was 27 seconds per order ($P<.01$) (Fig. 6).

The ordering process can be broken into small identifiable steps, which can be individually analyzed. For the written ordering process (see Fig. 2), the most time-consuming portion involves the unit secretary and transcription of the order into a form so that nursing, radiology, and laboratory may be notified. The process is initiated when a provider attempts to find a patient chart and

Mean	0:02:03
Median	0:00:43
Range	0:30:01
Minimum	0:00:01
Maximum	0:30:02
Count	90

Fig. 4. Physician written order process. Time to find a chart in minutes. (*From* Stone WM, Smith BE, Shaft, et al. The impact of a computerized physician order entry system. J Am Coll Surg 2009;208:304–13; with permission.)

				Average time (h:mm:ss) from start of writing order to time entered in IDX for:						
	Patients	Orders	Average Write Time	Meds	Lab	Rad	Nurse	Diet	Other	Average
Routine Written Orders	86	319	0:00:43	0:45:14	0:41:33	0:56:56	0:47:35	0:55:04	1:01:59	0:51:24
Routine Verbal Orders	7	11	0:02:10	0:12:30	0:10:06	0:03:00			0:16:25	0:10:30
Admission Orders	4	110	0:00:21	0:43:48	1:06:06	1:28:40	0:57:03	1:12:29	1:03:31	1:05:16
STAT Written Orders	7	17	0:01:32	0:13:58	1:13:14	0:37:39		0:03:12	0:19:00	0:29:25
STAT Verbal Orders	3	6	0:00:53	0:06:23	0:00:25		0:06:21			0:04:23
Discharge Orders	1	4	0:01:15	0:26:41						0:26:41
Total / Average	108	467	0:01:09	0:24:45	0:38:17	0:46:34	0:37:00	0:43:35	0:40:14	0:38:24
Post-Op Orders										
Post-Op to Floor	5	132	0:00:16	7:02:05		7:56:58	7:56:18	7:49:58	8:26:08	8:02:20
Post-Op to PACU	1	2	0:00:16		6:43:28					
Sub-Total	113	601	0:00:16							
Pre-Op Orders										
	1	12	0:00:37							

Fig. 5. Measurement results for written orders. (*From* Stone WM, Smith BE, Shaft, et al. The impact of a computerized physician order entry system. J Am Coll Surg 2009;208:304–13; with permission.)

then transcribe an order for the unit secretary to process. The mean time for the provider to find a patient chart was just more than 2 minutes. The longest time for finding a chart was documented at 30 minutes. In the electronic environment, this process correlates to finding an electronic device to log on and activating a patient's medical record. This time was electronic device dependent but, even using the slowest device, the mean time to log on and patient record activation was just over 1 minute. The electronic order process had the advantage of not requiring the unit secretary input and thus saved approximately 38 minutes (Fig. 7). This unit secretary processing time included not only time required to input the particular orders but also, more importantly, time for clarification of the written order. Not only does poor handwriting necessitate frequent clarification but also medication dosing, allergies, and other factors frequently result in need for contact with the ordering physician. In addition, by removing the unit secretary from the ordering chain of events, human error potentially can be reduced. Our data, however, did not support that hypothesis.

The impact on patient care of this 38-minute efficiency gain with CPOE systems in the overall ordering process is difficult to quantitatively measure. In three reviews, CPOE was found to increase time in the ordering process [11,12,19]. Each of these three reviews evaluated physician time as the primary outcome measured, not the total time for the ordering process. These reviews did, however, show significant gains in efficiency (time) in pharmacy and in nursing services. Drug turnaround time, defined as the time from medication order entry to the time the medication was delivered to the ward, was measured and evaluated. This time, which is more consistent with our methodology for time and efficiency outcomes, was found significantly improved with implementation of a CPOE system.

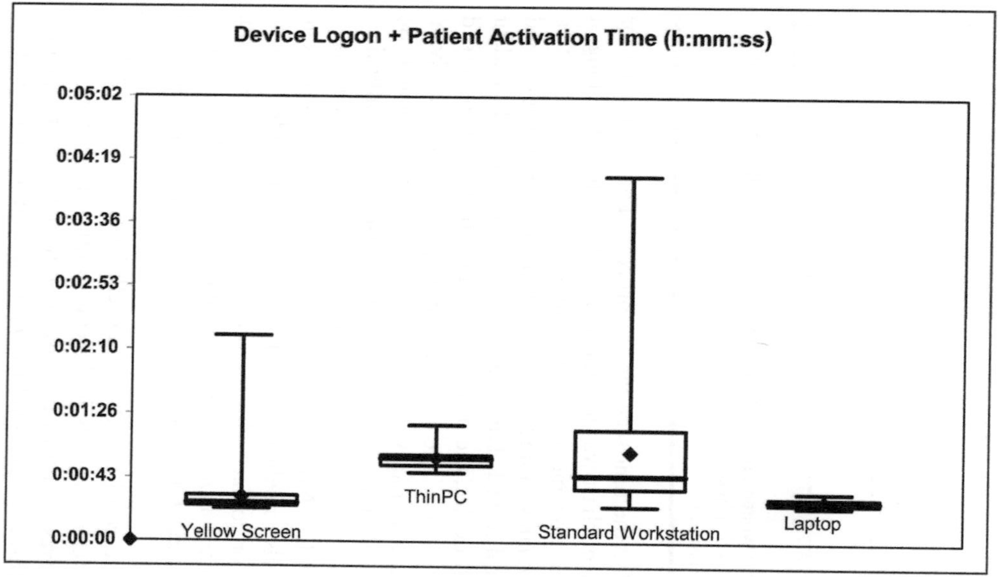

	Yellow	ThinPC	Standard	Laptop
Min(Actual):	0:00:22	0:00:47	0:00:24	0:00:24
1st Quartile:	0:00:24	0:00:52	0:00:36	0:00:26
Median:	0:00:26	0:00:57	0:00:45	0:00:28
Mean:	0:00:30	0:00:57	0:01:01	0:00:28
3rd Quartile:	0:00:31	0:00:59	0:01:16	0:00:30
Max(Actual):	0:02:19	0:01:19	0:04:08	0:00:34

Fig. 6. Device log-on and patient record activation times by device. (*From* Stone WM, Smith BE, Shaft, et al. The impact of a computerized physician order entry system. J Am Coll Surg 2009;208:304–13; with permission.)

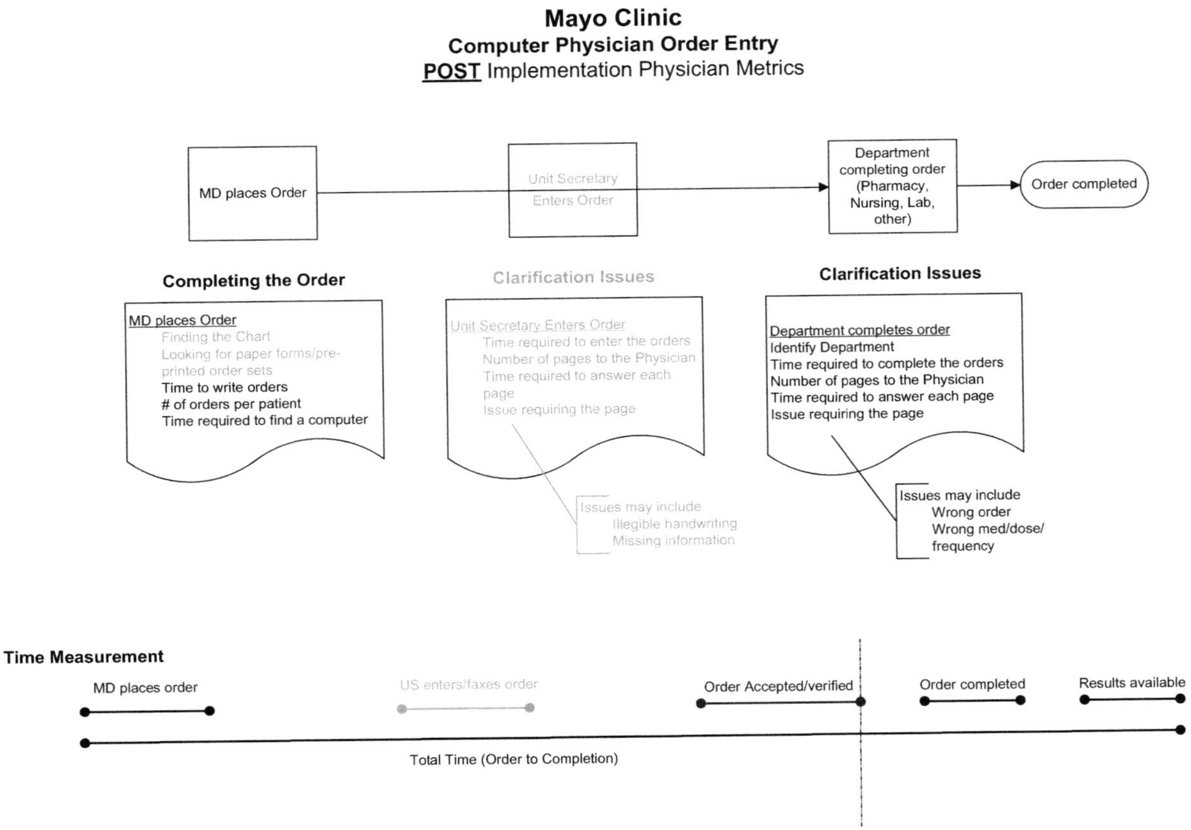

Fig. 7. Electronic ordering process (post-CPOE). (*From* Stone WM, Smith BE, Shaft, et al. The impact of a computerized physician order entry system. J Am Coll Surg 2009;208:304–13; with permission.)

PATIENT SAFETY

CPOE systems, as with any other disruptive technology, have specific, intended consequences. The addition of any new technology also has unexpected consequences, which may have a significant impact on patient care. Some of those unintended consequences are beneficial for patient care and others may be detrimental. The intended consequence of CPOE systems is to provide a safer environment for the ordering process, thereby decreasing medication errors. Most published reviews that have evaluated the impact of CPOE implementation have revealed beneficial effects on reduction of medication errors. Others, however, have demonstrated adverse consequences from the implementation of CPOE [20]. In our review, we found that there was no significant impact on the rate of medication errors or patient adverse events [18]. The total number of orders during the CPOE implementation process was 1,836,239. This consisted of 1,202,330 physician orders (66%), 589,196 midlevel practitioner orders (32%), 22,969 phone orders (1%), and 21,774 verbal orders (1%). Six months immediately before CPOE implementation, 6815 surgical procedures were performed in our multispecialty surgical practice. There were 15 medication errors identified (15/6815, 0.22%). No specific trends were noted in the etiology of these errors. After implementation of CPOE, 10 medication errors (10/5963, 0.16%) were identified with 5963 surgical procedures performed within the first 6 months. During the second 6 months after CPOE implementation, 6106 surgical procedures were performed with 13 medication errors identified (13/6106, 0.21%). When comparing pre- and post-implementation, medication errors were not statistically significantly different during any of these time periods. The patient safety score metric established by the Mayo Clinic Hospital in 2002 revealed no statistically significant change comparing pre- and post-CPOE scores (see Fig. 3).

Most of the outcome measures evaluated from implementation of CPOE systems have revolved around patient safety. Patient safety has primarily been investigated by measuring numbers of medication errors. Each study identifies and tabulates medication errors using its own distinct methodology. There is no consistent standard for the identification and tabulation of these errors. Some medication errors result in harm to patients (adverse drug events), and some result in no actual or potential harm. In a systematic review by Eslami and colleagues [21], 21 studies evaluating the impact of CPOE on medication errors, adverse drug events, and mortality were analyzed. In all studies, there was a statistically significant benefit on medication errors or a trend toward benefit. All trials reviewed were not performed in a prospective randomized fashion but did involve comparison between pre- and post-CPOE implementation. Although evidence is present to demonstrate the beneficial effect of CPOE on medication errors, little evidence is present to demonstrate its effect on adverse drug events. Bates and colleagues [22] performed a prospective, randomized, comparative study that was the first review to reveal a significant reduction in medication errors (55% reduction of serious medication errors) yet was not adequately powered to reveal any statistically significant difference in adverse drug events.

Although most reviews have found beneficial effects on medication errors, recent evidence suggests that drug event rates and mortality may be adversely affected. Koppel and colleagues [20] performed a qualitative and quantitative review of CPOE implementation using five differing focus groups. They identified 22 types of medication errors that were felt to be facilitated by the CPOE system. Although there were medication errors that were eliminated, these other additional errors were unintended consequences of the system. The potential errors that are unintended include orders on the wrong patient, errors of omission, nurses not knowing an order had been generated, desensitization to alerts, loss of information during care transitions, wrong medication dosing, and overlapping medication orders. In our review of CPOE impact on medication errors in the surgical practice, we noted no statistically significant difference in medication errors when comparing pre- and post-CPOE implementation. The capture and reporting of medication errors in our review was performed using a self-reporting process established in our inpatient hospital since its inception in 1998. Most reviews have used differing methodologies and definitions for medication errors. These definitions include wrong dosing, route and interval errors, drug interactions, drug allergies, wrong medication, formulary errors, illegibility, transcription errors, administration errors, dispensing errors, and contraindications.

Several factors may contribute to the lack of improvement in medication errors seen in our review of the impact of CPOE. The baseline rate of medication errors before CPOE implementation was low in our hospital. Sharek and Classen [23] found the incidence of medication-related harm in the inpatient pediatric population to be as high as 11.1 per 100 patient admissions. In addition, Dean and colleagues [24] found prescribing error rates of 0.3% to 39% of medication orders written in the adult inpatient setting. Unanticipated errors with CPOE implementation could have offset any gains made in the intentional aversion of errors. Some of these unanticipated events included new types of medication errors. These involve systems errors, such as medication discontinuation and renewal errors, and human errors, such as the wrong patient or medication selection [25].

Because our system of medication error is self-reported, there could have been increased vigilance in reporting and capturing of these errors after implementation of CPOE. For purposes of our review, we tabulated medication errors as "any medication error that may cause or lead to inappropriate medication use or patient harm, while the medication is in the control of the health care professional, patient, or consumer. Such event may be related to professional practice, health care products, procedures and systems including: prescribing, order communication, product labeling, packaging, and nomenclature, compounding, dispensing, distribution, administration, education, monitoring and use." The results, therefore, could have been influenced by behavioral change in our organization, but we are possibly not significantly different from other institutions that do not find a significant decrease in medication errors. A group of articles from the University of Iowa revealed that most error reports are inaccurate and the rationale in error reporting varies widely [26–28]. They suggest that providers must recognize the error, believe it is of significance, and overcome personal emotional feelings to report an error. Kaushal and colleagues [29] reported, however, that 74% of medication errors and 79% of potential adverse events occurred during the ordering stage of clinical care. Patient safety is not simply reducing the number of medication errors. Obtaining treatment more efficiently also should improve patient outcomes and possibly reduce costs. Several other measures that CPOE had an impact on have been reported, including adherence to guidelines, time, costs, efficiency, and satisfaction. All of the reviews to date have evaluated the impact on a pediatric or medical specialty practice.

FINANCIAL IMPACT

The overall financial impact of CPOE implementation has been reported to have a positive effect on the net operating income of an institution [5]. Costs of information technology systems can be divided into capital and operating expenses. The costs identified in our review were substantial ($2.9 million capital, $2.3 million operating during implementation phase); however, the full financial effect has not been evaluated and may not truly be objectively quantifiable [18]. Unlike some technologies, such as CT scanners, laboratory tests, or new clinical programs, developing an objective return on investment is somewhat elusive. It is difficult to place a price on patient safety and its ramifications.

Most reports have established a financial benefit to CPOE in at least one parameter studied. These were primarily focused reviews, however, without establishment of overall impact. It seems that CPOE has a beneficial effect on hospital and pharmacy costs. Kaushal and colleagues [30] found the capital and operational costs of implementing a CPOE system were $11.8 million over a 10-year period. When factoring the overall gains in efficiency and personnel, implementation of CPOE systems was felt to have an overall positive financial impact. In our institution, both of these costs were significant. The lead-up phase before implementation of CPOE was approximately 28 months. This includes assuring that all support was available for the providers (additional laptops, additional thin PCs, educational modules, and so forth) and that adequate technical support and buildup of the CPOE system was in place. Our inpatient hospital has used electronic medical records since its inception in 1998. Before implementation of the inpatient hospital CPOE system, an outpatient CPOE system was introduced and experience had already been gained in this process. Although overall costs seem easier to obtain than overall financial impact, the efficiencies gained are even more difficult to quantify. Personnel changes have occurred as a consequence of workload redistribution (eliminated 11 of the 56 unit secretarial positions or 19.6% of the positions). This resulted in a financial gain of $445,500 per year for our institution. The overall financial impact of this redistribution and efficiency gain has not been established.

CPOE systems have been proved to increase the capture rate for charges incurred in the inpatient hospital setting. Krohn [31] found that there was a 12% increase in charges with additional increased accuracy when CPOE was used. Improvement in compliance with hospital formularies has been shown to occur with these electronic systems [16,17]. Agrawal [6] has shown a correlation with improved compliance to hospital formulary and pharmacy cost savings.

Since its introduction in 1969, only 5% of medical facilities to date have instituted some form of a CPOE system [32]. Based on the most optimistic of predictions, it seems as though diffusion across the United States will take at least 20 years to reach as many as 50% of the medical facilities. Rogers' diffusion of innovations model suggests five patterns of adoption for any new technology [33]. He identified innovators, early adopters, early majority, late majority, and laggards as the five patterns of adoption. In light of the high costs, complexity, and physician skepticism, it is doubtful that the CPOE systems will gain much traction in the next few years. The marketing of adoption of CPOE can be used to enhance the notion of providing the highest quality of care by the investment in cutting edge technology. This may provide a competitive advantage for these few institutions [7]. If direct and indirect cost savings are realized, however, more institutions will likely show increased acceptance to implementation. This increased acceptance will result from the perceived cost savings and may also be offset by the recent economic downturn and significant decreases in available capital funds to purchase and implement the system. Furthermore, if regulatory agencies, such as the Joint Commission or Centers for Medicare & Medicaid Services, mandate electronic ordering systems, all institutions will most likely quickly migrate to implementation.

References

[1] Institute of Medicine. Preventing medication errors: quality chasm series. Washington, DC: National Academy Press; 2007.

[2] Kohn LT, Corrigan JM, Donaldson MS. To err is human: building a safer health system. Washington, DC: National Academy Press; 1999.

[3] Institute of Medicine. Crossing the quality chasm: a new health system for the 21st century. Washington, DC: National Academy Press; 2001.

[4] Birkmeyer JD, Birkmeyer CM, Wennberg MP, et al. Leapfrog safety standards: potential benefits of universal adoption. Washington, DC: The Leapfrog Group; 2000.

[5] Eslami S, de Keizer NF, Abu-Hanna A. The impact of computerized physician medication order entry in hospitalized patients—a systematic review. Int J Med Inform 2007;77: 365–76.

[6] Agrawal A. Return on investment analysis for a computer-based patient record in the outpatient clinic setting. J Assoc Acad Minor Phys 2002;13(3):61–5.

[7] Menachemi N, Brooks RG. Reviewing the benefits and costs of electronic health records and associated technologies. J Med Syst 2006;30:159–68.

[8] Tierney WM, Miller ME, Overhage JM, et al. Physician inpatient order writing on microcomputer workstations. Effects on resource utilization. J Am Med Assoc 1993;269(3):379–83.

[9] Ostbyte T, Moen A, Erikssen G, et al. Introducing a module for laboratory test order entry and reporting of results at a hospital ward: an evaluation study using a multi-method approach. J Med Syst 1997;21(2):107–17.

[10] Evans KD, Benham SW, Garrard CS. A comparison of handwritten and computer-assisted prescriptions in an intensive care unit. Crit Care 1998;2(2):73–8.
[11] Shu K, Boyle D, Spurr C, et al. Comparison of time spent writing orders on paper with computerized physician order entry. Medinfo 2001;10(2):1207–11.
[12] Bates DW, Boyle DL, Teich JM. Impact of computerized physician order entry on physician time. In: Proceedings of the Annual Symposium Computer Application in Medical Care; 1994. p. 996.
[13] Yamauchi K, Ikeda M, Suzuki Y, et al. Evaluation of the order entry system by end users—a step to the new hospital information system. Nagoya J Med Sci 1994;57(1–4):19–24.
[14] Weiner M, Gress T, Thiemann DR, et al. Contrasting views physicians and nurses about an inpatient computer-based provider order-entry system. J Am Med Inform Assoc 1999;6(3): 234–44.
[15] Amusan AA, Tongen S, Speedie SM, et al. Time saver: a time-motion study to evaluate the impact of EMR and CPOE implementation on physician efficiency. J Healthc Inf Manag 2008;22(4):31–7.
[16] Teich JM, Merchia PR, Schmiz JL, et al. Effects of computerized physician order entry on prescribing practices. Arch Intern Med 2000;160(18):2741–7.
[17] Dexter PR, Perkins S, Overhage JM, et al. A computerized reminder system to increase the use of preventative care for hospitalized patients. N Engl J Med 2001;345(13):965–70.
[18] Stone WM, Smith BE, Shaft JD, et al. The impact of a computerized physician order entry system. J Am Coll Surg 2009;208:304–13.
[19] Banet GA, Jeffe DB, Williams JA, et al. Effects of implementing computerized practitioner order entry and nursing documentation on nursing workflow in an emergency department. J Healthc Inf Manag 2006;20:45–54.
[20] Koppel R, Metlay JP, Cohen A, et al. Role of computerized physician order entry systems in facilitating medication errors. JAMA 2005;293(10):1197–203.
[21] Eslami S, Abu-Hanna A, de Keizer NF. Evaluation of outpatient computerized physician medication order entry systems; a systemic review. J Am Med Inform Assoc 2007;14: 400–6.
[22] Bates DW, Leape LL, Cullen DJ, et al. Effect of computerized physician order entry and a team intervention on prevention of serious medication errors. JAMA 1998;280:1311–6.
[23] Sharek PJ, Classen D. The incidence of adverse events and medical error in pediatrics. Pediatr Clin North Am 2006;53(6):1067–77.
[24] Dean FB, Vincent C, Schachter M, et al. The incidence of prescribing errors in hospital inpatients: an overview of the research methods. Drug Saf 2005;28(10):891–900.
[25] Campbell EM, Sittig DF, Ash JS, et al. Types of unintended consequences related to computerized provider order entry. J Am Med Inform Assoc 2006;13:547–56.
[26] Wakefield BJ, Wakefield DS, Uden-Holman T, et al. Understanding why medication administration errors may not be reported. Am J Med Qual 1999;14:81–8.
[27] Wakefield BJ, Wakefield DS, Uden-Holman T, et al. Improving mediation administration error reporting systems. Why do errors occur? Ambul Outreach 2000;16–20.
[28] Wakefield BJ, Wakefield DS, Borders T, et al. Understanding and comparing differences in reported medication administration error rates. Am J Med Qual 1999;14:73–80.
[29] Kaushal R, Bates DW, Landrigan C, et al. Medication errors and adverse drug events in pediatric inpatients. JAMA 2001;285:2114–20.
[30] Kaushal R, Jha AK, Franz C, et al. Return on investment for a computerized order entry system. J Am Med Inform Assoc 2006;13:261–6.
[31] Krohn R. In search of the ROI from CPOE. J Healthc Inf Manag 2003;17(4):6–9.
[32] Ford EW, McAlearney AS, Phillips MT, et al. Predicting computerized physician order entry system adoption in US hospitals: can the federal mandate be met? Int J Med Inform 2008;77(8):539–45.
[33] Rogers EM. Diffusion of innovations. New York: Free Press of Glencoe; 1962.

Advances in Surgery 44 (2010) 361–365

ADVANCES IN SURGERY

INDEX

Note: Page numbers of article titles are in **boldface** type.

0065-3101/10/$ – see front matter
doi:10.1016/S0065-3411(10)00034-5

C

D

E

F

Printed and bound by CPI Group (UK) Ltd, Croydon, CR0 4YY
08/05/2025
01864676-0001